"John McDougall, MD, has once again produced an outstanding book with recommendations gleaned from his decades of medical experience and strongly supported by the scientific literature. The information in this book can provide the reader the power needed to lose weight and regain health." —Alan Goldhamer, DC, director of TrueNorth Health Center and coauthor of *The Pleasure Trap*

"I personally know many people who have found the McDougall program to be the key to vastly improved health for themselves and their families. This book lays it out clearly and without compromise." —John Robbins, author of *No Happy Cows*, *The Food Revolution*, and *Diet for a New America*

"This time the Star McDougaller is John himself, joining with Mary in creating a masterfully crafted nutrition guide that destroys harmful myths and enhances the enduring capacity of whole food plant based nutrition as the foundation to our long overdue health revolution." —Caldwell B. Esselstyn, Jr., MD, author of *Prevent and Reverse Heart Disease*

"'Eat all you want; any time you want.' Statements that sound too good to be true usually are . . . too good to be true. But *The Starch Solution*, richly referenced for science, but gracefully written for consumers, just might be both good and true." —George D. Lundberg, MD, editor-at-large of *MedPage Today*

"Great news! Thank you John! Now we can eat carbs guilt-free and maintain our figures." —Elizabeth Kucinich, director of public affairs for the Physicians Committee for Responsible Medicine (PCRM)

"John McDougall has done it again. This time, clarifying the issue of starches and the important role they play in human nutrition, improving our health and the health of the planet." —Jeff Novick, RD, vice president for Executive Health Exams International and lecturer at the McDougall Program

"I love the book. It should be required reading for all medical students and doctors." —Craig McDougall, MD, internal medicine specialist at the McDougall Program

"The option is pretty simple. Meat and potatoes and later angioplasty and bypass or a plant-based (starch diet) and procedure-less and medicine-less health and happiness. This book shows the way. It is highly recommended."
                              —William C. Roberts, MD, editor-in-chief of
                    The American Journal of Cardiology and executive director of the
            Baylor Cardiovascular Institute of Baylor University Medical Center, Dallas

"Dr. John McDougall is on a mission to make us healthier. Read *The Starch Solution*. It may save your life and your brain."
                              —Dennis Bourdette, MD, chairman of the department
                              of neurology at Oregon Health & Science University

"*The Starch Solution* is an easy and powerful way to achieve the very best of health. Dr. McDougall's unparalleled knowledge and experience have brought us the best possible way to help people lose weight, lower their cholesterol and blood pressure, boost their energy, and change their lives."
            —Neal Barnard, MD, founder and president of Physicians Committee for
                              Responsible Medicine (PCRM)

"You'll be doing the happy dance when you read this book! Hallelujah, and bring on the pasta!"   —Kathy Freston, author of *The Veganist*

"Bold, honest, and ringing with truth, *The Starch Solution* will show you exactly how to reclaim your health and your life. Nobody has ever delivered this message so clearly. Dr. John McDougall's contribution is destined to become a classic."

                              —Douglas J. Lisle, PhD, coauthor of *The Pleasure Trap*

"*The Starch Solution* is a viable approach to solving many health problems, including obesity, heart disease, and type 2 diabetes, and will have a positive impact on our environment. I highly recommend it."
                              —Congressman Dennis J. Kucinich

"*The Starch Solution* is a thorough and absorbing explanation of the health benefits and nutritional excellence of a plant-based diet. In addition to being healthy, the food is delicious and satisfying."
                              —Robert A. Rosati, MD, coauthor of the
                              New York Times bestseller *The Rice Diet Solution*

The
Starch
SOLUTION

EAT THE FOODS YOU LOVE, REGAIN YOUR HEALTH, AND LOSE THE WEIGHT FOR GOOD!

JOHN A. McDOUGALL, MD,
AND MARY MCDOUGALL

RODALE.

© 2012 by John A. McDougall

Trade hardcover first published by Rodale Inc. in March 2012.

Rodale books may be purchased for business or promotional use or for special sales. For information, please write to:
Special Markets Department, Rodale, Inc., 733 Third Avenue, New York, NY 10017

Printed in the United States of America
Rodale Inc. makes every effort to use acid-free ♾, recycled paper ♻.

Illustrations by Lisa Kahn
Book design by Christina Gaugler

Library of Congress Cataloging-in-Publication Data

McDougall, John A.
    The starch solution: eat the foods you love, regain your health, and lose the weight for good! / by John McDougall and Mary McDougall.
        p.   cm.
    Includes bibliographical references and index.
    ISBN 978-1-60961-393-8 hardcover
    ISBN 978-1-62336-027-6 paperback
    1. High-carbohydrate diet.   2. Complex carbohydrate diet.   3. High-carbohydrate diet—Recipes.   4. Complex carbohydrate diet—Recipes.   5. Cookbooks.   I. McDougall, Mary A. (Mary Ann)   II. Title.
    RM237.59.M33   2012
    641.5'638—dc23   2011047107

Distributed to the trade by Macmillan
        16   18   20   19   17   paperback

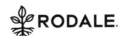

We inspire and enable people to improve their lives and the world around them.
www.rodalebooks.com

CONTENTS

Part I: Healing with Starch

Part II: The FAQs about Food

Part III: Living the Solution

To our grandchildren—
may the Starch Solution brighten your futures.

ACKNOWLEDGMENTS

The Starch Solution is the result of 44 years of personal care of thousands of patients, most of whom once suffered from dietary diseases. From these people we have learned our most valuable lessons. Many medical and nutritional pioneers, including Russell Henry Chittenden, PhD; Harold Percival Himsworth, KCB; William Rose, PhD; Walter Kempner, MD; Denis Burkitt, FRS; Nathan Pritikin, and Roy Swank, MD, laid the scientific foundations for the materials in this book.

Our grateful appreciation to:

Carole Bidnick, literary agent, for securing a powerful publisher.

Shannon Welch, Ursula Cary, Marie Crousillat, and Marilyn Hauptly for editing for success.

Cathy Fisher and Jennie Schacht for their help with writing.

Lisa Kahn for crafting the illustrations.

Star McDougallers for sharing their stories.

McDougall followers for contributing ideas and recipes.

The National Library of Medicine for providing access to the basic science.

Note to the Reader

Diet is powerful medicine. Do not change your diet or start an exercise program if you are seriously ill or on medications unless you are under the watchful guidance of a health care provider knowledgeable about nutrition and its effects on health and about the medications you are taking. The people in this book are real and their names are used with their permission. If you do as they have done, you should expect similar results. Although no treatment gives ideal outcomes for everyone, in most cases the Starch Solution provides an opportunity to remain free from common illnesses and to regain health and appearance. (Benefits with cancer recovery are real, but less common and well established.)

The McDougall Diet is based on starches with the addition of fruits and vegetables. If you follow this low-fat vegan plan strictly for more than 3 years, or if you are pregnant or nursing, then take a minimum of 5 micrograms of supplemental vitamin B_{12} daily.

Contact Information

Dr. McDougall's Health and Medical Center
PO Box 14039
Santa Rosa, CA 95402

Telephone: (707) 538–8609
Fax: (707) 538–0712

E-mail: drmcdougall@drmcdougall.com
On the Web: www.drmcdougall.com

Residential programs: (800) 941–7111 / (707) 538–8609

Book and DVD orders: www.drmcdougall.com/books_tapes.html

PREFACE

S tarch has unlocked the door to good health for thousands of my patients over the last four decades, allowing them to lose excess weight and heal from diet-related illnesses, like high blood pressure, heart disease, diabetes, and inflammatory arthritis. More than 5,000 people have taken part in the McDougall residential programs, the vast majority forever altering the course of their lives. One and a half million others have purchased my previous 11 books. The longer I practice medicine, the more crystal clear the solution becomes.

The Starch Solution shares what I have learned and teaches what you can and must do to regain control of your health and appearance. With intuitive information backed by scientific proof, an easy-to-follow plan, and nearly 100 simple and satisfying recipes to pave the way, *The Starch Solution* shows you how to reclaim your life, all by enjoying your favorite foods.

Whatever you are doing now is not working. That's why you've picked up this book. Most likely, you've tried other diets—probably many of them—but they have failed you. That's because most diets make losing weight easy if you stick with them—but because they ask you to suffer a life of deprivation, or make you feel ill, they are not sustainable. Instead, you lose weight, then you lose interest, quickly gaining all the weight back and more.

The Starch Solution is different because it offers a way of eating that keeps you feeling satisfied. You won't feel hungry or deprived, because starches are not only healthy, they're also comforting and filling. This is a plan you can follow indefinitely—even when you stray by not following it 100 percent—and its benefits will be with you for a lifetime. In other words, this is not an all-or-nothing approach.

Beyond shedding excess weight almost effortlessly, you will look better, feel better, function better, and live better. For the majority of people, blood pressure and cholesterol will drop and digestion will finally work the way it should. In most cases, you will be able to get off and stay off prescription and nonprescription medications and supplements, saving a bundle and enjoying good health naturally. Once you try it and see the results, you will know for certain that the Starch Solution is the answer you have been searching for your whole life. If you wish, skip ahead to test the plan yourself by using the 7-Day Sure-Start Plan in Chapter 14, while you continue to read and learn how and why the Starch Solution works.

You will have questions along the way, but fear not; I have heard most of them before and I have answered them here for you. You needn't worry about getting sufficient protein, calcium, vitamins, or other nutrients. These ingredients are naturally built into the foods. With an informed mind you will be able to evaluate health claims in product advertising, diet books, and public health messages. You will even learn why, if this approach holds such great promise, you have not heard this information before.

As you read this book, you will come to understand that the very same solution that helps you also benefits the environment. With just a simple U-turn in your diet to bring it back in line with healthier diets of long ago, you can help heal the world around you as you slim down, improve your health, save money, and change your life.

Introduction

My Personal Journey to the Starch Solution

One of my earliest life lessons was about honesty. As a child, I was a mischief magnet. I didn't mean to be. I was just a curious kid. When I was 7, the police caught me "breaking and entering" into the vacant house across the street. I thought I was exploring. The following year, I killed my pet hamster—it was an accident. At 9, I set the living room sofa on fire while conducting experiments with my dad's cigarette lighter and lighter fluid. I was sorry about that. My parents were wise. They knew that punishment ran the risk of turning their well-intentioned little troublemaker into a disaffected, rebellious teen. They reasoned that the more I told them about my antics, the better chance they had of gently guiding my energies toward more productive outlets. So, instead of yelling at me, they showed me that truth was the best way out of trouble. Finding and telling the truth has been my credo ever since.

I am a passionate person, with a larger-than-life, type A personality. I have lived with this high enthusiasm, for better or worse, every single day of my life. I don't just value truth, I seek it obsessively. At times, people find me brash, undiplomatic, and too direct. I can live with that. Speaking up is the single most effective way I know to awaken people from the falsehoods that are making them sick and teach the truths that can bring them health.

That information is what I seek to share here, in *The Starch Solution*. What you will find on these pages is the truth about food, health, misinformation campaigns, and our planet. I'm laying it all out so that you may form your own opinions, and live your life fully aware of the impact of what you eat on you, your family, and the world around you. Sharing what I have learned over the last 44 years of studying and practicing medicine is all I can do. The rest is up to you.

UNGUIDED WEALTH STOLE OUR HEALTH

My medical education started long before I became a doctor. At age 18, in 1965, I suffered a massive stroke that completely paralyzed my left side for 2 weeks. My recovery was slow and incomplete. Forty-seven years later, though I windsurf every day that I can, I still walk with a limp—a lifelong reminder of the path that led me to illness and then to newfound health.

My parents lived through the Great Depression of the 1930s. During those hard times, my mother's family survived on beans, corn, cabbage, parsnips, peas, rutabagas, carrots, onions, turnips, potatoes, and bread, which they bought for 5 cents a loaf. A little hamburger once a week was their only meat. My mother's painful memories caused her to promise herself never to let her children suffer as she had. Her children would enjoy the best foods money could buy. Ironically, her well-intentioned promise ended up causing more harm than good. It turns out the Depression-era diet was the healthier one!

I grew up eating bacon and eggs for breakfast, sandwiches stuffed with meat and slathered with mayonnaise for lunch, and beef, pork, and chicken at the center of the plate every night at dinner. All three meals were washed down with glassfuls of milk. Starches? Those were side dishes at best (and covered with butter). Except in refined breads and cakes, they rarely found their way into our home.

I didn't realize it then, but the best food money could buy nearly killed me. As far back as I can remember, I suffered daily stomachaches and brutal constipation. I was frequently sick with colds and flu, and when I was 7, out came my tonsils. I was always in last place in gym class, and my teenage face was oily and pocked with acne. At age 18 it became clear that something was terribly wrong when I suffered a stroke, something that I thought happened only to old people. I had no idea this had any connection to my indulgent diet—nor did the doctors in the hospital suggest anything of the sort—so I kept on eating the very same way. By my early twenties I was 50 pounds overweight.

I don't blame my mother. She fed us based on the best nutritional advice available at the time. Who knew that much of this advice came from the meat and dairy industries, which exalted protein and calcium as our most essential nutrient needs? Even as concerns began to surface about the adverse effects of animal foods, they were largely dismissed by food industry–funded scientists as unimportant.

I was raised in a lower-middle-class family in the suburbs of Detroit. My parents worshipped medical doctors as if they were exceptional beings possessing godlike qualities. I was just an ordinary person, at best; I never even dreamed of pursuing a career in medicine—at least until my fateful hospitalization for my stroke. My exalted view of doctors shifted radically during my 2 weeks between those hospital walls. I became a medical curiosity, attracting some of the area's top specialists to look in on me and review my case. As a patient, and a teenager eager to return to school, I asked each doctor who examined me, "What caused my stroke?" "How will you make me better?" "When can I go home?"

The typical response was nonverbal. They shook their heads and walked out of my room. I remember thinking to myself, "Well, I could do that." When it became clear to me that no doctor could answer even one of my three basic questions, I walked out of the hospital against medical advice. Returning to college at Michigan State University, I felt for the first time a fierce sense of direction and determination. I entered medical school in 1968 and pursued medicine with a great passion.

I also became passionate about a surgical nurse I met during my senior year in medical school as I assisted with a hip replacement.

Mary and I married and escaped to Hawaii, where I took my first year of post–medical school residency training, my internship, at The Queen's Medical Center in Honolulu. Over the next 3 years I worked as a general practitioner at the Hamakua Sugar Company on the Big Island. There, as a general doctor to 5,000 sugar laborers and their families, I delivered babies, signed death certificates, and did everything in between. The nearest specialist was a 42-mile drive away to Hilo. My patients were relying on me to do it all.

When I treated acute problems, like sewing up injuries suffered in the fields, casting broken bones, or dispensing antibiotics for infections, I enjoyed the satisfaction of seeing my patients heal. What frustrated me were the chronic problems. Despite my best efforts, I simply could not help patients suffering from devastating illnesses like obesity, diabetes, heart disease, or arthritis. When a plantation worker came to me with one of these complaints, I would do the only thing I was taught in school: prescribe medications. As they walked out the door, I would invite my patients to return if the pill I gave them didn't work. They would return. We'd try another pill. I never ran out of pills to try, but eventually the patient would stop coming.

Convinced that my failure resulted from my own shortcomings, after 3 years on the sugar plantation I left the Big Island of Hawaii, returned to Honolulu, and enrolled in the University of Hawaii Medical Residency Program. A little more than 2 years later, I left this intensive training experience still wanting answers to the same questions I entered with. I did learn one valuable lesson: It might not be my fault after all that my patients' health did not improve. Even some of the world's top medical scholars got no better results than I did. Like mine, their patients remained riddled with chronic disease; at best, a few of my peers temporarily controlled symptoms.

I graduated, took an exam, and received my board certification in internal medicine. But neither study nor that designation made me a good doctor. For that, I had to think back to my time on the plantation.

More Lessons from My Patients

People, including doctors, have an expectation that we will get fatter and sicker as we age. Children are the healthiest, their parents less healthy, and the eldest generation suffers from severe and chronic diseases.

What happened with my patients on the sugar plantation challenged that expectation. There, the elderly immigrant generation remained trim, active, and medication free into their nineties. They had no diabetes, no heart disease, no arthritis, and no cancers of the breast, prostate, or colon. Their children were a little heavier and not as healthy. But what really threw me was seeing the youngest generation—the grandchildren of these immigrant families—suffering from the most profound health problems, the same ones I had spent my years learning about during my medical training.

What could be causing this reversal of fortune? I took a careful look at the way these families lived. I considered their lifestyles, the work environment on the plantation in Hawaii, and their behaviors. After considering every aspect of their lives, I noticed an interesting trend. These families had gone from a traditional diet in their countries of origin to fully adopting an American diet. Had they lost the protection from obesity and common chronic diseases afforded by their native foods?

My elderly patients on the plantation had immigrated to Hawaii from China, Japan, Korea, and the Philippines, where rice and vegetables had been the foundation of their diet. They continued to eat the same way in their new American homes. The second generation, their Hawaiian-born offspring, began to incorporate Western foods into their parents' traditional diet. The third generation cashed in the life-sustaining starch-based diet of their grandparents for a diet rich in meat, dairy, and processed foods.

I grew up hearing the steadfast agreement among the government and every other source that the healthiest diet was a well-balanced one, taken from the four food groups: meat, dairy, grains, and fruits and vegetables. Yet on the plantation I watched elders thriving late into their senior years sustained by grains and produce—just two of the four food groups—while each successive generation got sicker and sicker as they increased their reliance on the other two groups—meat and dairy.

Over and over again, I saw this shift in diet over two, three, and four generations, and its reflection in my patients' declining health. Finally, something shifted in me as I awakened from the false promises of my medical education. My patients brought me the insight I had been searching for since age 18, when I was hit by that awful stroke and could not get answers to the most basic questions about what might have caused it and what those doctors planned to do to improve my health going forward.

My medical training had taught me nothing about the impact of food on health. Nutrition was almost never mentioned in medical school, my textbooks, or during my internship or residency. There were very few questions about it on my board exam. Yet it was this one simple insight that now allows me to take patients off ineffective pills, protect them from risky surgeries, and offer them a simple, effective pathway to health and longevity and permanent loss of excess body weight.

A WORLDWIDE PHENOMENON

Wondering whether this trend might apply beyond this small population in Hawaii, I began looking into traditional diets around the world. What I learned on the plantation was confirmed, over and over again. Diet was, indeed, the missing ingredient—and the most fundamental one—in human health.

The full potential of practicing dietary medicine became apparent only after I did additional research into what was known about the effects of diet on health. Sifting through stacks of scientific journals in the Hawaii Medical Library at The Queen's Medical Center, I learned I wasn't the first physician or scientist to come upon this discovery of a starch-based diet's potential for healing. Others before me had found that potatoes, corn, and whole grains led to robust health, while meat and dairy led to persistent, life-threatening diseases.

I also learned through those medical journals that people already sickened by disease could reverse the processes and recover, simply by no longer eating the foods that made them sick and instead supporting their natural healing processes with a starch-based diet. There wasn't just one lonely article saying so; study after study described weight loss, as well as the relief of chest pain, headaches, and arthritis, owing to a change in what people ate. Kidney disease, heart failure, type 2 diabetes, intestinal distress, asthma, obesity, and other troubles were also reversed by healthy eating. Volumes of research in these journal pages written over the previous 50 years showed me how my patients, with their chronic, seemingly intractable conditions, could be cured with one simple solution: a diet based on starch supplemented by vegetables and fruits. No pills or surgery needed.

I could hardly wait to share the discovery that what I had observed on the plantation—a simple change in diet to improve health and relieve much suffering—was already scientifically documented. I was certain my revolutionary breakthrough would be widely welcomed, that some fluke had prevented others from seeing this truth and shouting it out to a world of people eager to heal themselves from pain and suffering.

THE MCDOUGALL RESIDENTIAL PROGRAMS

Over time, I tested, documented, and systematized my plant-food, starch-based therapy into the McDougall Program. When St. Helena Hospital in California's Napa Valley asked me to implement it into their lifestyle residential program in 1986, I accepted. Their Seventh-Day Adventist faith, which endorses a vegetarian diet and a healthy lifestyle, seemed like a good match.

Working at St. Helena Hospital, one of the nation's leading heart surgery centers, gave me lots of exposure to surgeons and cardiologists. I offered to send these specialists my patients for a second opinion if they would reciprocate by sending me theirs. However, in my 16 years at St. Helena Hospital, though I referred many patients out for a second opinion or for other types of treatment, I never once received a referral from one of these doctors. Interestingly, when I occasionally cared for the hospital's own physicians, or their spouses or children, they commended my protocols. They just didn't seem to want the same simple, sensible treatments for their patients.

Still, I knew my approach was working: The radiologists assured me of this as they monitored my patients' repeat angiograms. They reported that their arteries were opening up and healing. This was all the reinforcement I needed.

Over my years there, I saw thousands of people helped by St. Helena Hospital's talented and caring staff. My lifestyle residential program, however, never flourished, even as my best-selling books, along with top television and radio programs, brought us international exposure. Maybe a hospital was not the best venue for a program focused on achieving health through diet rather than through a traditional medical approach. At $4,000 for my primarily educational program compared with $100,000 for bypass surgery, perhaps it just wasn't bringing in enough revenue for the hospital.

The opportunity to improve my census came when Dr. Roy Swank, the former head of neurology at Oregon Health & Science University who designed a dietary treatment for multiple sclerosis (MS), invited me to open up my live-in McDougall Program to treat patients with MS at St. Helena Hospital. I anticipated an enthusiastic response from the hospital administration, but after lengthy discussions, they decided that associating themselves with MS patients might stigmatize the hospital since these patients never seemed to get better. I also wondered whether the limited opportunity for profit might have been a consideration.

When my contract came up for renewal in 2002, I turned it in with VOID written over the front page. I was told later that they had thought that I would not be able to leave them, because without the organization they provided, the McDougall Program could not exist. But I had run the McDougall Program without them in Minneapolis for the Blue Cross/Blue Shield insurance company, where we demonstrated the same remarkable results that we had experienced at St. Helena Hospital: reduced weight, cholesterol, blood pressure, and blood sugar levels, as well as relief from indigestion, constipation, arthritis, and other ailments. That program also showed a 44 percent reduction in health care costs in 1 year based on the insurance company's own claims data. I'd done the same thing for Publix Supermarket employees in Lakeland, Florida. In both cases, we ran the program out of a local hotel. I knew I could easily set up a 10-day McDougall Program in any US city within 72 hours. All I needed were my staff, space, patients, and a kitchen that could prepare food the way I wanted it. The hospital's nudge out its door was the best win yet, both for me and for my patients.

May 2002 marked our first McDougall Program at an upscale resort in Santa Rosa, California. By this time my wife, Mary, had developed an enormous repertoire of enticing recipes reflecting the program's philosophy that would satisfy the appetites of our patients. Mary's recipes are easy to prepare, not only in a professional kitchen, but also at home. (Nearly 100 of our favorites are included in Chapter 15.) The resort's kitchen quickly learned to turn out copious quantities of food that tasted good while nurturing our participants' health and well-being.

McDougall's Medicine Using the Starch Solution

I have often been asked, "You are a doctor, so why do you speak against the practices of fellow physicians?" The answer is simple: I never took an oath to protect the financial interests of the medical industry. I did, however, take an oath to care for the sick and to keep them from harm and injustice, and to never give a deadly drug or procedure. I fully realize that the views I advocate cause people with vested interests to dislike me. But I can live with that unfairness. Too many physicians and dietitians pay allegiance to the big businesses of food and pharmaceuticals rather than to their customers, the patients.

Although I believe that most of my medical colleagues are well intentioned, their ignorance of basic human nutrition inhibits their ability to heal their patients and protect them from harm. I understand this. I operated with this same colossal blind spot when I first practiced medicine, back on the sugar plantation where I was frustrated by my powerlessness to perform the most elemental function of a physician: to help my patients regain their lost health and appearance. In 2011, I authored Senate Bill 380 for the state of California. This directive, passed unanimously by the legislators and signed by the governor, requires medical doctors to learn about human nutrition—a long over-due step forward for patients. These days, medical care is changing for the better because millions of informed people are demanding improved health rather than just more procedures and pills.

The Starch Solution represents a giant step toward healing a sick system and putting easy, healthy choices within everyone's reach, and directly into your own hands. In this book I share what I have learned over the past 44 years about promoting health and healing illness. To help you get started, I've included a 7-Day Sure-Start Plan in Chapter 14, backed up by practical information on how to ready your kitchen, your family, and your life for this change in the way you eat. Chapter 15 gets the foods you love on the table with nearly 100 easy-to-prepare recipes to suit every taste. Before long you will find yourself coming up with starch-centered meals effortlessly on your own. All you need to do to get started is turn the page.

Part I

HEALING
WITH
STARCH

CHAPTER 1

Starch: The Traditional Diet of People

*H*ave *you had your rice today?*
    This Chinese greeting—the equivalent of our *how are you?*—reminds us that, for the Chinese, whether you've eaten rice is the ultimate measure of well-being. Rice is that essential to the Chinese diet. Throughout most of Asia, the average person eats rice two to three times daily. Rice is also an important food in the Middle East, Latin America, Italy, and the West Indies. After corn it is the second most produced food worldwide, and the world's single most important source of energy, providing more than 20 percent of calories consumed by humans around the globe.

In China, the word for rice and food are one and the same. Likewise, in Japan the word for cooked rice also means "meal." Buddhists refer to grains of rice as "little Buddhas," while in Thailand the call that brings the family to the table is "Eat rice." In India, the first food a new bride offers her husband is not cake but rice. It is also the first solid food that will be offered to her baby.

The story is the same the world over. Whether rice in Asia, potatoes in South America, corn in Central America, wheat in Europe, or beans, millet, sweet potatoes, and barley around the globe, starch has been at the center of food and nutrition throughout human history.

What Is Starch?

Plants use water, carbon dioxide, and energy from the sun to form simple sugars through a process called photosynthesis. The most basic carbohydrate is the simple sugar glucose. Inside the plant's cells, simple sugars are linked into chains, some of them arranged in a straight line (amylose) and others in many branches (amylopectin). When these sugar chains gather in large quantities inside a plant's cells, they form starch grains, also called starch granules (amyloplasts).

Plants store in their roots, stems, leaves, flowers, seeds, and fruits the starch they produce. The stored starch provides them with a source of energy when they need it later, keeping them alive through the winter and fueling their reproduction the following spring. It's what makes starchy vegetables, legumes, and grains so healthy to eat: Their high concentration of carbohydrates not only sustains the plants but also provides the energy needed to sustain human life.

Starch should be our primary source of digestible carbohydrate. The enzyme amylase in our saliva and intestine breaks down the long carbohydrate chains, turning them back into simple sugars. Digestion is a slow process that gradually releases these simple sugars from the small intestine into the bloodstream, providing our cells with a ready supply of energy.

Fruits offer quick-burning energy mostly in the form of simple sugars, but little of that slow-burning, sustaining starch. As a result, fruits alone won't satisfy our appetites for very long. Green, yellow, and orange nonstarchy perishable vegetables contain only small quantities of starch. Their most important role is to contribute flavor, texture, color, and aroma to your starch-based meals. They offer a bonus in the additional nutrients (such as vitamin A and C) that come along for the ride.

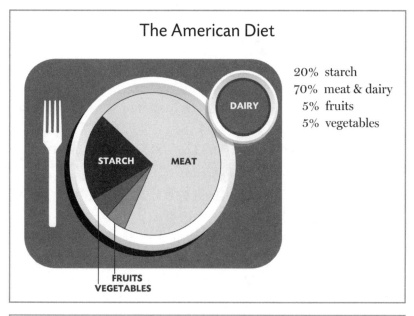

The American Diet

20% starch
70% meat & dairy
5%   fruits
5%   vegetables

STARCH • MEAT • DAIRY • FRUITS • VEGETABLES

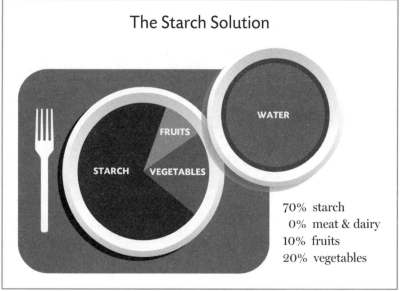

The Starch Solution

WATER • FRUITS • STARCH • VEGETABLES

70% starch
0%   meat & dairy
10% fruits
20% vegetables

Why then, here in the states and increasingly around the world, as all populations undergo economic development, have we become so afraid and ashamed of this most elemental food? And what price are we paying for shunning the most basic dietary staple known to humankind?

STARCH IS THE KEY INGREDIENT

Diet and nutrition advice is often focused on *how much* we ought to eat, and misses the point: More important than how much, how often, and when we eat is *what* we eat. Different kinds of animals require different types of diets. We humans are built to thrive on starch. The more rice, corn, potatoes, sweet potatoes, and beans we eat, the trimmer, more energetic, and healthier we become.

Starch? Really? Isn't that for laundry? Yes, but it's also the key to optimum health and satiety. We hear a lot about carbohydrates and whether or not we should eat them, but we don't hear enough about the most valuable type of carbohydrate, starch.

There are three basic types of carbohydrates—sugar, cellulose, and starch—each made up of carbon, hydrogen, and oxygen in specific configurations. The simplest of these—sugar—includes sucrose (the granulated sugar you bake into cookies), fructose (which makes fruit taste sweet), lactose (found in milk), and glucose (the simple sugar that comes together in chains to make cellulose and starch). Sugar provides quick and powerful energy because it is so efficiently broken down in the body. (You'll learn more about sugar in Chapter 12.)

The second type of carbohydrate, cellulose, is made up of chains of glucose bonded together by indigestible linkages. It is found in the cell walls of plants and in wood and other organic matter. Our digestive system doesn't have the enzymes to break down cellulose to use it for fuel, but termites do, which is why they can eat through the wood beams of your home. Although we get no energy from them, indigestible carbohydrates like cellulose are valuable to us for their dietary fiber.

The gold medal for the carbohydrate most beneficial to humans goes to starch. Like cellulose, starches are made up of long-branching chains of glucose molecules. Starch is valuable to us because we can break it down into simple sugars that provide us with sustained energy and keep us feeling full and satisfied. Starchy foods are plants that are

McDougall's Classification of Common Foods

STARCHES

Grains: Barley, buckwheat, corn, millet, oats, rice, rye, sorghum, wheat, wild rice

Legumes: Beans, lentils, peas

Starchy Vegetables: Carrots, Jerusalem artichokes, parsnips, potatoes, salsify, sweet potatoes, winter squashes (acorn, banana, butternut, Hubbard), yams

Green, Yellow, and Orange (Nonstarchy) Vegetables: Bok choy, broccoli, Brussels sprouts, cabbage, cauliflower, celery, chives, collard greens, eggplant, garlic, green beans, kale, leeks, lettuce, mustard greens, okra, onions, peppers, radishes, rhubarb, scallions, spinach, summer squashes, turnips, zucchini

Fruits: Apples, apricots, bananas, berries, cherries, figs, grapefruit, grapes, loquats, mangoes, melons, nectarines, oranges, papayas, peaches, persimmons, pineapples, plums, tangerines, watermelons

high in long-chain digestible carbohydrates—commonly referred to as complex carbohydrates. Examples include grains like wheat, barley, rye, corn, and oats; starchy vegetables like winter squash, potatoes, and sweet potatoes; and legumes like brown lentils, green peas, and red kidney beans. Starch is so important that an international scientific journal—*Starch*—is dedicated to its study. Starch is at the core of my health-enhancing diet. If you take away just one message from this book, it should be: Eat more starch. Basic to our human nature is the scientific fact that we are, and have always been, primarily starch eaters. According to the world-renowned anthropologist from Dartmouth College, Nathaniel Dominy, PhD, "A majority of calories for most hunter-gatherer societies came from plant-foods, not animal-foods, thus humans might be more appropriately described as 'starchivores.'" Think of yourself as a starchivore, like a cat is a carnivore and a horse is an herbivore.

You've probably heard about the benefits of a plant-based diet— one that reduces or eliminates animal foods like meat, dairy, and eggs. This concept does not go far enough. Without the addition of starch, a diet of low-calorie leafy greens like lettuce and kale, crucifers like broccoli and cauliflower, and fruits like apples and oranges will leave you feeling hungry and fatigued. Nonstarchy green, yellow, and orange vegetables are good for you to eat, but on their own do not give you enough calories to sustain your daily activities and keep you feeling satisfied. Your natural hunger drive may lead you to fill up on something else at the expense of your weight and health.

The Real Paleolithic Diet

Look at a globe—any region with a large population of trim, healthy people reveals the same truth: Healthy populations get most of their calories from starch. Eat a traditional meal in Japan, China, or most any Asian country and you will find your bowl filled with rice, possibly alongside sweet potatoes and buckwheat. The same truth dates back throughout recorded human history. The Incas of South America centered their diet on potatoes. The Incan warriors switched to quinoa for strength prior to battle. The Mayans and Aztecs of Central America were known as "the people of the corn." The ancient Egyptians' starch of choice was wheat. Throughout civilization and around the world, six foods have provided our primary fuel: barley, corn, millet, potatoes, rice, and wheat.

If the map hasn't convinced you, science documents it well: Over at least the past 13,000 years, starch has been central to the diets of all healthy, large, successful populations. In fact, new discoveries show evidence of starch-based diets even earlier.

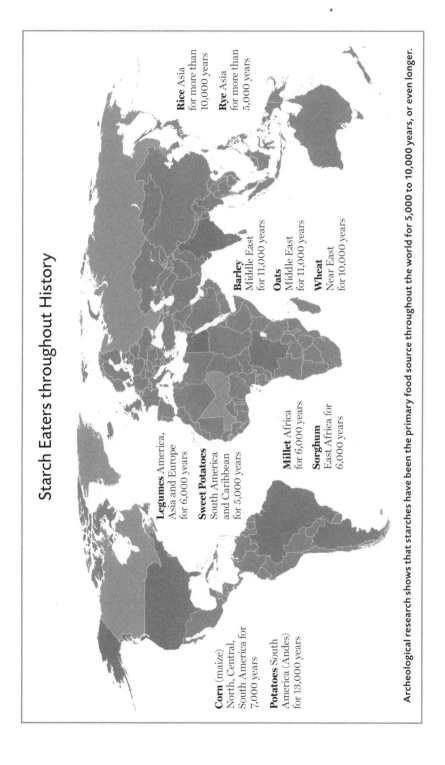

Starch Eaters throughout History

Rice Asia for more than 10,000 years

Rye Asia for more than 5,000 years

Barley Middle East for 11,000 years

Oats Middle East for 11,000 years

Wheat Near East for 10,000 years

Legumes America, Asia and Europe for 6,000 years

Sweet Potatoes South America and Caribbean for 5,000 years

Millet Africa for 6,000 years

Sorghum East Africa for 6,000 years

Corn (maize) North, Central, South America for 7,000 years

Potatoes South America (Andes) for 13,000 years

Archeological research shows that starches have been the primary food source throughout the world for 5,000 to 10,000 years, or even longer.

At Ohalo II, an Israeli site dating back 23,000 years, archeologists found wheat, barley, acorns, almonds, pistachios, berries, figs, and grapes among the huts, hearths, and a human grave.[1] Other documentation shows that bulbs and corms (an underground plant stem similar to a bulb; taro is an example) were a major food source for Africans almost 30,000 years ago.[2]

Countering the widely held belief that the European Paleolithic diet consisted predominantly of animal foods, starch grains from wild plants recently were found on grinding tools at archeological sites dating back to the Paleolithic period in Italy, Russia, and the Czech Republic. These findings suggest that processing vegetables and starches, and possibly grinding them into flour, was a widespread practice in Europe as far back as 30,000 years ago, or even earlier.[3] Other recent evidence suggests that those living in what is now Mozambique, along the eastern coast of Africa, may have followed a diet based on the cereal grass sorghum as long as 105,000 years ago.[4]

Recent studies show that even the Neanderthals ate a variety of plant foods; starch grains have been found on the teeth of their skeletons everywhere from the warm eastern Mediterranean to chilly northwestern Europe.[5] It appears they even cooked or otherwise prepared plant foods to make them more digestible.

THE DIETS OF WEALTHY ANCIENT EGYPTIANS

Proponents of a high-protein diet have suggested that reports showing heart disease in Egyptian mummies prove that their largely vegetarian diet was responsible for putting them in their graves.[6] Is this true?

CT technology uses multiple x-rays to give scientists a three-dimensional view of the body that's almost as good as peering inside. An April 2011 report in the *Journal of the American College of Cardiology: Cardiovascular Imaging* used CT scans to show that 20 out of 44 Egyptian mummies whose cardiovascular systems could be viewed had evidence of atherosclerosis, or hardening of the arteries.[7] The same kinds of calcification from atherosclerosis can frequently be seen in the CT scans of modern Americans and Europeans.

You would think that people in such early times, around 3,500 years ago, would have been reasonably healthy, with no fast food or tobacco and plenty of exercise. Yet the evidence shows that those selected to be embalmed as mummies ate a diet far richer than that of their less wealthy contemporaries.[8] In addition to atherosclerosis, these wealthy ancient Egyptians showed signs of other diseases we associate with modern diets, such as obesity, dental disease, and gallstones.[9–11] Spina bifida was found in a mummified child.[12] Since the spinal abnormalities typical of spina bifida result from insufficient folate in the womb, the child's mother likely ate a diet heavy in animal foods and lacking in folate-rich starches, fruits, and vegetables.

The gallstones are an interesting case: Stones typically form when there is too much cholesterol in the bile, owing to a diet rich in animal foods. Scientists who analyzed a mummy buried 3,500 years ago found bile acids that looked like those we see today.[11] Those aristocrats were indulging in the same rich foods.

The evidence indicates that only the wealthiest citizens—typically royalty and priests—became mummies. These privileged few were entitled to the most indulgent foods and, predictably, those foods produced diseases in the elite that were absent among the mainly vegetarian common folk. Hieroglyphics on Egyptian temple walls reinforce this finding with images of royalty feasting on beef, sheep, goats, wild fowl, rich breads, and cake. These foods have been excavated from the Egyptian pyramids, where they were buried alongside the deceased in hopes of providing for them in the afterlife. The diet of the elite has been conservatively estimated at more than 50 percent fat, much of it saturated, not unlike our typical modern Western diet.[8] Hair analysis of mummies (one of the most reliable indicators of diet, even long in the past) likewise shows their diet to be similar in composition to that of modern Westerners.[13]

The meticulously preserved Egyptian mummies provide unequivocal evidence that these highly placed individuals who ate the richest diet available suffered from heart and artery disease, obesity, and other illnesses, just as we do today. And for the same reason: a diet based on animal foods and deficient in starches. Fortunately for most ancient Egyptians, extravagant feasting was available only occasionally. If only we were so fortunate. Now, as then, a life of excess comes at great cost.

The Warrior's Diet

Throughout history, men and women who ate diets based on grains, vegetables, and fruits have accomplished history's greatest feats. The ancient conquerors of Europe and Asia, including the armies of Alexander the Great (356–323 BC) and Genghis Khan (AD 1162–1227), who conquered the known Western worlds during their respective times, consumed diets based on starches. Caesar's legions complained when they had too much meat in their diet and preferred to do their fighting on grains.[14]

The remains of 60 Roman gladiators who fought and died more than 1,800 years ago in Ephesus, in western Turkey, were recently found in a 200-square-foot plot along the road that led from the city center to the Temple of Artemis.[15] Analysis of their bones for calcium, strontium, and zinc showed that the world's fiercest fighters followed an essentially vegan diet. In contemporary accounts, the gladiators are sometimes referred to as *hordearii*, or barley men, since barley provided the bulk of the nutrients that gave their remarkably strong muscles and bones the strength and endurance to compete in the ultimate sport of life and death.

Our DNA Proves We Are Starch Eaters

Experts have long concluded that primates—humans included—are designed to eat a diet based on plant foods. Our anatomy and physiology require it. The natural diet of our closest relative, the chimpanzee, is almost purely vegetarian, made up mostly of fruits, leaves, and perishable vegetable matter. In the dry seasons, when fruit is scarce, chimps eat nuts, seeds, flowers, and bark.

Genetic testing has demonstrated that humans thrive best on starch.[16] Human and chimpanzee DNA is roughly identical; one of the minor differences is that our genes help us to digest more starch, a crucial evolutionary adjustment.

Studies of the gene coding for amylase, the enzyme that breaks down starch into simple sugars, found that humans have on average six copies of the gene compared to two copies in other, "lesser" primates.[16] This difference means that human saliva produces six to eight times more of the starch-digesting enzyme amylase. Their limited ability to utilize starch confined chimpanzees and other great apes to tropical jungles around the equator, where they found abundant fruits and perishable vegetables all year long to meet their caloric needs. It was our ability to digest and meet our energy needs with starch that allowed us to migrate north and south and inhabit the entire planet.

Nonfood Uses of Starch

The term "starch" comes from the Middle English word *sterchen:* to stiffen. In its pure form, starch is a white, odorless, tasteless powder. Starch granules don't dissolve in water, but heat causes them to swell and turn gelatinous. The starch gel cools into a paste that can be used as a thickener, stiffener, or glue. (Remember those flour-and-water paste projects in elementary school? Or papier-mâché? You might also have noticed that your cooked oatmeal or polenta turns stiff and gluelike after it cools.)

Starch is a principal ingredient in laundry products, medicines, cosmetics, and powders, with the largest nonfood use being paper production. The construction industry uses it to make gypsum wallboard, stucco, adhesives, and glues. Starch is a versatile substance in industry!

As early humans ventured north and south from Africa to colonize the rest of the planet, we relied on our ability to eat starchy tubers and grains for concentrated calories to last through the winter, after the fruits of summer and fall were gone. These starchy foods were widely available around the world and easy to gather from underground (roots, tubers) and aboveground (grains, beans). Starch's abundant calories also supplied the extra energy we needed to increase our brain capacity and size (threefold compared with that of lesser primates).[17]

RECLAIMING STARCH

With the exception of wealthy aristocrats, humans throughout history have derived most of their energy from starch. Life began to change with the colossal wealth created during the Industrial Revolution of the mid-1800s. As we began to successfully harness fossil fuels, millions and then billions of people began to eat from tables heaped high with meat, fowl, and dairy—foods that previously were eaten only by royalty. You can easily see the result: We've inflated to resemble the rotund images of aristocrats.

When we consume too much fat, the body looks for a place to store it, typically in the belly, buttocks, and thighs. The fat you eat is the fat you wear, quite literally. Starches provide energy and an abundance of nutrients without being stored visibly as fat. Quite the opposite: They fuel us with the proteins, essential fats, vitamins, and minerals that make our bodies run like the efficient machines they were meant to be.

Starches are a clean-burning fuel, with just a small fraction (1 to 8 percent) of their calories coming from fat. They have insignificant amounts of cholesterol. Unless they have come into contact with them from animal waste or tissue, they do not harbor pathogens like salmonella, E. coli, or mad cow prions (agents causing bovine spongiform encephalopathy). They don't store up poisonous chemicals from the environment, like DDT or methyl mercury. Unless they become contaminated by pesticides directly introduced by farmers, starches are squeaky clean.

Some starches, like potatoes and sweet potatoes, are complete foods: By eating these foods alone you will easily meet your basic nutritional needs with the exception of vitamin B_{12}. (We'll get into vitamins and supplements in more detail in Chapter 11.) Grains and legumes aren't quite so complete as potatoes, but add a small dose of vitamin A and C by eating a little fruit or green and yellow vegetables and you've got everything you need. No animal protein or dairy need be added for excellent and complete nutrition. (You will learn all about this in Chapters 7 and 8.)

Starches aren't just good for you, they're also satisfying. The abundant carbohydrates in starches stimulate the sweet taste receptors on the tip of the tongue, where gastronomic pleasure begins. Eat enough starches and your body will release hormones and go through neurological changes that ensure long-term satisfaction. Their naturally great taste and nourishing calories and the good feeling they give us during and after eating them are the reasons we refer to bread, rice, pasta, potatoes, corn, and beans as "comfort foods."

It is well accepted that starches are a great source of abundant calories, providing the energy athletes need to do everything from discus throwing to extreme skateboarding to running marathons. With all

---

E-MAIL TO DR. McDOUGALL

What I love best about your focus on starch is that it's much simpler for me to understand than focusing on carbs, proteins, and fats. I know what a starch is; I can recognize that food easily. And I can grow starchy foods in my gardens. But how do I grow a protein, a carb, or a fat? Those explanations were always too far removed from what I see on my plate.

Caroline Graettinger

---

those efficient calories, you would think that starches would promote excess weight gain, but they don't. That's because your body efficiently regulates the use of the carbohydrates you get from starch: Even if you consume them in excess, the body will burn them off as heat and energy rather than store much of them as fat.[18]

The Truth Is Well Known

Despite the drone from big business seeking to deafen our ears to it, sound advice to eat more vegetables, fruits, and whole grains—and less fat from meat and dairy products—has been given since the 1950s. In the introduction to a 1977 report from the US Senate Select Committee on Nutrition and Human Needs, Dr. D. Mark Hegsted of the Harvard School of Public Health wrote, "I wish to stress that there is a great deal of evidence and it continues to accumulate, which strongly implicates and, in some instances, proves that the major causes of death and disability in the United States are related to the diet we eat. I include coronary artery disease, which accounts for nearly half of the deaths in the United States, several of the most important forms of cancer, hypertension, diabetes, and obesity as well as other chronic diseases."[19]

In 2002, the World Health Organization published a report explaining that the shift toward refined foods, foods of animal origin (meat and dairy products), and increased fats was behind the global epidemics of obesity, diabetes, and cardiovascular disease. The report predicted that by 2020 two-thirds of the global burden of disease will be attributable "to chronic noncommunicable diseases, most of them strongly associated with diet."[20]

Our unwillingness to respond to this vast base of knowledge, from ancient to modern, has resulted in the greatest health crisis known to humankind. Worldwide, 1.1 billion people are overweight and 312 million obese, 18 million die of heart disease annually, more than 197 million have diabetes, and half of all people following a Western diet will develop life-threatening cancers.[21]

It's not just individuals who are suffering. Alongside escalating human sickness we are experiencing environmental catastrophes that are due in large part to abandoning a diet based on starches in favor of putting meat at the center of the plate. As you will see in Chapter 6, livestock are among the top two or three contributors to every one of our most serious environmental problems, including climate change.[22]

As you will learn throughout *The Starch Solution*, your change to a starch-based diet will do far more than heal your body. You will be making a contribution to changes that ripple out far beyond the foods on your plate. This shift, if adopted widely, will drastically shrink the pharmaceutical and medical industries by preventing and curing common illnesses, including obesity, heart disease, type 2 diabetes, arthritis, and intestinal disturbances ranging from heartburn to constipation.

The Starch Solution can help you to lose weight and feel and look better, and—with no extra effort—help to heal the world around you, reducing global warming and making our planet healthier and more sustainable for future generations. The only way to find out if a starch-based diet holds all these promises for you is to give it a try.

CHAPTER 2

People Passionate about Starches Are Healthy and Beautiful

My wife, Mary, and I sat at a table by the bay enjoying steamed sweet corn tamales with a side of black beans at Guaymas restaurant in Tiburon, California, just north of the Golden Gate Bridge. At the next table were three elegantly dressed women, ample in size. Over the course of our meal, I watched each make her way with great difficulty to the restroom and back.

I looked at Mary and thought, "These women are at least a decade younger than you are and all three are physically disabled." For what pleasure? Food? As the seaward breeze carried the greasy, fishy aroma of their deep-fried clams and shrimp to our table, I couldn't help but think that the McDougall Diet could make their lives easier. I wished I could have handed them my business card, or a copy of one of my books, without offending them.

Where have all the pretty women and handsome men gone? People spend thousands of dollars on clothes, cars, makeup, perfume, and plastic surgery to achieve what they believe to be more pleasing appearances. And yet, at the same time, they sacrifice their well-being for the sake of unhealthy foods they have developed a preference for, remaining in denial that these foods cause dependency and illness in much the same way that cigarettes, alcohol, and narcotics do. Too few people know that for free they can have all the health and beauty that money can't buy.

THE TRUTH IS SIMPLE AND EASY TO UNDERSTAND

Most people have been ingrained with the false notion, "Don't eat starches, because starch turns to sugar, which turns to fat, making you gain weight." If this were true there would be an epidemic of obesity among the 1.73 billion Asians living on rice-based diets. After moving west and replacing their starch-based diet with animal foods, people from Japan and the Philippines would become trimmer and healthier looking. But that's not so. In fact, the opposite happens.

Potatoes are fattening, right? Then why, during our McDougall Adventure trip to Peru—where potatoes are the staple food—were the residents so trim and strong? Consider the populations around the world that look the youngest, healthiest, and trimmest. Many are in Japan, China, Korea, Thailand, Indonesia, and the Philippines, eating mostly rice with some vegetables. In rural Mexico, we find people eating corn, beans, and squash. No one is overweight or on a diet there. The men, women, and children of central Papua New Guinea are nourished almost entirely by sweet potatoes. They have no need for Weight Watchers or Jenny Craig. In rural Africa, statuesque men and women thrive on starchy staples such as yams, cassava, millet, and beans. Worldwide, populations with the highest consumption of starch are the most trim and fit.[1,2] Delving deeper, we discover that they have extremely low rates of diabetes, arthritis, gallbladder disease, constipation, indigestion, multiple sclerosis, heart disease, and cancers of the breast, prostate, and colon. Their diets are centered around copious quantities of starch, and they are healthy.

Starches Generate Fitness

The body's metabolism is genetically encoded to run most efficiently on starch. No amount of willpower, dieting, or wishful thinking will change that fundamental fact. The one simple solution to health and beauty is to eat the diet we were designed for. In addition to being healthful, a diet based on starch offers a multitude of rewards.

Starches Satisfy the Appetite: The hunger drive keeps us alive. You cannot fool hunger by pushing yourself away from the table, putting down your fork between bites, eating from a small plate, or counting calories. You will never train yourself not to experience the discomfort associated with hunger, even if you practice until you are 90 years old.

The control you do have is over the foods that fill your plate. Meat, dairy, animal fats, and vegetable oils lead to excess weight gain and illness. Starches, vegetables, and fruits support a trim, fit body and a lifetime of excellent health.

You may have heard that all calories are the same when it comes to body weight. That's not true, especially when it comes to satisfying the appetite and accumulating fat. Three components of food provide the fuel we know as calories: protein, fat, and carbohydrate. Starches like corn, beans, potatoes, and rice offer abundant carbohydrates and dietary fiber and are very low in fat.

Satisfying the appetite begins with filling the stomach. Compared to cheese (4 calories per gram), meat (4 calories per gram), and oils (9 calories per gram), starches contribute only about 1 calorie per gram. They help you to feel full for just a quarter of the calories in cheese and meat, and one-ninth of those in oil.[3] Plus, they offer a great deal of satisfaction. Research comparing the way carbohydrates and fats appease the appetite shows that carbohydrates lead to hours of satiety, whereas fats have little impact. In other words, when you fill up on starch you stay full for a long time, whereas when you fill up on fats and oils you still want to eat more.[4,5]

Before I understood the importance of a starch-centered diet, my meals consisted of red meat (no carbohydrates), chicken (no carbohydrates), fish (no carbohydrates), cheese (2 percent carbohydrates), and animal fats and vegetable oils (no carbohydrates). After finishing a full plate of these foods I still found myself ravenous. My second plate left my belly feeling a sense of physical fullness, yet I was still yearning for more. After my third plate of carbohydrate-deficient foods, I finally received the signals that it was time to stop eating: I felt overstuffed and in pain. Still, because I remained unsatisfied, I remember thinking, "If I had room, I would stuff in one more pork chop, I'm still so hungry." At times, I wondered whether I might have emotional issues with food. After all, I had just downed large quantities and I was still starving. It wasn't until I began eating sufficient amounts of appetite-satisfying carbohydrates that I realized my "mental illness," commonly known as obsessive-compulsive overeating, was completely cured by this simple shift in my diet.

Excess Starch Does Not Turn to Body Fat: A widely held myth holds that the sugars in starches are readily converted into fat, which is then stored visibly in our abdomen, hips, and buttocks. If you read the published research, you will see that there is no disagreement about this whatsoever among scientists, and that they say that this is incorrect![6–14] After eating, we break down the complex carbohydrates in starchy foods into simple sugars. These sugars are absorbed into the bloodstream, where they are transported to trillions of cells throughout the body for energy. If you eat more carbohydrate than your body needs, you'll store up to 2 pounds of it invisibly in the muscles and liver in the form of glycogen. If you eat more carbohydrate than you can use (as your daily energy) and store (as glycogen), you'll burn the remainder off as body heat and through physical movement other than sports, such as walking to work, typing, yard work, and fidgeting.[10,14,15]

Turning sugars into fats is a process called *de novo lipogenesis*. Pigs and cows use this process to convert carbohydrates from grains and grasses

E-MAIL TO DR. McDOUGALL

I was talking to my neighbor and he noticed that I had lost weight. My coat now buttons! His comment was that I looked great and to keep up the good work and lay off the mashed potatoes. We both have some great recipes for mashed potatoes. Of course I said nothing to the contrary, but those mashed potatoes have been my daily main course many days with a side of vegetables. There's so much misinformation about starches. No wonder people are so fat and fail on other diets.

One thing I noticed after a couple weeks on the diet is that my intense cravings for meat, dairy, and oil are gone. I switched from coffee with cream and honey to hot lemon water. Bingeing thoughts are gone. I had a couple of stress-filled days this past week and instead of eating everything in sight to soothe myself, I just ate some mashed potatoes and broccoli, spinach, and corn. That was filling, my favorite foods, and that was it. No more stress or over-eating. Great plan.

Sincerely,
Suzanna Browne

into calorie-dense fats.[6] That's what makes them so appealing as a food source. Bees do it, too, converting honey (simple carbohydrate) into wax (fatty acids and alcohols).

We humans, on the other hand, are very inefficient at converting carbohydrate to fat; we don't do it under normal conditions.[6-15] (The cost for this conversion is 30 percent of the calories consumed.[12]) Subjects overfed large amounts of simple sugars under experimental laboratory conditions, however, will convert a small amount of carbohydrate to fat. For example, both trim and obese women fed 50 percent more calories than they usually ate in a day, along with an extra 3☐ ounces (135 grams) of refined sugar, produced less than 4 grams of fat daily

---

The "Eat More Starch" Challenge

In the seventies, researchers from the Food Science and Human Nutrition Department at Michigan State University (my alma mater) asked 16 moderately overweight college-age men to add 12 slices of white bread (at 70 calories a slice) or high fiber bread (at 50 calories a slice) to their diet daily.[16] On average, subjects eating the extra white bread lost 14 pounds (6.26 Kg) and those adding the high fiber bread lost 19 pounds (8.77 Kg) during the next 8 weeks. Appetite-appeasing breads worked by replacing the easy-to-wear fats found in the meats, dairy products, and vegetable oils, causing them to spontaneously, without any additional conscious thought or effort, lose the weight. The general health of these college students also improved as reflected by a very large and rapid reduction in their blood cholesterol levels (by 50 to 80 mg/dL).

This is my challenge to you if you are one of the few people who is not yet fully convinced about the power of the Starch Solution: Simply eat more starch without intentionally giving up

---

(less than $^1/_8$ ounce).[11] That's just 36 extra calories stored as fat per day. You'd have to overeat all of those extra calories and table sugar every day for nearly 4 months just to gain 1 pound of extra body fat.

The warning about carbohydrates turning to body fat is a myth and nothing more: In humans, even substantial quantities of refined and processed carbohydrates contribute only a trivial amount to body fat.[6–15] The same is not true of animal and vegetable fats, however. A passenger on a cruise ship gains an average of 8 pounds on a 7-day voyage—caused by dining on buffets of meats, cheese, oil-soaked vegetables, and high-fat desserts.

So, where does all the belly fat come from? It bears repeating: The fat you eat is the fat you wear.

---

anything else in your current diet. This commitment means adding daily any one (or a mixture) of the following to your regular diet:

4 cups of steamed rice

4 cups of boiled corn

4 mashed potatoes

4 baked sweet potatoes

3 cups of cooked beans, peas, or lentils

4 cups of boiled spaghetti noodles

12 slices of whole grain bread

Simply add this extra 600 to 900 calories (divided throughout the day) of your choice of grains, legumes, or starchy vegetables to what you are already eating in order to see remarkable benefits, just as the college-age men did.

Fat Is the Metabolic Dollar Saved for the Next Famine:
After you eat dairy, meat, nuts, oils, and other high-fat foods, you
absorb their fat from your intestine into the bloodstream. From there,
it is transported to billions of adipose (fat) cells for storage. This is a
very efficient process: It uses up only 3 percent of the calories you consume to move the fat on your fork and spoon to your body fat.[12] This
storage takes place almost effortlessly after every fat-filled meal. If you
have your body fat chemically analyzed, it will reveal the kinds of fats
you commonly eat.[17-20] Margarine and shortening, for example, result
in high proportions of trans fats in stored body fat. A diet high in cold-
water marine fish shows omega-3 fats. The saying "from my lips to my
hips" expresses the real-life effect of the Western diet. Fortunately,
starches contain very little fat for you to wear.

Starches Help Us to Radiate Vitality: Every year, millions of people lose weight without necessarily improving their
health. In fact, these weight-loss methods often cause illness.
The best example of this negative effect of dieting is the once-
popular Atkins-type, low-carbohydrate, high-protein approach.
These diets work by severe carbohydrate deprivation, which causes a
state of illness (with the common outcome of ketosis). When people
become sick they lose their appetite and lose weight. This method for
losing extra pounds is analogous to the weight loss seen in people taking
cancer chemotherapy drugs.[21] To the careful observer, people following
low-carbohydrate diets look and act sick, too.

A starch-based diet, on the other hand, brings radiant health along
with the loss of excess body fat. Endurance athletes know the benefits of
"carbo loading." In addition to enabling peak performance, a starch-
based diet improves blood flow to all tissues in the body. The skin glows
with a clear complexion from the improved circulation. A welcome by-
product of eating low-fat starches is the elimination of oily skin, black-
heads, whiteheads, and acne. From weight loss and the resulting relief
from arthritis, people on a starch-based diet feel active, agile, and more
youthful.

Health Is Attractive

I learned the facts of life from my father many years ago. We were close and discussed all matters frankly. As we walked down a busy street one day, he noticed my eyes drawn to many of the young women passing by. He said, "The reason you find some of these girls especially attractive is that they look healthy." My hormone-fueled boyish response was, "That's not what I am looking at, Dad." It took me many years before I understood how right he was. Health is attractive, by natural design, for the preservation of the species. Sexually, we are drawn to healthy people because those are the ones we want to mate—and share our genetic material—with. This characteristic of human nature enhances the chances that a loving relationship between man and woman will result in the highest quality offspring. Overweight, and even more so, obesity, is a glaring sign of malnutrition and poor health. Youth is associated with health; this is one reason young people are so attractive. As we age, our health deteriorates along with our good looks. One important benefit for people following the Starch Solution is graceful aging and preservation of the attractive spark of life.

In platonic relationships health is also a magnet that pulls people together. In times past, villages depended on the strengths of their individual members in order to survive. Physically fit people could hunt, gather, and defend on behalf of all members in the community. The sick were a burden, and often banished. These same principles transfer to the business world of today. Appearing healthy means you are more likely to add to the common goals of the company. Hearty employees work harder, for longer hours, more cleverly, and more efficiently—they are valuable contributors. Good health radiates your worth to others, resulting in personal advancement. *The Starch Solution* provides you the best opportunity to be healthy and attractive.

(continued on page 30)

Cloudy Rockwell, Director of Finance and Administration, Palmer, Alaska

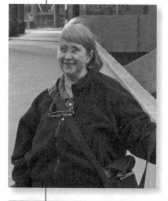

I have been heavy most of my life, but until I began this way of eating, I did not realize that I had been obese for almost all of my adult life. I did Weight Watchers twice, the Fit for Life diet of the mid-80s; I tried the South Beach Diet and many others. I was losing no significant amounts of weight, even after being very compliant, and gaining it all back each time. I know better than to fail like that! I'm a smart, educated woman; what is the matter with me?

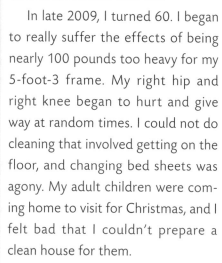

In late 2009, I turned 60. I began to really suffer the effects of being nearly 100 pounds too heavy for my 5-foot-3 frame. My right hip and right knee began to hurt and give way at random times. I could not do cleaning that involved getting on the floor, and changing bed sheets was agony. My adult children were coming home to visit for Christmas, and I felt bad that I couldn't prepare a clean house for them.

Somehow, I was lucky enough to find a link to some testimonials about Dr. McDougall. During the first shopping trip for groceries for his plan, I was in an agony of pain. It was enough to begin, though. I have to say that the first bite of brown rice, after 5 years of eschewing carbs, brought tears to my eyes! It was like welcoming back an old friend! The starch-based diet has been satisfying and filling. It is also easy to shop for, and meal planning is so simple.

There were two strategies that I found valuable. The first was to always be prepared. Every weekend, I would make a general food plan that I shopped and cooked for, making enough food for the week's lunches and dinners. I did this to keep myself from "poor me syndrome"—the condition of feeling that I am hungry and it will be so long until I can get to food, I had better eat whatever is at hand. I instead developed "enough syndrome"—I have had enough and there is food already prepared for me at home. Second, I developed an attitude toward non-plan food that told me: "It is not food." The chocolates in the jar in the office, the cheese in the drawer at home, the fried calamari on the table at the restaurant were no longer food to me—no more than the table linens or the candles were food. I knew what I was going to eat, and it would be available soon, and I was not about to start gnawing on "not-food" while I waited.

Within a month, the pains had begun to recede from my hip and knee. I am now at about 130 pounds, and I have lost more than 92 pounds. It took me about 18 months to lose the weight, averaging about a pound and a quarter per week. I have gone from a size 26 in jeans to a size 4 (not Levi's, I readily admit)! I have gone from a 3X to an XS. Buying new clothes has been the biggest expense on this journey! I went from being someone in denial about being obese, convincing myself that I was quite healthy simply because I didn't have a lot of reasons to visit the doctor, to someone who is actually vibrant with health. I can crawl on the floor to get iPhone pictures of my baby granddaughter in action, and then get back up again; I have brought down my cholesterol and blood sugars; I can run without tiring for 20 minutes. I went from being old before my time to a woman who is looking forward to all the years to come.

MODERATION IS IMPOSSIBLE FOR PASSIONATE PEOPLE

My great-grandmother, Laura Bristow, lived to be 106 eating a "well-balanced diet." I recall her telling me when I was a young child, "Johnny, you eat too much meat; it's going to make you sick."

Years later, when I was 31 and had given up almost all animal foods, and she was 102, she asked me to drive to McDonald's to buy her a hamburger—a 30-cent paper-thin patty of ground beef with two pickle slices and a blob each of mustard and ketchup, all hidden between two halves of an airy white bun. She cut the hamburger into quarters, shook one quarter in my face, and admonished, "If you ate a little more meat you would be healthier." She ate two of the quarters and put the rest away for later.

My great-grandmother picked at tiny platefuls of traditional American foods, drank a quarter cup of diluted coffee each morning, and had one small glass of red wine on holidays. Unlike me, she was the picture of moderation.

I am not a restrained person and neither are most of my patients. In my youth, I started the day with several mugs of strong coffee. I frequented all-you-can-eat buffets and fast-food restaurants, and I smoked two packs of Marlboros a day. Often, I unwound at the end of my stress-filled day with a whiskey or two. I paid a big price for this behavior: a cholesterol level of 335 milligrams per deciliter, 50 pounds of excess body fat, major abdominal surgery, and a debilitating stroke, all before the age of 25.

I realize most people are not as excessive as I am. But most do allow at least one of these overindulgences in their lives, and for many, that one extravagance is unending forkfuls of rich foods. For passionate people like us, any attempt at moderation results in continued dependence and recurring failures.

The phrase "everything in moderation" has been preached through much of human history. It didn't work in times past and it doesn't work for most people today. Have you ever met a smoker who quit by cutting down? An alcoholic who sobered up by switching to beer, or having just one drink a day? Westerners are addicted to their steaks, cheeses, and pies. Teasing us with a little bit of our most tempting vices is not a viable solution. Cutting down on the portion size of fried chicken, gravy, biscuits, and ice cream is slow torture for most, and is one of the primary reasons diets fail.

The startling observation that almost all people in Western societies are fat and/or sick with diseases that will wreck and shorten their lives should have health professionals up in arms, demanding an immediate and complete end to this senseless suffering, regardless of the expense and effort. Instead, the loss of a father or husband to a heart attack, the loss of a mother's breast to cancer, the blinding of a friend from diabetes are accepted consequences of our birthright to eat like aristocrats. To mitigate these food-induced tragedies, we are told to eat a little less of the same things.

Throughout my life I have been enthusiastic about everything: schoolwork, hobbies, sports. I was born that way, and scientific research establishes that, like the color of our eyes and hair, our personality traits are determined in part by genetics.[22,23] Early life experiences fostered my exuberant nature. So now, even if I wanted to, I could not become a moderate person. Still, I love life and do not want my high-spirited personality to kill me, as it almost did in my youth. This is one reason that motivated me to discover a solution that works.

I now direct that forceful energy toward supportive behaviors rather than destructive ones. I have learned to love healthy foods and I eat them without reservation. Windsurfing is one of my passions, and I eagerly anticipate long walks carrying my youngest grandchild in a backpack. My favorite drink is sparkling water—I drink a lot of it. In short, there is no limit to the good things I passionately pursue in life.

Excess and health need not be mutually exclusive, so long as you take a little time to learn which excesses are health enhancing rather than destructive. The Irish poet and dramatist Oscar Wilde once said, "Moderation is a fatal thing. Nothing succeeds like excess." I encourage you to take these words to heart and live life enthusiastically, with health-supporting behaviors.

CHAPTER 3

Five Major Poisons Found in Animal Foods

The benefits of a starch-based diet go far beyond controlling weight and improving personal appearance. Choosing starch over animal foods to meet your energy and nutritional needs protects you from a wide range of illnesses and injuries that come bundled with a typical Western diet. If I sound dramatic when I talk about the dangers of what you are eating it's because this is serious business, and I am by profession a medical doctor. The balanced diet most people take for granted as being healthy—and that is endorsed by medical experts and the USDA—is actually toxic to humans.

When we think about food being harmful, our first concern is that it will make us feel sick immediately after we eat. You probably learned the painful lesson as a child that it's not a great idea to go to a carnival and stuff yourself full of corn dogs and cotton candy, then take a ride on the Ferris wheel. If you travel, you may have taken along a pink bottle of Pepto-Bismol to ward off unfamiliar bacteria. Perhaps you follow the news and avoid foods that cause food poisoning from E. coli, Listeria, and salmonella that have been recalled due to contamination.

What you might not realize is that many of the foods you consume without suddenly feeling ill can be equally risky, or even more so over the long haul. Meat, poultry, fish, seafood, milk, and eggs are a slower type of poison, but they are every bit as dangerous as the ones that let you know right away you have made a big mistake. (A poison is a substance that causes injury, illness, or death, especially by chemical means.) You may never suspect these foods as the culprit when you become ill with heart disease, cancer, or inflamed joints as long as four decades later. The long lag between consuming these harmful foods and noticing the symptoms fools most people into believing they are safe. In fact, the overabundance of protein, fat, cholesterol, methionine (a sulphur-containing amino acid), and dietary acids in these foods leads us down a dangerous path from the moment we take our first bite.

Cause and Effect

What if the effects of the food choices we make were instantaneous? What if eating a plate of fried eggs caused excruciating chest pains? Or a stroke and paralysis followed a prime rib dinner? A cancerous lump appeared a week after eating a grilled cheese sandwich? Would you continue to eat those foods? Probably not. If the ill effects came quickly enough that we easily associated them with the foods that caused them, we would widely recognize animal foods for the real and serious risks they pose. Because the effects are not immediate, we have to dig a little deeper to understand how these foods affect us.

Choices about what we eat aren't very different from other lifestyle choices. If smoking a pack of cigarettes was followed by a week on a respirator, or if drinking a bottle of gin caused instant liver disease and coma, few people would make the choice to use these toxins. But choose them they do, because although they may have some unpleasant immediate effects, the perceived pleasure that people experience in the moment wins out over the damage that comes later.

There is one fundamental difference between the danger of animal foods and that of cigarettes and drinking. With tobacco and alcohol, the risks are nearly universally understood. We know the facts.

Meat, poultry, fish, seafood, cheese, milk, and eggs, on the other hand, are widely considered an appropriate, even essential part of a healthy diet. Most people eat these risky foods believing that they are nutritious and life sustaining. They may understand that eating too much fat or cholesterol, or too many calories, makes them vulnerable to health consequences, but that doesn't stop them from eating those foods. It may cause some conscientious people to relegate them to special occasions, or to substitute "leaner" versions of their favorite foods. We don't consider the danger inherent in eating these foods because nobody has told us how harmful they really are. We have been misled by medical doctors, dietians, and advertisements bought by the food industries. It's not a conscious effort to harm us and our families; it's "just business."

DISTRACT YOUR CUSTOMERS, THEN SLOWLY KILL THEM

Food companies use "unique positioning" to promote their products. Whether seeking to sell beef, cheese, eggs, or chicken, each industry positions its product by elevating some benefit it wants you to associate with it. This type of marketing has convinced us that milk and cheese build strong bones with their generous supply of calcium. Got beef? Then you've also got plenty of iron. Chicken on the menu? Great, that's an outstanding source of lean protein. Fish for dinner? What better way to get your brain-building omega-3 fatty acids? At least that's what these industries would have you believe. But are the claims true? Do they tell the whole story?

Marketing efforts by the meat and dairy industries have convinced us that calcium, iron, and protein are essential nutrients we should seek out in large quantities. In food and supplements, they are sold as a kind

(continued on page 38)

Jeff Armstrong,
Elementary School Art Teacher,
Sacramento, California

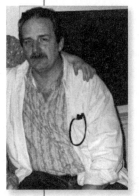

I grew up in the '50s and '60s when meat was cheap. In the late 1960s, steak was so cheap that my mom would serve it two or three times a week. I was able to maintain some semblance of slimness until I was about 19 years old. I never was one to be really athletic, and after age 19 I began to put on the pounds. My trim 190 on a 6-foot-4 frame became 220, then, in college, 240. I panicked and turned to Dr. Atkins. Within a few months of eating a pound of bacon for

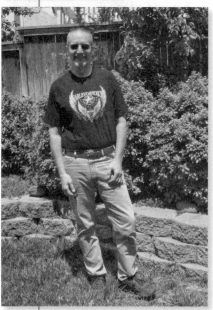

breakfast and "bunless" hamburgers for lunch and dinner I was able to drop about 35 pounds. It was a miracle. Only the miracle came at a price. My skin was greasy all the time. I had trouble sleeping. I felt nervous all day long. And at about the 3-month mark I started to get pains in my lower back. It was a while before I realized that the pain was probably my overworked kidneys. What a miracle. So I abandoned Atkins and within about 6 months gained back the weight I had lost and about 10 more pounds to boot. After several more of my failed attempts at dieting, my mother sent me some information about the McDougall Diet.

It's that time of year again, my birthday—time to take stock.

Tomorrow I turn 57, meaning that it was 10 years ago that I took the McDougall plunge. You said you never tire of hearing thanks, so I'm writing to say so again. Thanks to you I have lost 120 pounds from my high of 305 pounds. I'm now below my youthful trim weight of 190. Thanks to you, my cholesterol has plummeted from 271 to 127 milligrams per deciliter (mg/dL). (What a difference the order of those numbers makes!) Thanks to you, my favorite jeans fit better than ever. Thanks to you, I am finally at home in my body. My arthritis is gone. My sleep apnea is a past memory. I no longer experience lactose intolerance. My hiatal hernia has cleared up. No more atrial fibrillation. Even my ornery toenail fungus has cleared—is that a new one for you?

My friends and colleagues remain certain I am depriving myself, but I am not. I am perfectly happy with my simple regime of rice, beans, corn, greens, potatoes, and other veggies, mostly repeating the same combos over and over again. I walk 4 or 5 miles every day with my dogs, and I look forward to a workout at the health club three or four times a week. My doctor tells me that of all his patients he has seen only three or four accomplish what I have. But you and I know it is possible for anyone.

When my wife finally saw the light and jumped into the McDougall life with me she lost 40 pounds and now feels so much better. Her cholesterol is down 80 points and she is now a regular 5 days a week at the health club. She's been up to Santa Rosa for your 10-day program and back for tune-ups. In fact, we are constantly faced with so much nutritional misinformation that we've decided to come up for at least one McDougall Weekend a year, just to keep current and recharge our batteries.

of insurance policy against deficiency-caused illnesses. These nutrients are indeed essential, but what the animal product and pill marketers won't tell you is that illnesses from deficiencies of these nutrients are virtually unknown, and that common plant foods fully meet our calcium, iron, and protein needs. There actually is no known nutritional advantage to choosing red meat, poultry, dairy, or eggs for their high density of particular nutrients. In fact, high nutrient concentrations come at the expense of others: milk and cheese are deficient in iron, while red meat, poultry, and eggs (apart from the shells) provide almost no calcium. These cannot be considered balanced foods: When you eat them you end up with too much of some nutrients and not enough of others. The ones you get in excess pose real and well-documented risks.

In my 44 years of practicing medicine, I have never seen a patient sickened by eating potatoes, sweet potatoes, corn, rice, beans, fruits, or vegetables, except in rare cases where the foods were spoiled or contaminated, or where they triggered an uncommon allergy or food sensitivity.

What I do witness every day are serious diseases that stem from eating animal foods, including heart attacks, strokes, type 2 diabetes, arthritis, osteoporosis, and cancer. It doesn't matter whether those foods were processed by a large corporation using additives and chemicals, sold directly by a trusted organic farmer, or raised in your own backyard. All animal foods cause illness when consumed in amounts typically found in the Western diet. Why? Primarily because they are the wrong foods for humans.

ANIMAL FOODS ARE MORE ALIKE THAN DIFFERENT

All animal foods provide essentially the same nutrition and have roughly the same impact on your health. It doesn't matter whether you grill meat that comes from a cow, pig, sheep, lamb, or chicken, scramble eggs from a chicken or duck, or drink milk that comes from a cow,

Five Key Components of Selected Animal and Plant Foods

	BEEF	CHICKEN	CHEESE	EGGS	AVERAGE
Protein	37	46	25	32	35
Fat	57	51	74	61	61
Cholesterol	32	36	26	272	92
Methionine	268	335	162	251	254
Dietary acid	6.3	7.0	10	8.2	8

	BEANS	RICE	POTATO	SWEET POTATO	AVERAGE
Protein	27	9	8	7	13
Fat	4	8	1	1	4
Cholesterol	0	0	0	0	0
Methionine	98	66	50	41	64
Dietary acid	1	1	−5	−9	−3

Note: Protein and fat are expressed in percentage of total calories. Cholesterol and methionine are milligrams per 100 calories. Dietary acid is renal acid load per 100 calories (a negative number means the food is alkaline).

goat, or sheep. Industry-specific food marketers would have you believe otherwise, but in fact, these foods are so similar they are essentially equivalent as far as nutrition is concerned.

As you can see, animal foods are made up of large amounts of protein, fat, and cholesterol, with high levels of the sulfur-containing amino acid methionine and dietary acids. This is true whether you eat one of these foods on its own or combine them at mealtime in people's favorite blenders: their stomachs.

Except for the simple sugars in milk and honey, animal foods contain essentially no carbohydrate, and they never provide dietary fiber.

Comparisons of Levels of Potentially Harmful Substances in Animal Foods versus Starches (averages)

	ANIMAL FOODS	STARCHES	ANIMAL TO STARCH RATIO (ROUNDED)
Protein	35	13	3:1
Fat	61	4	15:1
Cholesterol	92	0	100:1
Methionine	254	64	4:1
Dietary acid	8	−3	10:1

Note: Protein and fat are expressed in percentage of total calories. Cholesterol and methionine are milligrams per 100 calories. Dietary acid is renal acid load per 100 calories (a negative number means the food is alkaline).

Like animal foods, starchy plant foods as a group behave essentially identically to one another. Plant foods are high in carbohydrate and fiber, low in fat and dietary acids, and have no significant amount of cholesterol. They also have sufficient, but not excess, amounts of protein on average. In other words, they provide considerably more of what is good for you and little to none of what makes you sick.

FIVE COMPONENTS OF ANIMAL FOODS THAT ARE POISONING YOU

Your body can handle only so much protein, fat, cholesterol, sulfur-containing amino acids, and dietary acids. When you take in more than your body can use, metabolize, neutralize, and/or eliminate, those excess amounts act as poisons. On a typical Western diet, these toxic by-products build up in your system on a daily basis. As you can see in the previous tables, compared with starches, animal foods burden us with inflated levels of these dietary components.

As if ingesting these toxic substances isn't bad enough, their effects are additive and cumulative. Taking in too much protein, methionine, and dietary acid weakens our bones over time. Excess dietary fat and cholesterol clog the arteries and increase the risk of cancer. In fact, these five elements—all found in animal foods in quantities far greater than we are able to use and excrete—harm us in many ways. Let's look at each of these potential toxins a little more closely.

Toxin: Protein

When we keep eating protein after we've met our daily requirement, the body seeks to eliminate the excess. The primary route is through the liver and kidneys. Some people may notice the strong smell of urea in their sweat and urine, one indicator of protein overload. (This isn't the only amino acid you can identify by smell: Most of us know the familiar scent of asparagine in urine that follows a meal with asparagus.)

Excess protein takes its toll, even when we are strong and healthy. On average, we lose a quarter of our overall kidney function over 70 years of life just from consuming a diet high in animal protein.[1,2] For those with already compromised livers and kidneys, excess protein speeds up the processes that lead to organ failure.[3-7] Protein overload also harms the bones; each time we double our protein intake we increase the amount of calcium excreted in the urine by 50 percent, escalating our risk for osteoporosis and kidney stones.[8]

Toxin: Fat

A 2007–2008 report on the epidemic of obesity in the United States found that 68 percent of adults were overweight, with a body mass index (BMI) over 25 compared to normal levels of 18.5 to 24.5.[9] More than one in three (33.8 percent) were obese, with a BMI over 30.9. (BMI is calculated by dividing a person's weight in kilograms by the square of his or her height in meters.)

The body stores dietary fat quite effortlessly as body fat.[10] We also store surplus fat in our liver, heart, and muscles. The accumulation of fat in these organs is a hallmark of a condition referred to as insulin resistance, which in turn contributes to heart disease, stroke, and type 2 diabetes.[11]

Carrying around excess weight also puts stress on the joints, leading to osteoarthritis in the hips and knees. Excess dietary fat and body weight alter your entire cellular metabolism and can stimulate the development of certain cancers.[12]

Toxin: Cholesterol

Cholesterol is found nearly exclusively in animal products; plants contain only insignificant quantities.[13] Like all animals, we produce all the cholesterol we need for our own uses. Unfortunately, our bodies are not very efficient at eliminating the excess; we excrete only a little more than the amount we make ourselves. When we add to our cholesterol load by eating animal foods, the excess accumulates in our skin and tendons, as well as in the arteries where it is a major contributor to vascular diseases of the heart and brain, leading to heart attacks and strokes.[14] Cholesterol also facilitates cancer development.[15]

Toxin: Methionine

The sulfur-containing amino acids found in large amounts in meat, poultry, fish, eggs, and cheese act as a culprit in a wide range of problems. Perhaps most noticeable is the familiar stink of sulfur we associate with rotten eggs. In the body, sulfur causes bad breath, body odor, and foul-smelling gas and stools.

When we take in the sulfur-containing amino acid methionine by eating animal foods, we metabolize it into another amino acid, homocysteine, which is a known risk factor for heart attack, stroke, arterial diseases of the legs, blood clots in the veins, dementia, Alzheimer's disease, and depression.[16] Sulfur feeds cancerous tumors and is known to be toxic to the tissues of the intestine, causing severe colitis.[17,18]

We eventually metabolize sulfur-containing amino acids, methionine included, into sulfuric acid, one of the most potent acids found in nature. These potent dietary acids dissolve the bones and cause the kidneys to produce calcium-based stones.

Toxin: Dietary Acid

Animal foods are loaded with dietary acids. After we eat them, our bones release the alkaline materials carbonate, citrate, and sodium from their generous storehouse to neutralize the acids, maintaining the body at the precise pH level needed to sustain life.[19–23] Over time, this process weakens the bones, leading to osteoporosis. Acids from animal foods also raise body levels of the steroid cortisol,[24] triggering bone loss. Thus, the chronic overconsumption of dietary acids from meat, poultry, fish, and cheese essentially causes you to pee your bones into the toilet.

THE PATH TO DETOXIFICATION IS PAVED WITH STARCH

Reducing or eliminating the animal foods in your diet immediately relieves the burden on your body from these five dietary poisons, and at the same time greatly reduces your risk of exposure to infectious bacteria, viruses, parasites, and prion diseases (like those that cause mad cow disease).[25,26] The best way to cut out these toxic foods is to replace them with whole grains, legumes, and starchy vegetables— foods that provide all of the nutrition you need, along with sufficient calories and substance to give you energy and keep you feeling satisfied. Even if you are already showing signs of sickness from the excesses of meat, dairy, and eggs, there is hope. Starch has an immense ability to allow your body to naturally heal itself.

CHAPTER 4

Spontaneous Healing on a Starch-Based Diet

Three-quarters of the illnesses suffered by people living in industrialized countries are long-standing, chronic conditions, such as obesity, heart disease, type 2 diabetes, arthritis, and cancers. What do people in these regions have in common? A diet dominated by meat, dairy, fat, and processed foods. Understanding the problem points to a simple solution: By replacing these body-burdening foods with healthful starches, vegetables, and fruits, we can reduce or eradicate the enormous personal, social, and economic burden of chronic disease.

Starches support your body's intrinsic ability to heal by providing a perfect balance of carbohydrate, protein, fiber, fat, vitamins, and minerals, along with a balance of antioxidants and other plant-synthesized phytochemicals. Unlike the foods that are making you sick, starches contain no significant amounts of dangerous cholesterol, saturated or trans fats, animal proteins, dietary acids, chemical toxins, or disease-causing microbes.

THE KEY TO RECOVERY: STOP THE CYCLE OF INJURY

If your health is deteriorating, do not assume that your body is failing you. Its efforts to heal never stop, not even for a second. However, by the time I meet most of my patients they will have endured tens of thousands of repeated injuries to their arteries, joints, and tissues, simply because of what they eat. For disease to progress, injury must outpace healing.

For healing to occur, the opposite must happen: Healing must outpace injury. It's a simple matter of allowing your body to take two (or more) steps forward for every step back. Or better yet, to stop all regressions by very clean living.

Understand, however, that if you continue injuring your body for too long, the disease-causing forces will eventually do irreversible damage. Your body will no longer be able to work its healing magic completely. Fortunately, most of us are not in that much trouble. There is still hope, and the solution is in our own hands. If you want to reverse your body's disease processes, all you need do is stop the damage. In almost all cases this means changing to a health-supporting starch-based diet. In this manner the five dietary poisons—protein, fat, cholesterol, sulfur-containing amino acids, and dietary acids—that were identified in the previous chapter are removed. With the same shift in food choices, essential nutrients that support healing are provided by a perfect design found in plant foods.

The Body Seeks Health

There are plenty of examples of the body's ability to heal from repeated injuries we inflict on ourselves by our bad habits. A cigarette smoker inhales toxic fumes many times each day, inflaming the lungs with every puff. The lungs fight back by making the smoker cough and produce mucus in an effort to expel the poisons. Because the nicotine in tobacco is addictive, we assault our lungs over and over again, hour after hour and year after year. Eventually, parts of the lung die and are replaced by scar tissue. The result is diminished lung capacity from emphysema. Chronic injury can also lay the foundation for lung cancer. But serious lung disease is not inevitable. Many smokers find the strength to quit before the damage becomes irreversible. The lungs heal to the best of their capacity and the former smoker once again breathes in full, deep, restorative breaths of air.

Toxic liver damage from alcohol and skin damage from overexposure to the sun are other examples of harm resulting from our habits and behaviors. In these cases, too, the first sign of the body's spontaneous attempt to mend is inflammation, an essential step in recovering from injury or infection. Our tissues become hot, swollen, and painful as plasma and white blood cells move from the blood into the injured areas to do their healing work. The immune system takes over with a cascade of biochemical events that eventually lead to improved health. The sooner you stop the hurtful behavior, the more quickly and completely you can recover.

A Colossal Example of Spontaneous Healing

As a medical doctor I have had the opportunity to observe self-generated, spontaneous healing thousands of times. Yet nothing makes a greater impression than the miraculous recovery that follows massive trauma. During my early years of medical training at The Queen's Medical Center in Hawaii, a young man mangled by a motorcycle accident was pushed through the emergency room doors one evening. A splintered bone poked out through his left thigh. A 12-inch gash across his left forearm streamed bright red blood. The skin on his left cheek and forehead were scraped off from his slide across the pavement. X-rays showed a skull fracture and many broken ribs. I feared he would not survive.

The young man's bones were straightened and his wounds cleaned and sewn right there in the ER. But it was his body's ability to repair this massive damage that ultimately allowed him to heal.

The healing processes began almost immediately after the accident. Platelets and blood-clotting proteins coagulated his blood and plugged thousands of leaking vessels. During the hours that followed, his white blood cells migrated into his open wounds to defend them against

(continued on page 50)

Robert Cross, Attorney, Sacramento, California

I was nervous as the day for my follow-up radioactive heart scan approached. The previous year's test showed a large area where too little blood was flowing into my heart. I had chest pain while taking 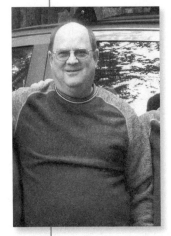 the treadmill test at that time, and I could barely get my heart rate up to 85 percent of the predicted maximum for my age of 62. My doctor recommended medication, an angiogram, and a type of heart surgery called angioplasty. Hoping to avoid the surgery and possible additional harm, I put myself on Dr. McDougall's low-fat, starch-based diet after reading about it on the Internet.

From almost the first day, I ceased having chest pain, even when I exercised. A year later I am off my cholesterol meds and my total choles-

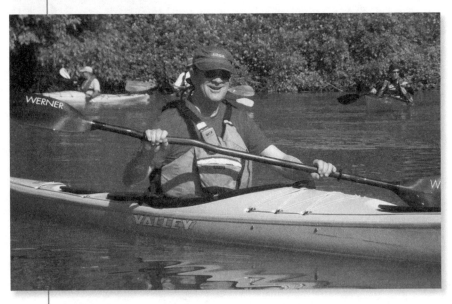

terol went from 294 milligrams per deciliter (mg/dL) to 160 mg/dL and my "bad" LDL cholesterol has dropped from 212 to 60 mg/dL. I'm also off my blood pressure medications, and at the doctor's office my blood pressure was perfectly normal at 110/75 millimeters of mercury (mmHg). I stopped my diabetes medications, too, and my last hemoglobin A1C—a blood sugar test for the long-term control of diabetes—was normal at around 6 percent. Also I have lost more than 60 pounds over this past year, as well.

It's a huge relief to have my numbers back under control and to be off those drugs. My newfound energy and sense of lightness have made me feel a decade younger. Still, I was nervous about my follow-up test.

During my second heart scan I had no pain on the treadmill, even though I got my heart rate all the way up to 160 beats per minute, beyond the highest the doctor expected I could go. When I stopped I still felt like I had more in me. The large areas in my heart that had not been receiving sufficient blood were almost completely functional now, leaving behind only a small deficiency my cardiologist called minor. He didn't go so far as to say the results were perfectly normal, but he did say they had improved dramatically and were now only mildly abnormal. I think he was afraid if he told me I was altogether normal I would stop the dietary changes that got me well. He needn't have worried. I see clearly now that what happened had everything to do with what I was eating. I would like to add that after almost 4 years, I have maintained my gains. My total cholesterol is now 139. I am another 5 pounds lighter and have had no further health problems or required any medications.

infection. Fluids collected in his torn flesh and around his broken bones. Swelling in his thigh, shoulder, and face lasted for weeks, helping to hold his bones in place. Pain kept him still, preventing movements that could cause further injury.

Soon, the damaged tissues began to restore themselves. Cells called fibroblasts laid down new structural material in the soft tissue, with osteoblasts doing the same for his broken bones. Over the coming months, replicator cells produced new muscle, skin, bone, and scars, remodeling his wounds so that his body would look and function nearly as it had before the accident.

Within a week of his near-death incident, this brave young man was up and walking on crutches. After 10 days, the stitches came out of his thigh and arm. In about 6 weeks, the scabs fell off his face, revealing delicate pink skin with new hair follicles filling in his beard. His broken ribs were stable and painless after 7 weeks, and after 3 months he was walking on his own without a limp. The pain had mostly passed, but the memories were still raw; he sold the motorcycle to avoid risking a repeat of his massive injury.

The patient's 3-month journey—from broken, bleeding, and near death to nearly completely restored—was nothing short of miraculous. His injuries were due to a single collision of immense force. With the chronic diseases I treat, the damage is the result of thousands of micro-pinprick-size injuries to the arteries, joints, and other tissues over prolonged periods. However, although acute and chronic conditions differ with regard to the force, frequency, and means of impact, the mechanisms of repair are largely the same.

I reasoned at that time, and I understand now, that if a body can heal from an enormous assault on its systems as I witnessed with this motorcycle rider's recovery, given the chance, it can heal from most anything—even serious, chronic diseases like heart disease, arthritis, and sometimes even cancer. I've seen it over and over again with my patients. Watching the body spontaneously recuperate from these conditions seems like a miracle each and every time.

Spontaneous Healing from Heart Disease

Followers of the McDougall Diet are often eager to inspire others by sharing their success stories. The case studies presented over the following pages look at successes battling heart disease, inflammatory arthritis, and cancer. Other examples throughout the book illustrate specific challenges my patients and followers have faced and overcome. You will find many more inspiring stories of weight loss and healing, as well as photographs and video interviews, at the Star McDougaller section of my Web site (www.drmcdougall.com/star.html). As you read these stories, you will notice not only our bodies' astounding ability to heal from the gravest diseases, but also the great pride that comes from taking an active role in self-healing.

Robert, whom you met on page 48, ate meat, poultry, and dairy foods over six decades which caused his disease. Those foods prompted the formation of little pimplelike sores covering the interior walls of his arteries. Some of these pimples ruptured, causing blood clots to form. The scar tissue that formed around the sores and ruptures as they healed added to the blockages in the arteries, reducing the flow of blood through his heart. Before his tests, he didn't know this was the reason his chest hurt when he exercised. What he did know was that

---

Common Inflammatory Diseases of Arteries

Aortic aneurysms	Heart attacks
Bowel and other infarctions	Impotence
Claudication (legs)	Kidney failure
Degenerative disks of the spine	Macular degeneration
Gangrene	Strokes
Hearing loss	

Juliea Baker, College Student, Bay Area, California

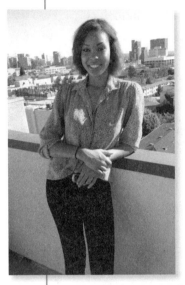

One morning when I was 15 years old I awoke with severe jaw pain. My doctor found no reason for it, and the pain disappeared as mysteriously as it began. Soon one shoulder was sore. Then the other. Again, the pain left. When it came raging back in my knees, my mom took me to the pediatrician. A year into my illness, the doctor put me on medication. By the following Christmas my knuckles were so swollen I could not get a size 10 ring over them. It hurt just to shake hands. I became depressed.

As my rheumatoid factor spiked and antibody markers rose, my doctor diagnosed juvenile rheumatoid arthritis. My body was on the attack—against itself. He prescribed a low dose of the cancer drug methotrexate to suppress my immune system. As I researched the drug I was so frightened by its side effects I refused to take it. Mom agreed.

Mom and I happened to be reading a book on veganism at the

his cholesterol, blood pressure, and blood sugar levels were rising. His cardiologist worried about his risk for heart attack and stroke.

Robert saw profound changes after he replaced animal foods with starches, vegetables, and fruits. His cholesterol, blood pressure, and blood sugar returned to normal. He could exercise more vigorously without feeling chest pains. He also got off the drugs he once needed to keep his test results in check. All that just from changing what he ate.

time, *The Kind Diet,* by Alicia Silverstone. The book referenced several doctors who believed arthritis could be cured through diet, among them Dr. John McDougall. My mother e-mailed him and he replied, recommending articles and books to read and a diet eliminating all meat, dairy, eggs, wheat, and soy. He said I should expect to feel better in about 4 months.

Within 2 months I felt 90 percent better. The pain was gone except for slight swelling in my knuckles. When soreness returned, Dr. McDougall encouraged examining my food more closely. My mom finally found the culprit: a packaged food I ate for breakfast that contained egg whites. It turns out that, for me, eggs and dairy trigger joint pain and inflammation overnight.

I now know firsthand that rheumatoid arthritis can be cured through diet. Were it not for the starch-based diet Dr. McDougall recommends, I would be suffering with terrible pain and disfigured joints, and taking a horribly toxic drug that might have destroyed my liver. Instead, I am a healthy 18-year-old college student, living a joy-filled life with a bright, healthy future in front of me.

Spontaneous Healing from Inflammatory Arthritis

Juliea, above, suffered from the hot, swollen, painful joints characteristic of inflammatory arthritis. As her immune system was compromised through years of eating a diet based on animal foods and vegetable oils, it should be no surprise that changing her diet improved her condition. That the improvement came so quickly—within just a few days—attests to the powerful effect of what we eat on the way we feel

Common Autoimmune Diseases

Ankylosing spondylitis

Crohn's disease

Dermatomyositis

Diabetes (type 1)

Lupus

Multiple sclerosis

Nonspecific inflammatory arthritis

Pernicious anemia

Polymyositis

Psoriasis

Psoriatic arthritis

Rheumatoid arthritis

Scleroderma

Thyroiditis (resulting in hypothyroidism)

Ulcerative colitis

Uveitis

Vitiligo

and the spontaneous healing performed by a healthy body.

When the animal proteins were eliminated from Juliea's diet, her body immediately stopped producing the antibodies that were attacking her joints. I've seen it over and over again. The result is almost instant relief from pain and swelling. The body continues to heal, with the painful inflammation beginning to subside within 4 to 7 days. Within 4 months of avoiding free oils (oils that have been separated from the foods that originally contained them), like olive and corn oil, and eliminating animal foods from the diet, more than 70 percent of people with inflammatory arthritis are dramatically improved or cured altogether.

Ruth Heidrich, Triathlete, Hawaii

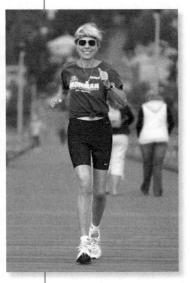

For my first 47 years of life, everything went well. I felt perfectly healthy. I ran daily for 14 years, including three marathons, and ate what I considered to be a very healthy diet, with plenty of lean chicken, fish, and low-fat dairy. What I didn't know was that cancer was growing in my right breast; that is, until it grew to the size of a golf ball.

When the lump was detected I was rushed off to surgery to have it removed. Recovering from the surgery, I was given the bad news: The tumor was malignant. Later, the doctor informed me that the cancer had spread throughout the breast and into my bones and one lung. The prognosis did not look good.

While paging through the newspaper during my recovery I saw a call for volunteers for a breast cancer study involving diet. I signed up. After meeting with Dr. McDougall in 1982 as part of that study, I left his office with instructions to follow a low-fat, vegan diet. That diet changed my life. I am now cancer free.

Since my diagnosis three decades ago, I have completed the Ironman Triathlon six times, run 67 marathons, won more than a thousand racing trophies, and been declared "One of the Ten Fittest Women in North America." At age 74 I had a "fitness age" of 32. I've even written a book about my recovery: *A Race for Life: A Diet and Exercise Program for Superfitness and Reversing the Aging Process.*

Spontaneous Healing from Cancer

Cancers begin and are spread by unhealthy components of a meat- and dairy-centric, oil-laden Western diet. Vegetarians are generally healthier and have lower cancer rates compared with others living in the same communities.

The problem is the same as with heart disease and rheumatoid arthritis: Repeated injuries from unhealthy foods trigger further injury, followed by attempts to recover through inflammation, which, when chronic, is implicated in all stages of cancer: initiation, promotion, and progression.

Explanations for the micro-pinprick injuries that initiate and promote cancer focus on radiation and chemicals, as well as substances found in tobacco products and foods. Thankfully, however, the fact that a cancer has formed doesn't mean that the body will abandon its attempts at spontaneous healing. Cancer is not a time for losing hope. It is a time for heeding the body's message and taking action. Ruth's recovery from cancer is an important example of how the body never ceases in its efforts to heal and stay healthy, even after very serious damage.

Reported Spontaneous Regressions (Healing) of Common Cancers

Brain	Kidney
Breast	Melanoma
Colon	Prostate

Chronic Disease Does Not Have to Be Forever

Unhealthy eating habits, along with smoking, drinking coffee and alcohol, and taking drugs, have been known since antiquity to be at the root of many human maladies. The challenge comes in recognizing these lifelong behaviors and habits as the source of repeated injury to the body, then putting a stop to them, once and for all.

Change can be challenging, but understanding the source of suffering makes it considerably easier. It all begins with a simple understanding of one basic truth: The diet that best prevents disease, best supports the body's innate healing mechanisms, and best promotes sustained weight loss is a low-fat diet based on starches, with added vegetables and fruits, and with no animal products or free oils (like olive or corn oil). A giant step toward health and spontaneous healing is yours for the taking. You should expect big results after making these big changes to a starch-based diet.

You will find more than a hundred similarly fascinating Star McDougaller stories and the science that supports such remarkable healing on my Web site, www.drmcdougall.com.

Spontaneous Healing of Other Diseases

Acne	Constipation
Asthma	Diabetes (type 2)
Cholecystitis (gallbladder pain and inflammation)	Diarrhea (chronic)
	Hypertension
Cholesterol (high)	Obesity

The list goes on. You will not be disappointed with your body's abilities to heal. Give it a chance.

CHAPTER 5

The USDA and the
Politics of Starch

As Americans, we place our trust in the United States Department
of Agriculture to help us choose foods that will keep us healthy.
But does it really have our best interests in mind?

In 2011, the USDA enacted two policies that limit the nation's consumption of starchy vegetables and grains, the very foods that offer the
best hope for addressing our current epidemics of obesity, diabetes,
and heart disease as well as a host of other medical challenges. These
are the foods that have provided the bulk of human sustenance
throughout recorded history, that continue to nourish large populations around the globe that cannot afford to put meat, dairy, and processed foods at the center of their plates, and that place the lowest
demand on our environment.

THE USDA RECOMMENDATIONS

In its January 2011 report, *School Meals: Building Blocks for Healthy Children,* the USDA Committee on Nutrition Standards for National School
Lunch and Breakfast Programs recommended reducing starchy vegetables, like potatoes and corn, to 1 cup per student per school week.[1]
Instead, children are encouraged to eat turkey sausages, cheese omelets,

beef egg rolls, hot dogs, hamburgers, pepperoni pizza, roast beef, deli ham, chocolate milk, and margarine. It doesn't take a nutrition degree to see there's something terribly wrong here.

The second policy prevents needy families from using WIC coupons to purchase potatoes.[2] The Special Supplemental Nutrition Program for Women, Infants, and Children (WIC) provides vouchers that mothers use to buy food for their families. Only WIC-approved foods may be purchased with the coupons, and the new regulation specifically excludes potatoes from the list. A WIC recipient could use the coupons to load butter, sour cream, and cheese on her baked potatoes, then wash it down with a glass of whole milk, but could not use the coupons to purchase the only healthy part of that meal: the potato itself.

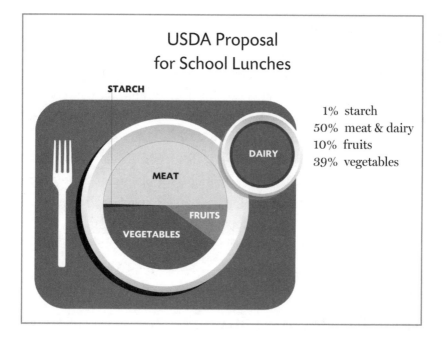

USDA Proposal
for School Lunches

1% starch
50% meat & dairy
10% fruits
39% vegetables

The Problem with the Recommendations

These two policies suggest that limiting access to starches will encourage greater consumption of green, yellow, and orange vegetables. That might seem admirable on its own merits; the more colorful the vegetable, the more vitamins and antioxidants it might contain, and therefore the healthier it might be to eat. But that simplistic argument masks a more complex reality.

Eating more very low-calorie vegetables and fewer starches leaves people feeling hungrier. (Think of a plateful of broccoli, cauliflower, lettuce, kale, and pea pods for breakfast.) They will need to eat something else to make up the rest of the calories they need and satisfy their hunger. The easiest way to do that under the USDA recommendations is with meat, dairy, eggs, processed foods, and oils. Not only are these foods at the center of our nation's worst health problems, but they also are among the most expensive in the supermarket. With a diet high in nonstarchy vegetables, meat, and dairy, families in need won't have an easy time stretching their food budget to the end of the month.

A national food policy promoting healthy starches would fuel schoolchildren with comforting, familiar foods that please their palates and satisfy their bellies. Instead of filling up on fatty, processed meats and sugary flavored milks, they would fill their bellies with whole grains, beans, and potatoes (starchy vegetables), setting them on a path toward healthy eating for the rest of their lives. Promoting these foods to WIC recipients would provide the same benefit to families, and would help assure their ability to put food on the table for the entire month. As a nation, we would save money through increased productivity and reduced health care costs. It's an undeniable win-win.

If we are not benefiting from these USDA policies, who is? What's the motivation for taking the healthy, filling, widely enjoyed potato and other starches out of the equation and essentially replacing them with foods that have been well established to cause illness?

Whether by design or as an unintentional side effect, the key beneficiaries of these policies are the beef, poultry, egg, and dairy industries that benefit from increased consumption of their products.

To make sense of all this, you need to understand something about the USDA.

WHO'S DRIVING THE USDA'S TRACTOR?

When Congress created the US Department of Agriculture in 1862, Abraham Lincoln dubbed the USDA the "People's Department": At the time, farmers and their families made up roughly half of our nation's population. (By comparison, less than 1 percent of the US population now claims farming as its occupation.) The agency's role was expanded when Congress passed the Food and Drugs Act of 1906 in response to the uproar following publication of *The Jungle*, Upton Sinclair's exposé of the filthy and brutal meatpacking practices of the time.

The number of US farms peaked at 6.8 million in 1935. The nation's population totaled more than 127 million at the time, meaning that there was one farm for approximately every 19 Americans. By 2005, the US population had more than doubled, and just four companies (Tyson, Cargill, Swift & Company, and National Beef Packing Company) controlled the processing of 84 percent of the country's beef.[3] Three of these same four, along with one other, processed 64 percent of the nation's pork. Processing of chickens and turkeys is also limited largely to four companies.[3]

Instead of representing the common interest, the agency has been corrupted by its sanctioned allegiance to agribusinesses into ignoring scientific evidence that goes against industry interests. The USDA's conflicting allegiances and responsibilities are at the core of our inability to address the costly epidemics of obesity and other diet-related illnesses. No matter how easy and obvious the solution may be, we will never get to it so long as big agriculture and public health are represented by the same federal agency.

THE DIETARY GUIDELINES FOR AMERICANS

It wasn't until the 1970s that the USDA took control of food assistance programs to become the nation's leading authority on dietary recommendations. Beginning in 1980, and every five years since, the USDA and the US Department of Health and Human Services (HHS) have jointly published dietary guidelines that drive much of the nation's nutrition and health policy, funding, and activities. The HHS's Office of Disease Prevention and Health Promotion and the USDA's Center for Nutrition Policy and Promotion coordinate development of the guidelines.

A major factor influencing the nation's dietary policies is the revolving door that shuttles industry leaders into roles as legislators and government regulators, then back into industry. Members of the USDA have had known associations with the National Cattlemen's Beef Association, the National Pork Board, the National Livestock and Meat Board, the American Egg Board, ConAgra Foods, the National Dairy Council, and Dairy Management Inc.[4,5] In other words, health care, nutrition policy, and agribusiness are all tucked cozily together in a king-size bed.

As part of its expanded role, today's USDA is responsible not only for overseeing the safety of our food supply, but also for tackling the nation's growing epidemic of obesity. Still core to its role, however, is supporting and promoting agriculture. The USDA's twin roles

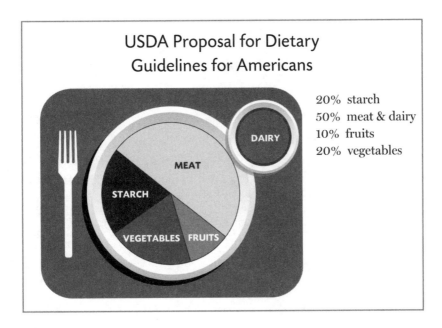

USDA Proposal for Dietary Guidelines for Americans

20% starch
50% meat & dairy
10% fruits
20% vegetables

representing these two often opposing concerns, compounded by corporate lobbying that is widely known to corrupt our food and health care systems, are a conflict of interest that calls into question the agency's motives and credibility, as well as its conclusions and recommendations. How can a consumer really know, for example, whether cheese and dairy are recommended because they are truly good for our health or because they support businesses the USDA is charged with protecting?

For the most part, we cannot know the motive behind a particular dietary recommendation or piece of proposed legislation; the USDA's reports do not pick apart its conflicting interests. However, what is in the best interest of agribusiness is often not in the best interest of your and your family's health. We are on our own in interpreting its recommendations. Based on nearly 40 years of helping patients improve their health through diet, I think the interpretation is pretty clear: Although the USDA was created to represent our farm-based population, 150 years later the agency has morphed from the "People's Department" into the "Agribusiness Industries' Department," primarily serving the interests of giant, consolidated, politically influential food production and distribution corporations.

THE 2010 DIETARY GUIDELINES FOR AMERICANS: A BIG STEP FORWARD

In July 2010, I responded to the USDA's call for written comments on its Dietary Guidelines for Americans, suggesting that it look at starch's long and positive history of contributing to good health and evaluate its biased views of the scientific literature and factual errors that favor the livestock industries.[6]

The following January, I was heartened to learn that the USDA had revised its Dietary Guidelines for Americans to something less industry friendly and more in keeping with the interests of the people.[7] Americans were told to "emphasize nutrient-dense foods and beverages—vegetables, fruits, whole grains, fat-free or low-fat milk and milk products, seafood, lean meats and poultry, eggs, beans and peas, and nuts and seeds." If its interests were purely in our health, it would have left out the seafood, meat, poultry, eggs, and dairy. Still, the 2010 Guidelines emphasize the importance of whole grains, all vegetables (both starchy and nonstarchy), legumes, and fruits. They also discuss the DASH (Dietary Approaches to Stop Hypertension) and Mediterranean diets as well as the benefits of vegetarian and vegan diets. This is indeed a step in the right direction.

The Guidelines suggest: "Enjoy [y]our food, but eat less." That may work well as a sound bite, but is it advice people can and will follow? If we were all so easily able to control the quantity of food we put into our mouths, would we see food continually being supersized into jumbo and colossal portions? Would so many people be overweight? What we *can* recommend to assure that the population remains healthy is that we eat less of foods that are harmful and instead fill up on foods that are satisfying, comforting, and filling: starches.

The new USDA report includes no discussion of the important role of starch in satisfying the appetite without the harmful effects of meat, poultry, dairy products, and fat. Healthy and filling calories that cause no harm are the cornerstone of any successful diet, and starch fits the bill perfectly. For the most part, however, the report shrouds starches in negative connotations, mentioning "refined starches" that need "to be minimized or excluded along with solid fats, sugars, and sodium." The recommendations are so noncommittal that they can easily be interpreted to support a low-carbohydrate, high-protein (Atkins-type) diet, which is an exceedingly dangerous one.

Doctors Chime In

I sit on the advisory board of the Physicians Committee for Responsible Medicine (PCRM; www.pcrm.org), a Washington, DC–based nonprofit promoting ethics and effectiveness in preventive medicine. PCRM filed a lawsuit against the USDA and HHS over their 2010 Guidelines, stating:

The problem is word choice. For healthful foods that people should eat more of, the Guidelines are clear. They encourage readers to eat more fruits, vegetables, and whole grains. But when it comes to foods people need to eat less of (e.g., meat and cheese), the Guidelines resort to biochemical terms instead of listing specific foods, apparently out of fear of upsetting food producers. That is, the Guidelines call for limiting 'cholesterol,' 'saturated fat,' 'solid fat.' Similarly, while dairy products account for more than 30 percent of the saturated ('bad') fat in the American diet, the Guidelines disguise this fact by splitting dairy products into many categories, including cheese (8.5 percent), butter (2.9 percent), whole milk (3.4 percent), reduced-fat milk (3.9 percent), dairy desserts (5.6 percent), and pizza (5.9 percent), so their contribution to ill health is harder to see.[8]

PCRM urged that portions of the Guidelines be rewritten using terms that make clear the risks of consuming meat and dairy products. The suit also raises concerns about members of the Dietary Guidelines Advisory Committee having ties to the meat and dairy industries, including one member who served on an advisory council for McDonald's, and another who worked for the Dannon Institute.[8]

This isn't the first time PCRM has challenged the USDA and its ties to agribusiness. In 2001, the organization won a lawsuit against the USDA, bringing national attention to the heavy influence of the meat, dairy, and egg industries in the development of our nation's food policies. US District Court Judge James Robertson ruled that the USDA violated federal law by withholding documents revealing bias among members of its advisory panel.[9] The organization has exposed other inconsistencies and conflicts, including that the federal government spends about *$16 billion* every year on agricultural subsidies, the majority of which support foods it has suggested we consume less of.[10]

PCRM has developed its own version of the USDA's original 1956 Basic Four Food Groups recommendations that were later reformulated into its familiar Food Guide Pyramid.[11] PCRM's New Four Food Groups recommends five or more daily servings of whole grains, four or more of vegetables, three or more of fruits, and two or more of legumes. These guidelines reflect current knowledge and research on the importance of fiber, the health risks of cholesterol and fats, and the disease-preventing power of many nutrients found exclusively in plant foods. They also note that plant foods are an excellent source of protein and calcium, previously believed to come primarily from meat and dairy products. In other words, these animal foods are no longer recognized as a necessary part of a healthy diet; in fact, they are contrary to a health-promoting diet because of the cholesterol, fat, chemicals, microbe contaminants, and other harmful components they contain.

There is still much work to be done before the USDA cycles back from serving as the "Agribusiness Industries' Department" to its original role as the "People's Department."

THE TIDE IS TURNING

Concerns about financial influence, politics, and some problematic wording aside, the 2010 Dietary Guidelines have ended any doubt about which foods most support our health and which contribute to harmful and sometimes fatal illnesses. They establish a clear direction for restoring our nation's health and reducing its exorbitant medical bill.

The new guidelines bring to the public's attention a message I have been communicating for nearly four decades. From 1983 until the early 1990s, my books promoting simple dietary solutions to complex health problems were major bestsellers. In the early 1990s, my publisher suggested it was time to change my writing style. An editor told me that my books supporting a starch-based diet were out of date, and that diet books now must focus on increasing meat and protein and decreasing carbs. "Dr. McDougall," she advised, "we would like you to make this change in your future books to reflect the new trend." I reminded the editor that essentially all respected science corroborates that eating animal products results in heart disease, cancer, diabetes, and obesity, while research over the last 70 years has shown that a diet based on starches, vegetables, and fruits makes people healthy. I reminded her that I was not in the book business simply to make money, but to help people improve their health. With six national bestsellers under my belt, and more than a million copies in circulation from this company alone, I parted ways with the publisher. History confirms that my editor was right: Diet books were indeed headed in the direction she predicted. History also has proven me right: Those diets made people sick, while my approach made them healthy.

I am heartened to see the tide turning back at long last, with the USDA promoting vegetables at the core of a healthy diet. It is your job and mine to keep steering this ship in the right direction so that we can, at long last, heal our ailing nation and put funds now wastefully directed at agribusiness and unnecessary health care expenditures to better use.

CHAPTER 6

We Are Eating the PlSanet to Death

*T*he Starch Solution is meant to assure your health and well-being through a relatively simple shift in the way you eat. But how well can we really feel in the face of devastating environmental destruction? In addition to epidemics of obesity, diabetes, and other weighty health concerns, we find ourselves facing climate change and ecological damage of epic proportions. Moreover, vast swaths of the world population suffer from malnourishment and starvation while those of us living in prosperous western nations indulge in our favorite foods.

As luck would have it, the very same actions that can save your health and that of your loved ones will also mitigate the monumental environmental and food access problems that plague the world we live in. It is the ultimate win-win: Improve your health and you will be doing your part to heal the world, with absolutely no added effort.

Our Food Choices Are Not So Personal

The decision to pile our plates high with meat, poultry, seafood, eggs, and dairy does not just threaten our personal health. What may seem like very personal choices about what we eat day in and day out have an enormous impact, with dramatic effects that go far beyond our own enjoyment and well-being. Consider these consequences of our food choices that affect all beings living on Earth, and the planet itself:

- We are suffering from rampant and increasing chronic illnesses from overindulging in foods that put our health at risk. Most critically, we consume too much protein, too much fat, and too much cholesterol. (We may also consume too much sugar and salt, but this is not nearly as critical a concern as eating animal foods.)

- At the same time, we fail to benefit from the widely available nutritional elements that can improve our health—chief among them dietary fiber and complex carbohydrates (found only in plant foods).

- We are faced with enormous national debt, in part due to the spiraling public health costs of caring for a population that is sick and getting sicker as a result of what we eat.

- Animal foods are one of the primary contributors to climate change, otherwise known as global warming. Climate change is exacerbated by the way animals are raised, slaughtered, and prepared, in addition to their production of ozone-killing methane gas.

- The production of animal foods takes an enormous bite out of resources that could secure sufficient food for all of the world's populations that now face starvation. It takes about 7 pounds of edible, healthy grains to produce just 1 pound of beef, 4 pounds for a pound of pork, and 2 pounds for a pound of chicken.[1,2]

OUR GLOBAL HEALTH CRISIS

We are in the midst of a pandemic health crisis. More than 1.1 billion people are overweight, nearly as many (1 billion) are hypertensive (have high blood pressure), 312 million are obese, and 197 million are diabetic.[3] As a result of these chronic conditions, 18 million people die from heart disease every year. Yet because these diseases generally come in for the kill only after the victims have passed through their reproductive years, the seeds of further destruction are firmly planted in the unhealthy habits passed along to the next generation. If ever there was a vicious cycle . . .

One would hope that the world's leaders would have banded together by now to address this catastrophic human suffering, but they have not even acknowledged one of the primary causes—our worldwide dependence on meat and dairy products. Why? Because political and commercial interests profit from brushing that reality under the carpet. In fact, so little attention is devoted to educating the public about this problem, and to making the changes required to address it, that you could easily get the impression that the science about animal foods and human illness is inconclusive. But the science is conclusive, and it is frightening, and it doesn't take a medical education to understand it, as you are seeing over and over again throughout this book.

ENVIRONMENTAL DEVASTATION

Tied to our rising levels of chronic illness are continuing and escalating environmental catastrophes. You see it everywhere: Weather is becoming more erratic, more intense, and more destructive, as witnessed not only in new highs (and lows) of the thermometer, but also in the swell of hurricanes, tornadoes, severe flooding, and droughts. Many of our most prized plant and animal species are threatened with extinction. Diseases are spreading. Crops are failing. We are burning the candle at both ends, pushing extremes of heat and cold, fire and ice. Without intervention, many scientists predict our planet Earth will become inhospitable to human life, and then to any form of life at all.[4,5]

Some say our only chance for salvation is a radical reduction in the Earth's population, currently bulging at seven billion people. Fatalists say this will come about by nuclear war or a viral pandemic. But is that our only choice? Or is it worth testing less severe measures to improve our lot, such as dramatically reducing our dependence on animal foods? That one change would at least give us time to address other pressing problems, such as our dependence on fossil fuels.

LIVESTOCK AND GLOBAL WARMING

It is no longer news that livestock are a major contributor to global warming, accounting for 18 percent of global warming gases, more than the 14 percent contributed by all forms of transportation combined.[6] So why are we putting our focus in the wrong place? Why are we not discussing this elephant in our global living room?

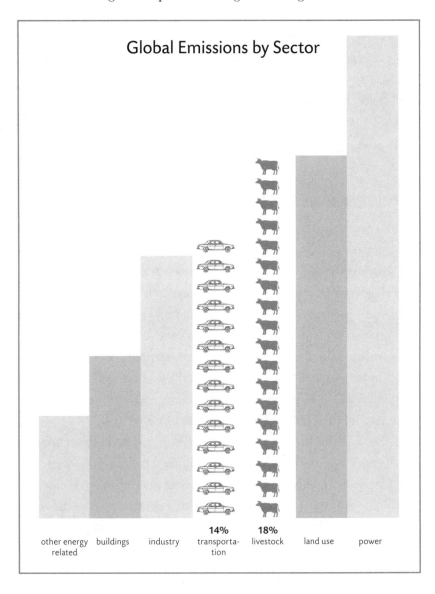

The 2006 United Nations report *Livestock's Long Shadow: Environmental Issues and Options* concludes, "Livestock have a substantial impact on the world's water, land and biodiversity resources and contribute significantly to climate change."[6] Yet this 407-page report mentions the term *vegetarian* a shy four times and avoids any meaningful discussion of this obvious answer to the dilemma it poses; the word *vegan* is MIA.

Based in Rome, Italy, Henning Steinfeld was in 2006 the head of the livestock sector analysis and policy branch of the Food and Agriculture Organization of the United Nations. As an agricultural economist, Dr. Steinfeld has been working on agricultural and livestock policy for the last 15 years, with a special focus on environmental issues, poverty, and public health. He is also the senior author of the UN report *Livestock's Long Shadow*. You would think that, over the course of his career, Dr. Steinfeld would have developed some insight into the cause and effect of this worldwide problem. His comment? "Livestock are one of the most significant contributors to today's most serious environmental problems. Urgent action is required to remedy the situation. . . . Encouraging the global population to become vegans is not a viable solution, however."[7]

What Dr. Steinfeld fails to offer is any reason why this solution is *not* viable. Instead, the report's recommendations run from improvements in grazing, manure, and water management to a modified diet that reduces the toxic fecal and gaseous output of cows, pigs, and sheep. What?! We will change the livestock's diet, but heaven forbid we change our own? Indeed, this report won't offend many people, but neither will its recommendations have any significant impact.

(Please note: The United Nations estimate of an 18 percent greenhouse gas contribution from livestock was conservative. Calculations by the World Watch Institute concluded that over 51 percent of these global-warming gases are the result of raising animals for people to eat.[8])

Only 3.2 percent of the US population, or 7.3 million people, identify themselves as vegetarian, and most of these consume milk, cheese, and eggs.[9] About half of 1 percent of the population, or one million

Effects of Livestock Production on the Environment

- Animal agriculture produces 18 percent of the world's greenhouse gas emissions (carbon dioxide equivalents), compared with 14 percent from all forms of transportation combined.

- Livestock also generate other toxic gases, including nitrous oxide, methane, and ammonia.

- Nitrous oxide has 296 times the global warming potential, and methane 23 times, of CO_2.

- Ammonia contributes to acid rain and ecosystem acidification.

- Livestock are the identified culprit in 15 out of 24 important ecosystems that are reported to be in decline.

LAND DAMAGE

- Grazing livestock occupy the equivalent of 26 percent of the ice-free terrestrial surface of the planet, and one-third of all arable land is used in producing food for these animals.

- Forest clearing for new pastureland is a major source of deforestation. In Latin America, 70 percent of former Amazon rainforests has been given over to grazing. As the "lungs of the Earth," these forests are vital to removing greenhouse gases from the atmosphere.

people, are vegans, consuming no animal products. Another 10 percent of adults, or 22.8 million people, say they follow a largely vegetarian diet. It is well documented that increasing the number of people following a vegan or even vegetarian diet makes a *real and significant* impact.

This change is already happening with some of the world's most powerful leaders. What do Bill Clinton, Steve Wynn, John Mackey, and Mike Tyson have in common? These four powerful men have all declared themselves in favor of a vegan diet.[10] I know of no other

WATER DAMAGE

- The livestock industry is one of the heaviest users of our scarce water supply, and contributes to excessive growth of organisms in water, oxygen depletion of water, and the erosion of coral reefs.

- Livestock pollute our waters with their waste, antibiotics, hormones, chemicals from tanneries, fertilizers, and the pesticides used to spray the feed crops they consume.

- US livestock are responsible for 55 percent of soil erosion and sediment, 37 percent of pesticides, 50 percent of antibiotics, and one-third of the nitrogen and phosphorus polluting our freshwater sources.

- Widespread overgrazing disturbs water cycles, reducing their ability to replenish, both aboveground and belowground.

SPECIES LOSS

- The presence of livestock over vast land areas, coupled with their depletion of food crops, contributes to the loss of other plants and animals that are unable to compete.

Source: *Livestock's Long Shadow: Environmental Issues and Options,* United Nations, 2006[6]

similarities among this ex-president, hotel tycoon, supermarket entrepreneur, and ex–prize fighter. You might think that a public figure's declaration to not eat animals could be a reckless business decision. Traditionally, a vegetarian diet has been considered a sign of weakness, conjuring pale, listless hippies hanging out at the health food store. These four men must have found reasons not only to ignore this common stereotype but also to prove it wrong. My guess is that they were motivated in part by personal gain. A fountain of youth becomes especially important as health declines with age, causing people to make desperate changes—as radical as replacing burgers and bacon with barley and beans.

POPULATION EXPLOSION

Until just before the end of the 20th century, an estimated two billion people worldwide lived primarily on an animal-based diet, while twice as many—an estimated four billion—consumed a largely plant-based diet.[11] These figures are rapidly shifting. It has been predicted that by the middle of the 21st century, the global population will increase to about *nine billion people,* an increase of six million people every month. At the same time, incomes are rising in developing and middle-income countries, most notably in China, India, Brazil, and Argentina. As income rises, so does the consumption of expensive meats, dairy products, and processed foods. These foods are costly in more ways than one: In addition to being costlier to produce and purchase, they have a greater negative environmental impact and cause more medical problems.

The Earth can support an estimated one billion to two billion people living at the American standards of income, health, food consumption, personal dignity, and freedom.[12] The US share of this population would be 100 to 200 million. This compares with a current world census of seven billion and a US population of more than 312 million.

At the present growth rates, if every human being on Earth were to live according to American standards, including consuming the typical American or European diet, we would need four or more planet Earths to feed, house, and care for us all.[13]

We have three options for addressing worldwide overpopulation and the problems that result from it: population control (an unacceptable approach to most), increasing agricultural productivity to feed more people, and changing the way we eat.

In 1978, China implemented a one-child-per-family policy to alleviate the country's social, economic, and environmental burdens. An estimated 400 million births have been prevented by this policy over the past three decades.[14] Reducing the population in this manner worldwide would require a huge investment in reproductive health care and birth control services.

Even if the human species stopped reproducing altogether, it would take more than two generations to cut the world's population in half. Wars, starvation, and disease could force a more rapid decline, but naturally these are conditions we wish to avoid. On its own, elective population control would take too long to preserve the planet in its current state.

Couldn't we simply increase agricultural output to assure food for all? While we have made great strides in food production over the past 50 years, these improvements can't continue under the conditions caused by climate change. Fires in Russia have destroyed hundreds of thousands of acres of grain. Canada's wheat crop has been decimated by heavy rain. Drought in Argentina has devastated the soybean crop. Floods in Australia have destroyed much of the country's wheat. The growing unpredictability of our weather conditions makes any sustained agricultural efforts nearly impossible.

Adding to these food shortages are what we do with the food once it's grown. Currently, one-third of US-grown corn is diverted to produce ethanol fuel. We can and must continue to squeeze as many healthy calories as possible from our agricultural lands. But even with increased agricultural output, there is no possibility of keeping up with the increasing demands of animal production on our agricultural resources. We can run as fast as we can, but we will never catch up.

STARVATION DOESN'T KILL, PEOPLE DO

In recent times we have seen citizens in the Middle East, from Egypt to Libya, turning to revolt in an effort to remove their leaders from power. Their motivation is the primary challenge they live with every day: feeding themselves and their families on subsistence wages or less.

Starvation poses a threat to more than individual or even population health; it threatens global stability and security, affecting even those of us living far from these politically unstable regions.

The Middle East was once known as the word's breadbasket, yet millions of people living there no longer have enough to eat. In 2009, UNICEF reported that 30 percent of children in half a dozen countries throughout the Middle East and North Africa were suffering from stunted growth as a result of malnutrition.[15] The UN announced in 2011 that world food prices had reached record levels. Currently, nearly a billion people worldwide live at the edge of starvation as the prices of their staples—rice, corn, and wheat—rise beyond their meager income of about a dollar a day.

There is something seriously wrong with a world in which half of the population is severely underfed while the other half overfeeds itself into a state of illness and even death. You might think the most sensible thing for people to do would be for those with excess resources to share their bounty with those who are starving. If those enjoying the excess were to make the change to a starch-based diet, this would free up sufficient rice, corn, wheat, and potatoes (now going to animal feed) to allow the entire world population adequate or even bountiful food supplies.

In fact, reallocating land from animal to crop production would increase our food resources at least seventeenfold: Crops like potatoes can produce 17 times the calories as animals on the same piece of land.[16] There would be additional positive consequences of replacing animal foods in our diet with plants. Fossil fuels used in the production of food could be reduced fortyfold. Consider that about 2 calories of fossil-fuel energy are required to cultivate 1 calorie of starchy vegetable food energy; with beef, the ratio can be as high as 80 to 1.[17] We would also reduce the needless suffering from the health consequences of our lives of excess, including obesity, heart disease, type 2 diabetes, arthritis, and breast, prostate, and colon cancer, to name a few. We would reduce our national debt by vastly reducing the health care costs associated with these unnecessary illnesses. And we would free a great portion of the world from starvation.

THE QUEST FOR ANSWERS AND A SINGLE SOLUTION

Governments, businesses, local groups, and individuals are seeking answers to our environmental problems through reducing the use of fossil fuels—coal, oil, and natural gas—and by trying to get industrial waste under control. At the same time, we are waging a war on chronic diseases with strategies to reduce smoking, the use of alcohol and drugs, toxic environmental chemicals, and infectious diseases. But where is the effort to fix the food?

It would not take much for us to solve these individual and global problems in one fell swoop. All it takes is one big U-turn back to where we came from. Back to our roots. Back to what we once knew was healthy and natural: a diet based on starches and other plants, including fruits and vegetables. At the root of both human and environmental health is *what we eat*. Food is plentiful. We just need to choose the Starch Solution.

As you seek to achieve your personal goals of dropping a few (or even a hundred or more) pounds, bringing your blood pressure and blood sugar under control, weaning yourself from medications for high blood pressure or diabetes, battling cancer or staving off a recurrence of it, relieving your joints that ache from arthritis, easing your depression, increasing your energy, or simply slipping gracefully into your swimsuit this summer, consider your immense contribution to the world around you. As you switch to a starch-based diet, think about the positive impact of what you are doing will have on your children and grandchildren, and on generations yet to come. If you get stuck along your path and find yourself heading back to old eating habits, reflect on how far you have come and what a difference you have already made.

You are now helping billions of people beyond yourself. You are helping all of planet Earth.

Vote for a Better World at Your Dinner Table

Protest world hunger: Stop eating meat.

Protest environmental pollution: Stop eating dairy.

Protest destruction of the oceans: Stop eating fish.

PART II

THE FAQS ABOUT FOOD

CHAPTER 7

When Friends Ask: Where Do You Get Your Protein?

How much protein do we really need, and which types are best? These fundamental questions are at the core of endless debates about the best way to achieve enduring weight loss and optimal health.

For the past 150 years, the pendulum has swung to and fro, between recommendations that an ultra-high-protein regimen, or a diet low in protein, holds out the best promise for good health. Wrapped up in that discussion is a second question: Should you choose a diet rich in animal proteins or one based on vegetable sources?

While the debate rages on, a solid foundation of scientific evidence confirms the answer: A diet with adequate but not excessive protein, derived from plants, is best. But why let popular opinion stand in the way of facts? Pushing evidence aside, the meat- and cheese-craving public continues to invest great faith in the mythical benefit of a high-protein diet. Cadres of popular diet authors who promote that view continue to propagate the fallacy.

Have Advertising Dollars Bought Your Opinion?

An inherent taste preference for meat and dairy is not the real driver behind the protein myth. Sure, many people think these animal foods taste good, though they would not like meat so much if salt, sugar, and spices (in the forms of steak, barbecue, and ketchup sauces, which are used to disguise meat's bland taste) were taken away. Even more so than the seasonings that make it palatable, your appetite for animal protein has been influenced by billions of dollars spent by huge industrial machines to ensure your continued taste for beef, pork, chicken, eggs, milk, and cheese. Backing up industry muscle are government subsidies and advertising dollars, all working to convince you this stuff is healthy. Animal foods are big business, and proponents employ the same industry- and advertising-supported practices that have persuaded countless people to take up smoking against their best interest, and then made it nearly impossible for them to quit. How can the facts expect to win against those odds?

Popular Opinion Ignores Science

Protein intake, both the total amount and the source, varies widely around the world. People living in many rural Asian societies consume 40 to 60 grams of protein a day, mostly from rice, other starches, and vegetables.[1] On the Western side of the globe, food choices typically are centered around meat and dairy, with these foods providing 100 to 160 grams of daily protein, two to four times that consumed by rural Asians. Dieters on a high-protein diet of meat and dairy (such as the Atkins diet) could be consuming 200 to 400 grams of protein a day, similar to what Eskimos survived on with a diet that was, of necessity, focused on marine animals.[2] In other words, *those consuming the most protein are taking in nearly 10 times as much as those who remain healthy on the lowest levels.*

One of the earliest proponents of a high-protein diet was the distinguished German physiologist Dr. Carl Voit, who lived from 1831 until 1908.[3,4] After studying laborers who consumed about 3,100 calories daily, he concluded that people ideally should strive for 118 grams of protein per day. That number became known as the Voit Standard, and while it is in the range of what people on a Western diet consume, it is about twice what is typical for healthy Asians.

How did Voit reach his conclusion? He figured that the laborers he observed were able to work hard and maximize their incomes by instinctively selecting a diet with the right amount of protein, from the best sources, to achieve optimal health and productivity. Other famous scientists of the time, both in Europe and America, made similar observations about the eating habits of workingmen with incomes that allowed them to afford meat. They came to similar conclusions, recommending diets of 100 to 189 grams of protein per day.[1,3,4] This "science" was all based on the assumption that, given the opportunity, people innately make the right choices.

Of course these conclusions were based on observation and hypothesis, rather than a standard of research that would be acceptable today. No experiments were performed, and no comparison was made with the significant numbers of less wealthy Europeans and Americans leading healthy lives on low-protein diets based largely on plant foods.[1,4] Likewise, the healthy, active lives of hundreds of millions of less affluent people laboring in Asia, Africa, and Central and South America—whose diets provided less than half the amount of protein recommended by Dr. Voit (and which contained almost no meat or dairy products)—were entirely overlooked when the suggested protein levels were established.

If you believe his research methods are reliable, try doing your own Voit-style study by observing the quality of food people select at your local grocery store and in restaurants. What do more than one billion people choose? Ice cream sandwiches, donuts, and candy bars at the store, and McDonald's, Burger King, and Pizza Hut for a meal out.

Shall we assume these people have naturally gravitated toward the foods that best meet their nutritional needs? Should we base our national nutrition standards on the breakdown of the most popular foods consumed at these outlets? Our current epidemics of obesity, type 2 diabetes, heart disease, and cancer prove beyond a doubt that we are *not* predisposed to making food choices that are in our own best interest.

Most exasperating is that virtually all scientific research over the past century comes to a different conclusion from Dr. Voit's. Yet elevated protein standards based on centuries-old biases continue to drive health recommendations even today.

Russell Henry Chittenden Told the Truth a Century Ago

Voit's narrow-minded thinking in the late 1800s, echoed and amplified by his peers, should have been put to rest by 1904. That's when Russell Henry Chittenden, who was a professor of physiological chemistry at Yale University, published his scientific findings on human protein needs in his classic book, *Physiological Economy in Nutrition.*[4]

Professor Chittenden believed Dr. Voit had mixed up cause and effect: People did not become prosperous because they ate high-protein diets; rather, they ate meat and other expensive high-protein foods because they could afford them. Chittenden wrote, more than 100 years ago, "We are all creatures of habit, and our palates are pleasantly excited by the rich animal foods with their high content of proteid [protein], and we may well question whether our dietetic habits are not based more upon the dictates of our palates than upon scientific reasoning or true physiological needs."

Chittenden reasoned that science ought to establish once and for all the minimum protein requirement for good health. He further suggested that consuming protein beyond that requirement could cause harm, especially to the liver and kidneys. As he explained, "Fats and carbohydrates when oxidized in the body are ultimately burned to simple gaseous products . . . [and are] easily and quickly eliminated . . . proteid [protein] foods . . . when oxidized, yield a row of crystalline nitrogenous products which ultimately pass out of the body through the kidneys. [These nitrogen-based protein by-products]—frequently spoken of as toxins—float about through the body and may exercise more or less of a deleterious influence upon the system, or, being temporarily deposited, may exert some specific or local influence that calls for their speedy removal."

With these few words, Professor Chittenden encapsulated the damaging effects of a diet based on meat, poultry, fish, and dairy products, consequences too few practicing doctors understand today. (You can read more about protein and other dietary toxins from animal foods in Chapter 3.)

THE CHITTENDEN EXPERIMENTS

Professor Chittenden himself served as the subject of his first experiment to establish a minimum protein requirement. For 9 months, he consumed one-third of the protein level recommended by Dr. Voit, during which time his weight dropped about 10 percent, from 143 to 128 pounds. Chittenden's health remained excellent and he described his condition as having "greater freedom from fatigue and muscular soreness than in previous years of a fuller diet[ary]." He described how his previous knee arthritis disappeared, along with his periodically "sick headaches" and bilious attacks of abdominal pain. Chittenden maintained his normal mental and physical activity, all on about 40 grams of protein a day.

Chittenden went on to perform valid scientific studies by collecting daily dietary histories and urine analyses of his subjects (himself included) to understand protein utilization. Because he was contradicting the beliefs of his time, he conducted his experiments with extreme care. He organized three observational trials to test the adequacy of diets lower in protein than what was recommended at the time.

The first trial involved a group of five men connected with Yale University. These men led active lives but were not engaged in work with high demands on their muscles. On an average diet of 62 grams of protein daily for 6 months, the men all remained healthy and in positive nitrogen balance, an indication that they were taking in and absorbing adequate protein from their diet.

The second trial studied 13 male volunteers from the Hospital Corps of the US Army. These men were described as doing moderate work, with 1 day per week of vigorous activity at the gymnasium. The men remained in good health on an average 61 grams of protein daily.

Chittenden's final trial involved eight Yale student athletes, some of them with exceptional performance records. The students ate an average of 64 grams of protein daily while maintaining their activities, and found that their athletic performance improved by a striking 35 percent.

Chittenden concluded in 1904 that 35 to 50 grams of protein per day allowed adults to maintain their health and physical fitness. Studies over the past century have consistently corroborated Professor Chittenden's findings, yet you would hardly know it. Despite his groundbreaking studies, and later confirmation of them, people continue to believe that the more protein they eat, the better.

EXPERTS TODAY AGREE: 40 TO 60 GRAMS IS PLENTY

Professor Chittenden's conclusions more than 100 years ago remain right on target. We need protein in our diet to build new cells, synthesize hormones, and repair damaged and worn-out tissues. But how much do we need? We lose about 3 grams of protein each day through shedding skin, sloughing intestine, and other miscellaneous losses.[5] Add to this loss other physiological requirements, such as growth and repairs, and the final tally shows, based on solid scientific research, a *total daily protein requirement of about 20 to 30 grams.*[6,7] Plant proteins easily meet that need.[1]

Protein Values for Adults (g/day)

Atkins-type high-protein diet	200 to 400
Typical Eskimo diet	200 to 400
Voit Standard	118
Late 1800s scientists	100 to 189
Typical Western diet	100 to 160
USDA/WHO	33 to 71
Typical rural Asian rice-based diet	40 to 60
Chittenden	35 to 50
McDougall	30 to 80

The US Department of Agriculture, the World Health Organization, and all other international health organizations recommend protein levels ranging from 33 to 71 grams a day for adult men and women, very close to Chittenden's numbers. Yet even these policymakers, who are fully informed about our small protein need, remain confused about the issue of animal versus plant proteins.

PLANT VERSUS ANIMAL PROTEINS

Proteins are built from 20 amino acids that are connected into chains in varying sequences. It's a bit like the way all of our words in a dictionary are made up of combinations formed from the 26 letters in our alphabet. Plants and microorganisms are able to synthesize all 20 of these amino acids. Humans can synthesize only 12 of them, which we call *nonessential* because we needn't rely on food to get them already formed. The eight remaining amino acids are called *essential* because we must get them from the foods we eat.

(continued on page 92)

Donna Byrnes,
Retired Information Systems Project Manager,
Amelia Island, Florida

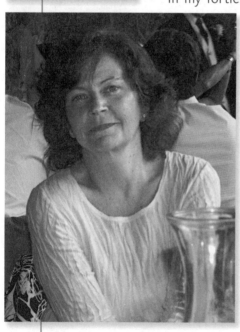

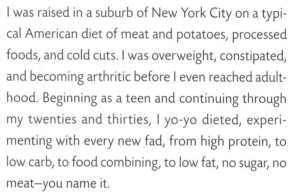

I was raised in a suburb of New York City on a typical American diet of meat and potatoes, processed foods, and cold cuts. I was overweight, constipated, and becoming arthritic before I even reached adulthood. Beginning as a teen and continuing through my twenties and thirties, I yo-yo dieted, experimenting with every new fad, from high protein, to low carb, to food combining, to low fat, no sugar, no meat—you name it.

In my forties my health took a turn for the worse, with problems snowballing until everything hurt. I had pain in my toes and arthritis in my knees; in bed, my hips ached; I had indigestion and gallbladder problems, headaches, costochondritis, hot flashes, and mood swings. My size kept increasing along with my health problems. As I dragged myself from bed each morning after a bad night's sleep I would survey my body for new aches. How could I feel so old in my forties? I turned to doctors, who suggested that I should eat less. They would not discuss diet and I would not agree to medicines. I felt like a physical wreck, and I was emotionally distraught.

I looked for help in many places. After landing on Dr. McDougall's Web site I knew at once that he was different. He didn't advocate dieting as a way to lose weight. Rather, he suggested that a plant-based, low-fat, whole foods regimen was the path to health. As I paged through images of potatoes, rice, pasta, vegetables, and fruit I thought, "I can do this!"

I started by giving up meat and alcohol, the easiest changes for me. Then I let go of dairy, then any added oils. My body responded immediately. My nagging health problems began dropping away and gradually I was feeling better and doing more. I was having whole pain-free days. I started sleeping peacefully through the night. My headaches and hot flashes disappeared. I stopped having gallbladder attacks, and my costochondritis cleared up. With each change came greater energy, happiness, and health.

As I lost those 77 pounds I began to exercise. Now, instead of feeling sluggish, I hop out of bed feeling refreshed and excited to greet the day. In February 2008, you could have found me zip-lining through the treetop canopies of Costa Rica on a McDougall Adventure, or more recently hiking along the Oregon coast. Next up: hiking and rafting through the Grand Canyon.

When we eat, our stomach acids and intestinal enzymes break the protein molecules back down into individual amino acids. The body absorbs these amino acids into the bloodstream, and then reassembles them to form new proteins. These newly formed proteins help us to maintain the shape of our cells, to create enzymes for biochemical reactions, to produce the hormones that signal messages between our cells, and to perform other life-sustaining activities.

Because they are such a rich source of complete proteins, plants alone meet the entire protein and amino acid needs of the Earth's largest animals, including elephants, hippopotamuses, giraffes, and cows, all of which are vegetarian. If plants can satisfy the demands of these enormous mammals, wouldn't you think they could easily meet our own protein needs? Indeed, they can and they do.

How Did We Get So Confused?

The misconception that protein from animal foods is of superior quality to that found in plants dates back to 1914, when Lafayette B. Mendel and Thomas B. Osborne published studies on the protein requirements of laboratory rats; specifically, the effects of animal versus vegetable protein sources on growth.[8]

Mendel and Osborne found that rats grew faster and larger from eating protein derived from animal sources than from vegetable sources. These and other animal experiments led to the classification of meat, eggs, and dairy foods as superior, or "Class A," protein sources. Vegetable proteins were relegated to inferior, or "Class B," status. Subsequent researchers suspected that the vegetable foods used in the study contained insufficient amounts of some of the amino acids essential to the growth of rats.

Studies in the early 1940s by Dr. William Rose of the University of Illinois found that 10 amino acids were essential to a rat's diet.[9] The removal of any one of these essential amino acids from the rats' food led to profound nutritive failure, accompanied by a rapid decline in weight, loss of appetite, and eventual death. Feeding the rats meat, poultry, eggs, and/or milk prevented this decline. Based on these early experiments with rats, the amino acid pattern found in animal foods was considered the gold standard.

Subsequent research affirmed what should have been obvious: Even though animal products supply the ideal protein pattern for rats, that does not mean the same is true for humans.[10] In fact, the dietary needs of humans and rats are quite different. One important difference is our relative rates of growth: Rats grow very rapidly, reaching their full adult size after just 6 months; humans take about 17 years to fully mature. Rapid growth requires high concentrations of nutrients, including protein and amino acids. Comparing the breast milk of these two species makes the differing nutritional needs crystal clear: Rat breast milk is 10 times higher in protein concentration than human breast milk.[11,12] Their rapid growth, with baby rats doubling in size in just $4\frac{1}{2}$ days compared to the 6 months required for a human infant, underscores the rat's need for that high-protein support.

WILLIAM ROSE DETERMINES THE PROTEIN AND AMINO ACID NEEDS FOR PEOPLE

In 1942, Dr. Rose turned his attention to people, studying amino acid requirements in healthy, male graduate students using essentially the same methodology he had used with the rats.[13] The students were fed a diet of cornstarch, sucrose, butterfat, corn oil, inorganic salts, and known vitamins. Their only protein came from mixtures of highly purified amino acids. They also received a large brown "candy" made of concentrated liver extract to provide any missing vitamins. The candy was sweetened with sugar and flavored with peppermint oil for a "never-to-be-forgotten taste."

Dr. Rose tested the students' need for each individual amino acid by removing one at a time from the diet. When an essential amino acid was given in insufficient quantity for approximately 2 days, all subjects complained bitterly of similar symptoms: nervous irritability, extreme fatigue, and a profound loss of appetite. The subjects were unable to continue the amino acid–deficient diets for more than a few days at a time.

Dr. Rose found that only eight of the 10 amino acids essential to rats were also essential to these young men. The other two amino acids essential to rats were *nonessential* to humans because we can synthesize them ourselves. Dr. Rose also identified the minimum required level for each of the eight essential amino acids. Because he found small amounts of variation in individual needs among his subjects, he included a large margin of safety in his final conclusions on minimum amino acid requirements: For each amino acid, he took the highest recorded level of need in any subject, then doubled that amount for a "recommended requirement," described as a "definitely safe intake."

Even Dr. Rose's inflated amino acid levels are easily met by a diet consisting of any single grain, legume, or starchy vegetable. Rice or potatoes alone supply all of the protein and amino acids both adults and

Essential Amino Acids of Selected Foods (g/day)

AMINO ACIDS	ROSE'S MINIMUM REQUIREMENTS	ROSE'S RECOMMENDED REQUIREMENTS	CORN	BROWN RICE	OATMEAL FLAKES	WHEAT FLOUR	WHITE BEANS
Tryptophan	0.25	0.50	0.66	0.71	1.4	1.4	1.8
Phenylalanine	0.28	0.56	6.13	3.1	5.8	5.9	10.9
Leucine	1.10	2.20	12.0	5.5	8.1	8.0	17.0
Isoleucine	0.7	1.4	4.1	3.0	5.6	5.2	11.3
Lysine	0.8	1.6	4.1	2.5	4.0	3.2	14.7
Valine	0.8	1.6	6.8	4.5	6.4	5.5	12.1
Methionine	0.11	0.22	2.1	1.1	1.6	1.8	2.0
Threonine	0.5	1.0	4.5	2.5	3.6	3.5	8.5
Total protein (g/3,000 calories of each selected food)	20	37 (WHO)	109	64	108	120	198

children need. All unrefined starches and green, yellow, and orange vegetables, it turns out, are perfectly calibrated by natural design to meet our protein needs, so long as we eat enough of them to satisfy our energy (caloric) requirements. These foods perfectly support peak human nutrition, as they have done for eons.

Other researchers have examined the capacity of plant foods to meet our protein needs and have found that children grow to be healthy and strong, and adults continue to thrive, on a diet based solely on a single type of starch.[14] No benefit is derived from mixing plant foods, nor from supplementing them with amino acid mixtures to make the combined patterns look more like protein from flesh, dairy, or eggs.[14]

THE AUTHORITIES DON'T GET IT

Despite the well-documented fact that humans can absorb or synthesize all of the amino acids needed to construct complete protein chains from

POTATOES	SWEET POTATOES	TARO	ASPARAGUS	BROCCOLI	TOMATOES	PUMPKIN	BEEF CLUB STEAK	EGG	MILK
0.8	0.8	1.0	3.9	3.8	1.4	1.5	3.1	3.8	2.3
3.6	2.5	3.0	10.2	12.2	4.3	3.0	11.2	13.9	7.7
4.1	2.6	5.2	14.6	16.5	6.1	6.0	22.4	21.0	15.9
3.6	2.2	3.0	11.9	12.8	4.4	4.3	14.3	15.7	10.3
4.4	2.1	3.4	15.5	14.8	6.3	5.5	23.9	15.3	12.5
4.4	3.4	3.5	16.0	17.3	4.2	4.3	15.1	17.7	11.7
1.0	0.8	0.6	5.0	5.1	1.1	1.0	6.8	7.4	3.9
3.4	2.1	2.7	9.9	12.5	4.9	2.7	12.1	12.0	7.4
82	45	58	330	338	150	115	276	238	160

Refer to *The McDougall Plan* for more details.[14]

plant food sources, many people continue to believe the misguided notion that one cannot get sufficient high-quality protein on a plant-based diet. This doesn't stop with popular opinion; even revered experts get the protein story wrong, believing that plant proteins are incomplete in amino acids and therefore cannot alone adequately support our protein needs.

Important authorities continue to toe this line, including scientists

---

Erroneous Statements by the Experts about Plant Proteins

Tufts Human Nutrition Research Center on Aging (2011): "Plant protein sources, although good for certain essential amino acids, do not always offer all nine essential amino acids in a single given food. For example, legumes lack methionine, while grains lack lysine."[15]

Tufts University School of Medicine (2011): "Single plant protein foods usually are lower in protein quality than most animal proteins because they lack significant amounts of various essential amino acids."[16]

Harvard School of Public Health (2011): "Other protein sources lack one or more 'essential' amino acids—that is, amino acids that the body can't make from scratch or create by modifying another amino acid. Called incomplete proteins, these usually come from fruits, vegetables, grains, and nuts."[17]

Feinberg School of Medicine, Northwestern University (2011): "Plant sources of protein (grains, legumes, nuts, and seeds) generally do not contain sufficient amounts of one or more of the essential amino acids. Thus protein synthesis can occur only to the extent that the limiting amino acids are available."[18]

The American Heart Association (2001): "Although plant proteins form a large part of the human diet, most are deficient in one or more essential amino acids and are therefore regarded as incomplete proteins."[19]

---

from Tufts University's Human Nutrition Research Center on Aging and its School of Medicine; registered dietitians, research nutritionists, and physicians at Northwestern University; and the Harvard School of Public Health. All of them are flat-out wrong about sufficiency of proteins in plant foods. It is a dangerous error. Following their advice predicts a lifetime of sickness, obesity, and premature death for countless people.

THE AMERICAN HEART ASSOCIATION GOT IT WRONG

In an October 2001 position paper published in the American Heart Association's journal *Circulation*, health care professionals from the AHA's Nutrition Committee of the Council on Nutrition, Physical Activity, and Metabolism wrote, "Although plant proteins form a large part of the human diet, most are deficient in one or more essential amino acids and are therefore regarded as incomplete proteins."[19]

I was alarmed to see this kind of misinformation quoted and published in such a respected journal, so I wrote a letter to the editor correcting this often-quoted but incorrect information. My letter was published in the June 2002 issue of *Circulation*.[20] However, the Nutrition Committee remained steadfast in its position, declining to cite a stitch of research to support the authors' original statement. Its denial of the scientific facts fueled me to write another letter, published in the journal's November 2002 issue.[21] Even after reviewing the evidence that refuted the Nutrition Committee's point of view, the head of the committee, Barbara Howard, PhD, still would not admit that her committee's findings were wrong. This time, she cited the research of the world's leading expert on protein, Dr. D. Joseph Millward, to defend her position.

In fact, Dr. Millward did not agree with the American Heart Association's position. Dr. Millward was an emeritus professor of human nutrition at the University of Surrey in England when he reviewed this professional confrontation between me and the American Heart Association. He e-mailed me, "I thought I had made my position quite clear in my published papers. In an article I wrote for the *Encyclopedia of Nutrition*[22] I said, 'Contrary to general opinion, the distinction between dietary protein sources in terms of the nutritional superiority of animal over plant proteins is much more difficult to demonstrate and less relevant in human nutrition.' This is quite distinct from the AHA position which in my view is wrong."[23]

I forwarded Dr. Millward's e-mail to the American Heart Association, but it remained silent for almost a decade before softening its position on amino acids. Currently (2011), the AHA makes the following two statements echoing the points I tried to make back in 2001:[24]

All-Potato Diets Provide All the Protein and Amino Acids for Men, Women, and Children

Many populations throughout history—for example, people in rural Poland and Russia at the turn of the 19th century—have lived in good health doing hard work with the white potato serving as their primary source of nutrition. In one landmark experiment carried out in 1925, two healthy adults—a 25-year-old man and a 28-year-old woman—ate a diet of white potatoes for 6 months.[25] (A few additional items of little nutritional value and empty calories were included, such as pure fats, a few fruits, coffee, and tea.) The final report of their experiences included two revealing statements about the value of potatoes: "They [the man and woman] did not tire of the uniform potato diet and there was no craving for change." Even though they were both physically active (especially the man) they were described as "in good health on a diet in which the nitrogen [protein] was practically solely derived from the potato."

The potato is such an excellent source of nutrition that it can supply all of the essential proteins and amino acids for young children, even in times of food shortage. Eleven Peruvian children,

---

You don't need to eat foods from animals to have enough protein in your diet. Plant proteins alone can provide enough of the essential and non-essential amino acids, as long as sources of dietary protein are varied and caloric intake is high enough to meet energy needs.

Whole grains, legumes, vegetables, seeds and nuts all contain both essential and non-essential amino acids. You don't need to consciously combine these foods ("complementary proteins") within a given meal.

ages 8 months to 35 months, recovering from malnutrition, were fed diets in which all of the protein and 75 percent of the calories came from potatoes.[26,27] (Soybean and cottonseed oils and simple sugars, neither of which contain protein, vitamins, or minerals, provided some of the extra calories.) Researchers concluded that this simple potato diet provided all the protein and essential amino acids to meet the needs of growing and small children.

Note: These two experiments are strong testaments to the abundance of nutrients in and the weight-loss benefits of the potato. After adding "empty calories" from oils and sugars, the basic potato still provided all the protein, amino acids, vitamins, and minerals required to maintain the health of very active adults and promote the growth of young children. The "empty calories" prevented undesirable weight loss in both experiments. Thus, the much-maligned potato is an ideal food for dieters—low in calories and high in nutrient density. And it is especially beneficial for people with type 2 diabetes, who can be cured by simply shedding a few extra pounds.

At last, the American Heart Association has accepted the scientifically proven conclusion that plant foods do, indeed, contain all of the essential amino acids we need to survive and thrive. Unfortunately, experts from Tufts, Harvard, Northwestern, and most other major universities and medical organizations have chosen to continue spreading incorrect information, the result being serious health consequences for billions of people worldwide.

What You Don't Know Can Make You Sick

The people we trust to educate our children and form our public policies appear to be ignorant about our basic nutritional needs. The result is disastrous: Millions of Americans are suffering from diet-related illnesses, including 18 million people with coronary heart disease, 25.8 million with type 2 diabetes, 400,000 with multiple sclerosis, and millions with inflammatory arthritis.

While there is ample evidence that a starch-based diet can help to drastically improve our nation's health and reduce our exorbitant health care bill, your doctor, or even the Surgeon General, probably will not tell you about this solution. One reason is the misguided fear that such a diet would bring about protein deficiency. But protein deficiency doesn't exist except alongside starvation, a condition under which all nutrients, including calories, are in inadequate supply.

That the experts promote this view translates to poor advice in the doctor's office. Suppose your loving spouse of 35 years has a massive heart attack. While your spouse recovers, both of you pledge you will do anything to avoid a repeat experience. On your first follow-up visit, you tell your doctor that your family plans to follow a low-fat, vegan diet—no meat or dairy—from here on out. Based on the information he has learned in medical school and from leading organizations, your doctor might say, "I would strongly advise you against that. Plant foods are missing essential amino acids and you will become protein deficient. I think it's a good idea to follow a healthy diet, but in order to be balanced you've got to include high-quality proteins, like those from meat, dairy, and eggs." His defense for this position? The opinion of a variety of nutritional experts that once included the Nutrition Committee of the American Heart Association.

STARCH PROVIDES PERFECT NUTRITION

In addition to protein, Mother Nature designed her plant foods with a perfect balance of fat, carbohydrate, vitamins, and minerals to support optimal health. So long as you have enough food to eat, the question of fulfilling specific nutrient requirements is a moot one; it's all right there.

How, then, have scientists, dietitians, physicians, diet gurus, and the general public gotten so fixated on a problem that doesn't exist? When they speak of protein, why is it assumed that the best sources are meat, poultry, fish, eggs, and dairy products when these foods have steered those who can afford them toward lives of ill health, from the earliest time in history right up to the present day? Is it because we confer a higher social status on those who indulge in meat? Do we consume meat as a way to elevate ourselves? To separate ourselves from populations that, it turns out, may be a lot more fortunate than us by enjoying the indigenous plant foods that surround them? Is it because high-protein foods reap high profits? Because billboards and television advertisements and best-selling books say it is so?

All the way back in 1904, Professor Chittenden had faith that knowledge and truth would prevail.[4] He wrote, "Habit and sentiment play such a part in our lives that it is too much to expect any sudden change in custom. By a proper education commenced early in life it may, however, be possible to establish new standards, which in time may prevail and eventually lead to more enlightened methods of living."

Sadly, the past century of declining health, most strikingly among those living in developed countries with adequate resources, has proved Chittenden wrong. But that does not mean it is too late to prove him right.

CHAPTER 8

When Friends Ask: Where Do You Get Your Calcium?

O nce you've convinced your friends and family that you will not perish from lack of protein on a starch-based diet, they will likely begin firing questions about other nutrients. The most common next question: How will you get enough calcium? Don't you need milk and cheese for that?

While you can get calcium from dairy, it is not your only option, and it most certainly is not your best option. In fact, there is no good argument for eating dairy products, and there are plenty of reasons to avoid them.

CALCIUM IN A GLASS

Milk is as pure white as fresh fallen snow and as familiar as a mother's warm touch. If this single food, as a sole source of nutrition, can sustain a newborn, surely it must be nature's perfect food. Our need for milk supposedly doesn't stop with infancy or childhood. Milk, we are told, strengthens and protects our bones in adulthood as well. These structural beams of the body are built with calcium, so it shouldn't surprise us that milk is essential to our strength and stability.

It turns out those "facts" are what the dairy industry would like us to believe. Please don't feel bad about having been gullible enough to believe this carton of untruths. I did, too, right up until I began to probe a little deeper into the science of calcium and milk.

Misinformation Builds Profits, Not Bones

The American cow-based dairy industries—milk, yogurt, cheese, ice cream, and the like—together make up a $100 billion-a-year business. That gives them plenty of income to support the approximately $202 million they have to spend on their own scientific research and other propaganda each year to spread the myth that dairy foods are not only a healthy choice, but are essential to avoiding illness.[1] The dairy industry tells us: "To meet calcium recommendations, increased consumption of calcium-rich foods such as milk and other dairy foods often is necessary. Unfortunately, few Americans consume sufficient calcium, thereby increasing their risk for major chronic diseases such as osteoporosis."[2]

The industry's fearmongering seems to be working: In 2011, the average American was consuming more than 620 pounds of dairy products annually, compared with 541 pounds in 1981.[3] Annual milk consumption among children ages 6 to 12 has increased to 28 gallons per child. Children under 18 years of age drink 46 percent, or nearly half, of all milk consumed.[4] This will come as no surprise when you learn that 18 percent of the industry's marketing budget is aimed at schoolchildren, an audience that does a keenly effective job of driving supermarket sales, but is ill equipped to evaluate what is best for its own health and well-being.

A Talking Cow Wouldn't Lie to You, Would She?

In my Midwestern youth, Elsie the Cow taught me that milk builds strong bones. When I moved to Hawaii as a young doctor, Lani Moo took over, assuring me that I would never outgrow my need for milk. As I settled in Northern California to develop my practice and raise a family, the torch was passed to Clo, who dispenses dairy-friendly advice from billboards lining Highway 101. When it comes to milk, it's hard to argue with an adorable, information-dispensing cow doing her best to ensure you don't fall victim to the dangers of dietary calcium deficiency.

But wait a second. Have you ever met someone suffering from calcium deficiency? Is calcium a key mineral found in copious quantities in the dairy industry's favorite product, without which our bones will fail to hold us upright?

Calcium Comes from Dirt, Not Cows

Where does the cow get her calcium from? Does her body produce it? No. Actually, she gets it from the soil. Calcium is a basic mineral element that is neither created nor destroyed. Plants absorb calcium and other

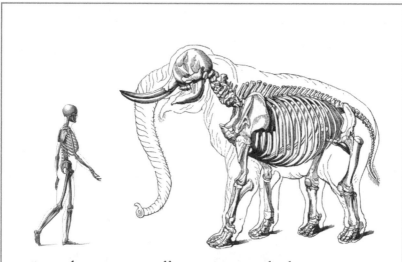

Since plants contain sufficient protein and calcium to grow giant animals, they will easily meet these needs for people.

minerals from the soil through their roots. As the plant grows, that calcium is built into its fabric from root to stem to fruit or vegetable to seed. The calcium gets into the cow when she eats grass and other calcium-rich plants. I recommend that you skip the cow altogether and go straight to the plant source for your calcium. Plants are the source of calcium and minerals that build strong bones for humans, cows, and the largest animals walking the earth—even horses and hippopotamuses—which eat no animal or dairy foods whatsoever.

If the giants of the animal kingdom can get all the calcium they need to support their massive bones, with no help from milk beyond their own mother's milk during their infancy, wouldn't you think plants would provide enough for us relatively small humans? In fact, they do: Until recent times, and still today in most parts of the world, people have grown into their adult skeletons with no help from milk except for when nursing as infants. They certainly had no need for or access to calcium supplements.

The problem is not finding a way to get enough calcium through what we eat; a plant-based diet of starches, vegetables, and fruits will always give you plenty of it. The problem is holding on to that calcium. Once you understand this, you can see that the logical answer is not to increase calcium intake through eating dairy or taking supplements. The best way to increase your calcium retention is to steer clear of animal proteins, including those found in hard cheeses and other dairy foods.

Calcium Is Good—We Just Don't Need So Much

I don't mean to suggest that calcium is unimportant. It is essential for all living things, from microbes to plants to animals. It is the most abundant mineral found in the human body, with the average adult carrying around 2.2 pounds of it, about 99 percent of which is stored as calcium phosphate salts in the bones. Calcium plays crucial roles, from

Bantu Women: An Example of Plants Supplying Abundant Calcium

The Bantu women of Africa consume no dairy products. Instead, they take in about 250 to 400 milligrams of calcium each day through vegetable sources. That's just a quarter to a third of the US Recommended Daily Allowance of 1,000 to 1,300 milligrams of calcium for reproductive-age women.

During her reproductive years, a typical Bantu woman will have 10 children and will breastfeed each of them for about 10 months.[5] With no dairy in their diet, a comparatively small calcium intake, no calcium supplements, and the tremendous demands of repeated pregnancies and breastfeeding, you would expect osteoporosis to run rampant. Yet it is virtually unknown among Bantu women.[5]

It isn't until rural African women migrate to cities or to Western countries and adopt richer diets—also rich in calcium—that osteoporosis becomes a problem.[6] Why the bone loss with additional calcium? Their new Western diet includes large quantities of animal proteins, which come loaded with dietary acids.[7] As discussed in Chapter 3, these acids accelerate the excretion of calcium and other bone materials into the urine. This increased calcium output outpaces the added calcium in their newly adopted Western diet, leaving these women with a deficit.

forming the skeleton to regulating the nervous system and blood vessel function.

Three organ systems very efficiently and precisely regulate the body's calcium balance: the gastrointestinal tract, the bones, and the kidneys. When you overindulge in calcium, your intestinal cells block out much of it, with the kidneys cooperating by eliminating any excess.

If your body didn't take these measures to avoid a buildup of excess calcium, the surplus would find its way into your heart, muscles, and skin in addition to your kidneys, eventually leading to heart and kidney failure and even death.

When you eat relatively little calcium, on the other hand, the intestine extracts more of it from your food, while the kidneys work to conserve the calcium already in your body. The body so efficiently utilizes this precious mineral that calcium deficiency due to a low-calcium diet is essentially unknown in human beings, even in those billions of people who consume calcium from no other sources than plants.

> **Disease due to calcium deficiency is essentially unknown in humans on natural diets.**

CAN YOU GET SICK FROM INSUFFICIENT CALCIUM?

A comprehensive review of the scientific literature on diets consumed around the world shows virtually no diseases related to calcium deficiency.[8–11] You have probably heard of rickets, a disease where the bones weaken, leading to fractures and deformity. Rickets is seen only in children, and nearly all cases result from inadequate vitamin D, from a lack of sunshine (see Chapter 11). While it is possible to get rickets from insufficient calcium—a condition called nutritional rickets—it is exceedingly rare and is found only with extremely restricted diets.[12] Even in these few cases the exact role that very low calcium intake plays is unclear.[13]

Even for children, contrary to the dairy industry's marketing campaign, the scientific literature has clearly documented that extra dietary calcium *does not* build strong bones.[14,15] A review in the March 2005 journal *Pediatrics* concludes that: "Scant evidence supports nutrition guidelines focused specifically on increasing milk or other dairy product intake for promoting child and adolescent bone mineralization."[15]

Industry-Funded Research Shows
Few Benefits of Dairy for Adults

According to the time-honored message from the National Dairy Council, milk and its by-products are important, if not essential, for the prevention of osteoporosis. However, this conclusion runs contrary to the scientific research on the effects of cow's milk on the bone health of women. In a review of 57 studies, more than half of the studies (57 percent) showed no significant benefit from dairy, 29 percent showed a benefit from consuming dairy, and 14 percent found that dairy products actually seemed to harm the bones.[16]

The review included seven randomized, controlled trials (a research design scientists consider most reliable), six of which were funded by the dairy industry. Yet they *still* could not make the case for dairy's benefit.

Just one of these randomized studies looked at the effects of drinking cow's milk on postmenopausal women.[17] The others looked at the effects of milk on adolescent and premenopausal women or those who used calcium sources other than the one most commonly consumed: milk. In this single study, the postmenopausal women who drank extra milk actually lost *more* bone than those who did not. The authors' interpretation: "The protein content of the milk supplement may have a negative effect on calcium balance, possibly through an increase in kidney losses of calcium or through a direct effect on bone resorption . . . this may have been due to the average 30 percent increase in protein intake during milk supplementation."

A 2006 editorial in the *British Medical Journal* confirms these findings, pointing out that: "Populations that consume the most cow's milk and other dairy products have among the highest rates of osteoporosis and hip fractures in later life."[18] As it turns out, the more calcium in the diet, the greater the risk of hip fractures worldwide.[19,20] Consuming dairy products may actually *harm* our bones. It's not surprising, since hard cheeses, like Parmesan, burden the body with the largest amounts of dietary acids of any commonly consumed animal foods.[21-26]

Nettie Taylor, Director of Religious Education for a Catholic Church, Lexington, South Carolina

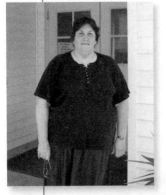

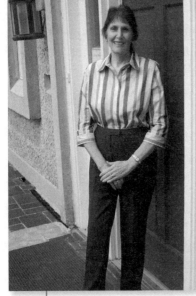

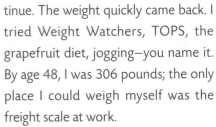

I began dieting before I reached high school, then took amphetamines in my teens to lose weight. I starved myself for a week in college to squeeze into an outfit. I continued on and off diets until my weight ballooned with pregnancy. When my second child was born, I weighed 200 pounds.

I lost weight eating meat and eggs for a year on the Atkins diet until I felt so sick I couldn't continue. The weight quickly came back. I tried Weight Watchers, TOPS, the grapefruit diet, jogging—you name it. By age 48, I was 306 pounds; the only place I could weigh myself was the freight scale at work.

When I came across Dr. McDougall, I decided to give this starch-based approach a try, stopping short of forgoing skim milk with my morning cereal. Meanwhile, my cholesterol hovered stubbornly around 200. It wasn't until I gave up the milk that my cholesterol levels dropped below 160. The McDougall Diet was surprisingly easy to follow, in large part because I could eat as much as I wanted. A little over a year later I weighed 146, 160 pounds below my peak. I went from being miserable, embarrassed, and nearly immobile to feeling happy and energetic. My new confidence helped me to leave a 23-year career for a job that made me happy.

There was a bump in the road when, after a breast cancer diagnosis and lumpectomy, I was given steroids to counter the side effects from chemo. My steroid-fueled appetite broke my resolve as I added sweets back to my diet, then meat. By age 58, I found myself in the parking lot of my favorite fast-food restaurant, crying out for help while stuffing down a sandwich, fries, brownies, and a Diet Coke. I was back up to 282 pounds.

My doctor prescribed drugs when my cholesterol shot back up into the 250s. He insisted on Fosamax for osteoporosis. Chest pains, along with numbness and tingling in my feet, pointed to potential heart problems and diabetes. Yet, despite a painful hip that kept me from sleeping, I refused to take prescription medications for fear of their health risks. My doctor referred me to a nutritionist but I refused to go. I knew what their advice would be: dairy products, "healthy" fats, and skinless chicken breasts. I also knew what I needed to do: get back on the McDougall Diet.

I bit the bullet, and less than 2 years later I'd lost 149 pounds to weigh 133. I bought my first pair of size 8 pants, ever. My blood pressure dropped from 146/86 to 105/64 millimeters of mercury and my cholesterol to 163 milligrams per deciliter. I now exercise daily and my hip no longer hurts. I feel younger and more energetic than ever. I am no longer depressed. And I've regained my self-respect.

Excess Protein and Acid in Dairy and Meat Cause Bone Damage

Worldwide, rates of hip fractures and kidney stones increase with increasing calcium intake. The United States, Canada, Norway, Sweden, Australia, and New Zealand have the highest rates of osteoporosis, while the lowest rates are found in rural Asia and rural Africa, where people eat the fewest animal-derived foods and also consume low-calcium diets.[19,20]

Osteoporosis is caused by several controllable factors, the most important being what we eat. The greatest risk comes from foods that are high in protein and dietary acids,[21–26] including meat, poultry, fish, seafood, and hard cheeses.

Acid Loads of Common Foods [21]

Cheddar cheese	10.0
Fish (cod)	9.3
Chicken	7.0
Beef	6.3
Peas	1.0
Wheat flour	1.0
Potatoes	−5.0
Apples	−5.0
Bananas	−6.0
Tomatoes	−18.0
Spinach	−56.0

Figures represent renal acid load per 100 calories. Foods are ordered from most acidic (highest positive number) to most alkaline (lowest negative number).

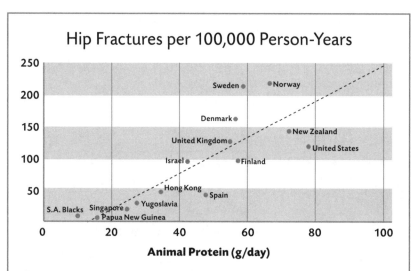

Hip Fractures per 100,000 Person-Years

Animal Protein (g/day)

This incontestable evidence shows the more protein a population consumes, the greater the risk of hip fractures.[19,20]

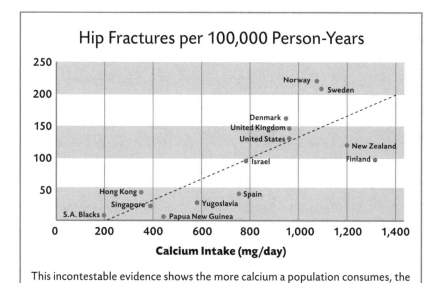

Hip Fractures per 100,000 Person-Years

Calcium Intake (mg/day)

This incontestable evidence shows the more calcium a population consumes, the greater the risk of hip fractures.[19,20]

Our bones neutralize the acids from the foods we eat, leaching calcium from them in the process.[21] Fruits and vegetables, which are alkaline by nature, help to neutralize acids as well, preserving the bones from being drained by this demanding work.

DAIRY FOODS CAUSE OTHER SERIOUS HEALTH HAZARDS

Milk labeling is notoriously misleading. Whole milk, advertised as 3.5 percent fat, may indeed have 3.5 percent fat by weight, but in terms of calories, half of them come from fat, most of it the saturated, artery-clogging kind. Even milk labeled low-fat or 2 percent (again, by weight) gets nearly one-third (32 percent) of its calories from fat. Cheese is the worst offender; roughly 70 percent of its calories come from fat. Fat is the major contributor to obesity, and from obesity comes type 2 diabetes.

Fat is highly publicized as a hazard of consuming dairy products. But dairy proteins and the milk sugar lactose also lead to common illnesses. Cancer is caused, at least in part, by both high- and low-fat dairy products, implicating other components of dairy products besides the fat.[27] The protein in milk increases growth hormones (like IGF1) that promote the development and growth of common cancers, such as breast, prostate, colon, brain, and lung cancer.[28-31] Dairy proteins are a major contributor to food allergies and more serious autoimmune diseases as wide ranging as rheumatoid arthritis, asthma, and multiple sclerosis.[32-34] Intolerance of the milk sugar lactose causes the majority of people worldwide to become ill with stomach cramps, diarrhea, and gas (lactose intolerance).

Although a case can be made against many of dairy's individual components (protein, fat, cholesterol, sugar, lack of dietary fiber or complex carbohydrates), such microanalyses distract us with oversimplification that misses the larger point: Dairy foods make people fat and sick. Plain and simple, dairy foods are not intended for, or tolerated by, children or adults. Cow's milk is for calves, and then only for the first 6 months of their lives, at most.

Illnesses Caused by or Associated with Consumption of Dairy Foods

BODY SYSTEMS AFFECTED	SYMPTOMS AND ILLNESSES
General	Loss of appetite, growth retardation
Upper gastrointestinal	Canker sores; irritation of the tongue, lips, and mouth; tonsil enlargement; vomiting; gastroesophageal reflux disease (GERD); Sandifer's syndrome; peptic ulcer disease; colic; stomach cramps; abdominal distention; intestinal obstruction; type 1 diabetes
Lower gastrointestinal	Bloody stools, colitis, malabsorption, diarrhea, painful defecation, fecal soiling, infantile colic, chronic constipation, infantile food protein–induced entero-colitis syndrome, Crohn's disease, ulcerative colitis
Respiratory	Stuffy or runny nose, inner ear infec-tions, sinus infections, wheezing, asthma, pulmonary infiltrates
Bone and joint	Rheumatoid arthritis (juvenile and adult), lupus, Behçet's disease, psoriatic arthritis, ankylosing spondylitis
Skin	Rashes, atopic dermatitis, eczema, seborrhea, hives, acne
Nervous	Multiple sclerosis, Parkinson's disease, autism, schizophrenia, irritability, restlessness, hyperactivity, headache, lethargy, fatigue, allergic-tension fatigue syndrome, muscle pain, mental depres-sion, bed-wetting
Blood	Abnormal blood clotting, iron deficiency anemia, low serum proteins, thrombocy-topenia, eosinophilia
Other	Nephrotic syndrome, glomerulonephri-tis, anaphylactic shock and death, sudden infant death syndrome (SIDS or crib or cot death), injury to the arteries causing arteritis, and eventually, atherosclerosis

Calcium Pills May Be Hazardous, Too

If the dairy industry has us wrapped around its milk glass, the supplement industry is no better. Taking calcium supplements may be dangerous, too. Calcium supplements interfere with iron absorption and cause constipation, and may cause even greater harm over the long term.[35,36]

Calcium supplements, given alone, improve bone mineral density but offer little benefit in reducing the risk of fractures, and may even increase fracture risk.[37–39] It is likely that any benefits they do provide are a result of the supplements' alkalinizing effects.[23] Antacids made from calcium carbonate are commonly taken for bone health. It is not the calcium that benefits the bone but the alkalinizing carbonate, which neutralizes dietary acids that result from eating meat, poultry, fish, and cheese. If not for the antacid, the bones would have to give up their carbonate and other neutralizing agents, eventually leading to bone loss. Other antacids, such as sodium bicarbonate, potassium bicarbonate, or aluminum hydroxide, offer a similar benefit by neutralizing dietary acids and preventing bone loss, even though they contain no calcium at all.[40]

A review in the July 2010 *British Medical Journal* found that calcium supplements (without added vitamin D) were associated with an increased risk of heart attacks.[41] The analysis included 12,000 participants from 11 randomized controlled trials, and found that calcium supplements were associated with an approximately 30 percent relative increase in heart attacks, as well as small increases in the risk for stroke and overall mortality. In their summary, the authors state that the " . . . treatment of 1,000 people with calcium for 5 years would cause an additional 14 myocardial infarctions, 10 strokes, and 13 deaths, and prevent 26 fractures."

There is no simple explanation for these findings. Undoubtedly, taking calcium as an isolated, concentrated nutrient causes imbalances in the body, which increases the risk of death and disease. (See Chapter 11 for a more detailed discussion of dietary supplements.)

Dairy Is a Dirty Word

Dairy products have been the foods most often recalled by the FDA because of contamination with infectious agents.[42] These foods are commonly tainted with disease-causing bacteria such as salmonella, staphylococci, Listeria, and deadly E. coli.[43] Dairy may also carry Mycobacterium paratuberculosis,[44] which may cause the life-threatening form of chronic colitis known as Crohn's disease. Dairy foods are also contaminated with viruses, including those known to cause lymphoma and leukemia-like diseases, as well as immune deficiency, in cattle.

The Animal and Plant Inspection Services division of the USDA reported in 2007 that the cattle in 89 percent of US dairy operations showed evidence of infection with bovine leukemia virus.[45-47] Spread of the virus within herds was commonly caused by factory farming practices that include passing contamination through shared syringes, dehorning instruments, rectal probing, tattooing needles, and pooled colostrum (milk for newborn calves that cows generate right before giving birth). Factory farms feed their sick and dying cows, called "downer cows," to chickens and pigs. They also feed the floor sweepings from chicken and pigs back to the cows, recirculating infectious microbes. These practices affect nearly our entire US milk supply; holding tanks used to collect milk from herds of 500 or more cows are found to be infected 100 percent of the time with these viruses.[45] Scientists have known about this health hazard since 1969.[47]

Bovine leukemia viruses are easily spread through cow's milk to other species of animals, such as goats and sheep, which can subsequently become infected and ill with leukemia.[45,46] In 1974 it was reported that two of six infant chimpanzees fed infected cow's milk died of leukemia within a year.[48] In December 2003, researchers from the University of California at Berkeley published their findings from a study that used state-of-the-art detection methods to discover that 74 percent of 257 people selected from their community had been infected with bovine leukemia viruses.[47]

Each year in the United States, about 45,000 new cases of leukemia and 74,000 new cases of lymphoma occur for what most doctors claim to be "unknown reasons." Although the dairy industry and others may consider research findings inconclusive when they connect these illnesses with bovine leukemia viruses, the burden of proof should lie with those selling this food to you and your family. It has not been proven safe to eat dairy infected with leukemia viruses, and the evidence is even more damning now that it is clear that these viruses infect the vast majority of people who eat meat and milk products.

THE DAIRY INDUSTRY REMAINS UNACCOUNTABLE

Nutritionally speaking, dairy products—whether in liquid or solid form—are similar to red meats. The difference is that most educated people are reasonably well aware that eating too much meat is unhealthy. However, with milk, we are more likely to believe advertising claims that it is strengthening our bones and, if it is represented as low in fat (despite that it generally is not), that it will help us to lose weight and become healthy.

The fact that billions of people the world over grow into normal adults with healthy bones without ever drinking a glass of milk or taking a calcium supplement should make it obvious that we do not need any more calcium in our diet than we get from eating plants. If milk is truly critical to building strong bones, why are humans the only species that continues to drink it after weaning, and the only animal that drinks the milk of other species? Causation and association have been documented between dairy products and any number of diseases. If you are willing to stop eating just one group of foods, you will experience the most profound improvement in your health and appearance by eliminating all dairy. Even though I feel very strongly about the ill effects of meat, poultry, and fish, and am so very passionate about the harm to health and the environment caused by eating them, I encourage you to send Elsie the Cow out to pasture, first and foremost.[49] You and your family will be much better off without her.

CHAPTER 9

Confessions of a Fish Killer

I fell in love with the ocean at age 5 in my kindergarten class while watching a 35-millimeter film depicting undersea life. The movie showed fish in a rainbow of brilliant hues, scraggly coral formations, giant clams, and hermit crabs.

When I was 12, my dad and I took up scuba diving. My early underwater explorations were limited to the murky, lifeless waters of nearby Michigan lakes. When I was in my early teens, our family vacationed in the Outer Banks of North Carolina, a chain of barrier islands that is home to the largest estuary system in the world. We hung our poles over the side of our small boat, catching and devouring deep-sea flounder, bluefish, and dorado.

My first open-ocean scuba experience was in 1969, during spring break from my first year of medical school at Michigan State University. This time I traveled to John Pennekamp Coral Reef State Park, an underwater park in the Florida Keys where thousands of colorful fish swarmed around me as I meandered through coral forests. I was so delighted with the experience that I brought my new bride, Mary, back there for a scuba-diving honeymoon 3 years later.

In 1972 we moved to Hawaii, where we collected small tropical fish with hand nets for our saltwater aquariums. Sadly, most of them landed belly up in their tank within a few days of capture, my first peek at a grim reality: My love of fishing, diving, and stocking our aquarium required that I kill the very fish I treasured. Over the next couple of decades, several times a year I would capture large, beautiful fish—mahimahi, tuna, salmon—in the waters off Hawaii and California using line or spear. I considered it my birthright to take these fishes' lives for my own enjoyment and sustenance. I reasoned that proteins and good fats were critical to my nutrition and that fish was one of the most healthful sources of both. It all seemed so natural. But I had so much to learn.

Since the blissful ignorance of childhood I have spent the last five decades directly witnessing the devastation of the lively ocean ecosystem I so greatly prize and had a hand in depleting. Since the 1950s,

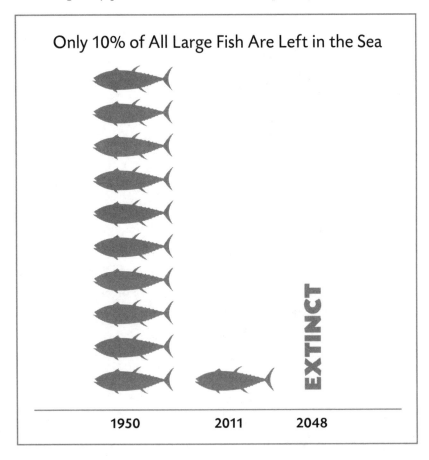

Only 10% of All Large Fish Are Left in the Sea

| 1950 | 2011 | 2048 |

90 percent of the world's fish stocks have been exhausted by the fishing industry.[1] More than a third of all sea life—bluefin tuna, Atlantic cod, Alaskan king crab, and Pacific salmon—have had their populations nearly decimated; 7 percent of all fish species have gone extinct altogether.[1]

Diminishing supply has caused the price of fresh, wild-caught salmon to triple over the past decade. Because of the rarity of bluefin tuna, the Japanese are now making some of their sushi with beef. In order to avert, or at least delay, the extinction of salmon, fishing for them in California waters is now often prohibited.

When I returned to my beloved coral reefs in the Florida Keys in 2002, I found them no longer brimming with life as I remembered, but rather bleached white and barren by the loss of coral and fish due to environmental stresses and the ocean's warming temperature. By the year 2048, we are warned, all fish and seafood species will have collapsed, meaning that they will be either extinct or on the precipice of extinction.[1]

We might justify eating sea creatures if it improved our health and saved our lives, even if doing so would devastate the oceans and kill off their inhabitants. But what if the opposite were true? What if eating fish in the amounts commonly recommended by health professionals posed a health hazard rather than a benefit to us?

PLANTS MAKE ALL OMEGA-3 AND OMEGA-6 FATTY ACIDS

Omega-3 and omega-6 fats are called *essential* because we need them but cannot manufacture them ourselves. That means we must get them through the foods we eat. These plant-derived fats have many important functions, such as forming cell membranes and synthesizing hormones. These fatty acids are named for their carbon-to-carbon double bond on a carbon chain; omega-3 fatty acids have their double bond at the third carbon position from the omega (methyl) end of the chain and omega-6 fatty acids have theirs at the sixth carbon position. What's important about this is that only plants are able make a double bond at the third or sixth carbon position. Neither fish nor animals nor humans can create their own omega-3 or omega-6 fats.

The basic omega-3 fat made by plants is alpha-linolenic acid, abbreviated ALA. Linoleic acid (without the second "n") is the basic plant-generated omega-6 fat. Small fish take in ALA by eating seaweed and algae, then converting some of it into long-chain fats, such as eicosapentaenoic acid (EPA) and docosahexaenoic acid (DHA), which they store in their body fat. You may have heard that humans need to eat fish to obtain these elongated fatty acids because we cannot manufacture sufficient amounts on our own, but that simply is not true. Research has demonstrated that men, women, children, and pregnant women convert small but perfectly adequate quantities of ALA into EPA and DHA without any help from fish.[2-9]

The omega-3 fatty acid DHA is highly concentrated in the nervous system, leading some people to believe that fish and fish oil can improve our mental health and protect us from neurological diseases. However, there is no evidence that dementia or any other condition of mental deficiency occurs in populations that take in all of their essential fats from plants and have a low intake of EPA or DHA from fish or supplements.[10-12] Furthermore, research shows that those who eat plenty of fish have about the same risk of developing dementia and Alzheimer's as those who eat no fish at all.[13,14] Consider this reassuring observation: People on vegetarian diets characterize themselves as being in a "better mood" twice as often as meat eaters, and are half as likely to suffer from dementia.[12,15]

Many nutritionists and doctors worry about meeting the needs of the unborn during early development. Infants born to mothers who have taken supplements of DHA during pregnancy have been found to show no improvement in neurologic function as assessed by their visual development early in life.[16] A critical review of the scientific literature on essential fats by John Langdon, a professor of biology and anthropology at the University of Indianapolis, concluded: "There is no evidence that human diets based on terrestrial food chains with traditional nursing practices fail to provide adequate levels of DHA or other [omega] n-3 fatty acids. Consequently, the hypothesis that DHA has been a limiting resource in human brain evolution must be considered to be unsupported."[5] Meaning that if we eat natural plant foods we will always, during all stages of life, get enough DHA and other omega-3 fats.

Something Fishy about Health Claims

The recommendation to consume more fish began with observations of populations worldwide that have traditionally favored fish. These populations have lower rates of heart disease than populations that eat primarily beef, chicken, or pork. The most notable fish-eating country is Japan. But are we certain that fish holds the key to their good health?

Look a little closer and you will find that the Japanese diet is based largely on rice. In fact, it is their significant consumption of this starch, not of fish, that explains their better health, trimmer figures, more active lifestyle, youthful appearances, and greater longevity. Look at a traditional Japanese meal and you will see that only small amounts of fish are eaten as a condiment atop a bowl of rice. In the United States, where Japanese restaurants serve a little rice with a large plate of fish instead of the traditional opposite, we lose these health benefits. This explains why Japanese people who move to the United States and slowly transition to a Western diet begin to lose their immunity, soon looking more like Americans; that is, fatter and sicker.

Health organizations worldwide, including the American Heart Association, the American Medical Association, the American Diabetic Association, the British Dietetic Association, and Australia's leading health research body, the National Health and Medical Research Council, among others, recommend that we eat fish primarily because it is a reliable source of the "good" omega-3 fatty acids. Yet these same groups warn about the hazards of methylmercury and other environmental contaminants in fish. This information has us stuck between a rock and a coral reef: In order to protect our hearts we must consume chemicals that put us at risk for brain damage and cancer.

While there is no danger in avoiding fish sources of omega-3 fatty acids, there is certain danger in consuming fish or fish oil.

Fish Are Toxic with Mercury

Eating fish and taking fish oil capsules exposes you to mercury, a natural element found in the earth and released as industrial pollution during certain manufacturing processes. As mercury is dumped into our rivers, streams, and oceans, it is converted into highly toxic methylmercury, which becomes ever more concentrated as it accumulates up the food chain. Fish at the top of the food chain have the greatest mercury contamination levels. Which fish swim at the top of the food chain? Freshwater pike, walleye, and bass are examples, along with saltwater tuna, salmon, swordfish, herring, mackerel, and sardines.

These saltwater fish are also the ones with the highest concentrations of EPA and DHA. In other words, the fish that give you the most of those fatty acids come packaged with the highest mercury levels. Not just the few specific species listed here, but all fish and shellfish are contaminated with potentially dangerous environmental chemicals.

Mercury-contaminated seafood is almost the sole source of chronic human mercury poisoning. Serious health risks from mercury poisoning include damage to the heart, kidneys, and immune and nervous systems. In the brain, mercury poisoning can cause motor dysfunction, memory loss, learning disabilities, and depressive behavior. Even if eating fish fat or taking fish oil supplements did reduce your risk of nervous and motor disorders (they do not), that benefit would be more than offset by the toxic effects of mercury. In addition to mercury, fish and fish oils contain other toxins that promote cancer and have damaging effects on the reproductive system.[17]

Cholesterol in Fish Compared with Other Foods

FOOD	CHOLESTEROL (MG/100 CAL)
Bass	60
Crab	55
Cod	53
Mackerel	51
Salmon	40
Egg	272
Chicken	36
Pork	28
Beef	32

Grains, vegetables, and fruits have no significant amounts of cholesterol.

FISH CAN INCREASE THE RISK OF HEART DISEASE

The fact that fish is high in blood-thinning omega-3 fatty acids has led to the belief that fish protects us from heart disease. After all, thinner blood reduces the chance of forming a clot in an artery leading to the heart, and thus prevents heart attacks. The mercury that can poison the brain and kidneys also affects blood vessels, causing the formation of free radicals, inflammation, blood clots, and muscle dysfunction of the blood vessel walls.[17–19]

In addition to the environmental chemical contamination problem, fish share similar nutritional qualities with other muscle-derived foods like beef, pork, and chicken. Muscles are high in protein, fat, cholesterol, methionine, and dietary acids, and contain no carbohydrate or dietary fiber. (See Chapter 3 to review the five major poisons found in animal foods.) Cholesterol in fish elevates blood cholesterol,[20] with even small doses of fish oils raising "bad" (LDL) cholesterol.[21,22]

THE SCIENTIFIC CONSENSUS

Research published in respected medical journals showing that fish offers no benefit to the heart, and may even be a step in the wrong direction, has failed to influence medical schools, doctors, dietitians, and health organizations to change their tune from promoting fish and fish oil supplements as a cornerstone of good health. Doctors are taught almost nothing about nutrition during medical school and rarely pursue it on their own, leaving them easily swayed by what they are told by individuals and organizations representing themselves as authorities.

Perhaps the animal food–centered diets of most doctors, dietitians, and scientists have clouded their perspective, too. Barraged by research findings suggesting that they shun beef, pork, chicken, eggs, and cheese due to their high levels of saturated fat and cholesterol, these learned professionals are left with just one animal food option that continues to be held up as healthful: fish.

You needn't look far to find an abundance of studies promoting a very different point of view from the one you may have heard in your doctor's office or read about in the papers. Following are a few to whet your appetite. (The italic emphasis is mine.)

- A meta-review (a review of multiple studies) of 15,159 articles— including 48 randomized controlled trials involving 36,913 participants taking fish oil or eating oily fish—in the 2006 issue of the *British Medical Journal* found *no health benefits:* "Long chain and shorter chain omega-3 fats do not have a clear effect on total mortality, combined cardiovascular events, or cancer."[23]

- A review in the May 2007 issue of the *American Journal of Cardiology* concluded: "The data supporting the inverse correlation of fish or omega-3 fatty acid (eicosapentaenoic acid plus docosahexaenoic acid) consumption and coronary heart disease are *inconclusive and may be confounded by other dietary and lifestyle factors.*"[24] The confounding factors are avoiding saturated fats (beef, cheese, and eggs), not smoking, and getting regular exercise—all of which are established heart-healthy choices made by people who would also choose to eat fish.

- The DART-2 trial of 3,114 men under age 70 with angina (chest pain from clogged heart arteries) advised one group of men to eat two portions of oily fish per week or take three daily fish oil capsules. The others were not given that advice. The men advised to eat oily fish, and particularly those supplied with fish oil capsules, had *a higher risk of cardiac death* compared to those who were not given this advice.[25]

- The OMEGA study of 3,827 patients treated within 3 to 14 days following a heart attack found *no difference* in the risk of sudden cardiac death, overall death, repeat heart attack, stroke, heart arrhythmia, or need for heart surgery between those taking fish oil and those given a placebo. Although not statistically significant, the rates of death, repeat heart attack, and stroke were actually higher in the fish oil group. Supplements contained 460 milligrams EPA and 380 milligrams DHA.[26]

- A double-blind, placebo-controlled trial published in the November 2010 issue of the *New England Journal of Medicine* of 4,837 patients who had had a heart attack found *no reduction* in the rate of major cardiovascular events after treatment with a supplement of EPA and DHA over 40 months.[27]

- A randomized placebo-controlled trial published in the November 2010 issue of the *British Medical Journal* of 2,501 patients with a history of myocardial infarction, unstable angina, or stroke found daily supplementation with omega-3 fatty acids (EPA and DHA) resulted in *no reduction* in cardiovascular disease over nearly 5 years of treatment.[28]

- A randomized, placebo-controlled trial of 663 patients at high risk for developing atrial fibrillation treated them with fish oil. The results, published in the December 2010 issue of the *Journal of the American Medical Association*, showed *no benefits* over 6 months of treatment.[29]

- Even direct studies show harm to the arteries. Patients with coronary heart disease documented by angiograms received either fish oil capsules or olive oil capsules for an average duration of 28 months.[30] The amount of closure (stenosis) increased by 2.4 percent and 2.6 percent, respectively. The authors concluded: "Fish oil treatment for 2 years does not promote major favorable changes in the diameter of atherosclerotic coronary arteries."

Two important studies show that elevated mercury in the body, primarily from eating fish, causes heart trouble.

- A study published in 2002 in the *New England Journal of Medicine* found that higher levels of mercury in toenail clippings predicted a *greater chance of future heart attacks.*[18]
- Another study found that high content of mercury in hair may be a risk factor for acute coronary events and CVD (coronary vascular disease), CHD (coronary heart disease), and all-cause mortality in middle-aged eastern Finnish men. The researchers concluded that any protective effects on the blood vessels and heart from the "good fats" in fish were *negated by the damaging effects of mercury.*[19]

One of the most recent reviews of the overall effects of recommending fish and fish oils, from the 2009 issue of the *Canadian Medical Association Journal,* came to this conclusion: "Until renewable sources of long-chain omega-3 fatty acids—derived from plant, algae, yeast or other unicellular organisms—become more generally available, it would seem responsible to refrain from advocating to people in developed countries that they increase their intake of long-chain omega-3 fatty acids through fish consumption. *The evidence for the comprehensive benefits of increased fish oil consumption is not as clear-cut as protagonists suggest.*"[31]

The research refuting any benefit to the heart from eating fish or taking fish oils is clear and convincing. If you are seriously contemplating these substances as a means for preventing or treating heart disease, it is worth your time to carefully consider the evidence.

More Dangers from Consuming Fish and Fish Oils

Studies show that fish causes or contributes to a variety of ills beyond heart disease.

- The fat you eat is the fat you wear and there is nothing especially attractive about *becoming overweight or obese* by eating fish fat.[32]

- Fish causes an *increase in blood cholesterol* similar to that caused by beef and pork.[20]

- Fish's highly acidic proteins accelerate calcium loss, contributing to *osteoporosis* and *kidney stones.*[33]

- The blood-thinning properties of omega-3 fats that may help prevent the formation of clots also *increase the chance of bleeding complications.*[34]

- The anti-inflammatory properties of "good fats" can *suppress the immune system,* increasing risk for cancer and infection.[35-39]

- Omega-3 fats *inhibit the performance of insulin,* increasing blood sugar levels and aggravating diabetes.[40,41]

- High intake of fish can prolong pregnancy and increase birth weight, prompting a greater chance of *fetal death, Caesarean section, and birth injury.*[42-46]

EATING FARMED FISH IS NOT GUILT FREE

The high cost of fresh, wild fish, coupled with concern about our oceans, causes many consumers to put farmed fish on the family table. Fed a diet of fish oils and fish meal made up of small fish taken from chemically contaminated seas, these farmed fish are loaded with concentrated toxins. They are also fed by-products rendered from cows, raising concern that the agent causing mad cow disease could be transmitted to the fish and those who eat them.[47]

Because fish meal boosted with "good fats" is expensive, fish farmers frequently opt for cheaper fish meal that contains palm, linseed, and canola oils. As with humans, the composition of a fish's body fat varies depending on its diet. With the cheaper oils, you may be eating fats that are far from heart healthy while thinking you are boosting your levels of healthy fish oils. As a result, your supposedly healthy diet of fish may be inflaming your arteries and increasing your risk of heart attack and stroke.[48,49]

Fish farming also raises serious environmental concerns. Waste from fish cages and chemicals used in farming contaminate the waters where they are dumped. Also, fish kept in close proximity breed disease. Robbing the ocean of herring and other small fish to feed farmed fish depletes the food supply for native ocean fish, including salmon, trout, tuna, grouper, and cod.

And, in case you were wondering, fish *do* have feelings.[50] I can only imagine that life for fish in a fish farm must be like living in prison, on death row.

I Will Never Eat Fish Again

My favorite place to visit is Cocos Island, more than 300 miles west of mainland Costa Rica. The trip from the mainland takes more than 30 hours by boat. In this national park, scuba divers can take a swim with large fish, including dozens of varieties of sharks and rays, whale sharks, humpback whales, swordfish, and tuna. Even though park rangers protect these waters, poachers have reduced the area's sea life by 70 percent over the last 20 years. It is predicted that within 3 years, no large animals will remain in the park; they will all have been caught and eaten by people who believe that a diet with plenty of fish will boost their health. It pains me to think that my grandchildren will never, ever experience the vibrant sea life I once frequently visited.

In my lifetime I have witnessed firsthand the destruction of our environment and its impact on the world's seas. While I once enjoyed fishing, now, even though I follow a vegan diet, I would eat a beefsteak before I would harm ocean life again. Whether I consume fish or another animal would have roughly the same effect on my health. Fish is not health food. If you believe otherwise, you'd better get your fill now, before the last 10 percent of the fish population is devastated by those who have been falsely convinced that fish equals healthy eating and minimal environmental impact.[1]

The situation is not entirely hopeless, however. Accurate information can fuel concerted efforts to change. We can make sensible choices, enjoying the enormous variety of delicious health-promoting starches and plant foods that surround us. The Starch Solution offers a chance to reverse the downward spiral of our own and our oceans' health, if only we can begin listening soon enough.

CHAPTER 10

The Fat Vegan

My first exposure to veganism—the practice of consuming no foods from animal sources—was in 1977, when I was working as a medical resident at The Queen's Medical Center in Honolulu. My young medical intern had gone vegan out of a personal commitment not to harm animals. If you didn't know this, you might think his nylon belt and plastic shoes were just frightfully bad fashion sense. I figured a diet of vegetables, fruits, and grains ought to make vegans healthier than meat eaters. So I was surprised that this young, vegan doctor was quite overweight, with an oily face pockmarked from acne.

It didn't take me long to discover the reason for his poor health: This busy intern's diet consisted largely of potato chips and Coca-Cola, both readily available in the hospital's dining room, gift shop, and vending machines. He was the ultimate junk food vegan. Sadly, it turns out he is not a point far off the curve. The fact that vegans are vigilant about what *doesn't* go into their mouths does not guarantee that they follow good eating habits. In fact, a great number of vegans are overweight and unhealthy.

On its own, a diet free of hot dogs, hamburgers, fried chicken, shrimp scampi, grilled salmon, mac 'n' cheese, eggs over easy, and ice cream does little to assure good health. Neither does going a step further, omitting honey (made by bees), sugar (which may involve using bone in processing), wine (which may be filtered with egg whites), and other foods in which animal products play a minor role in production.

That doesn't mean you should give up on the idea of a vegan diet. It only means you need to learn what makes up a *healthy* vegan diet. You won't be surprised that the answer revolves around obtaining the bulk of your calories from starches.

Old Habits Die Hard

Giving up favorite foods is terrifying. Swearing off meat and milk feels tantamount to risking starvation. Some people overcome those fears by making their dietary choices feel familiar and safe. They exchange animal foods with ersatz equivalents—foods made to look, feel, smell, and taste like those they replace. If before going vegan dinner was a burger, roasted chicken, hot dogs, or a cheese pizza, now it is soy burgers with painted grill marks and liquid smoke, "chicken" chunks sculpted from vital wheat gluten, tofu dogs, and fluffy white bread pizza topped with sweet tomato sauce and soy mozzarella.

Instead of replacing the meat with healthier alternatives, vegans too often fill their plates with meat equivalents crafted from highly processed soy proteins bathed in vegetable oil. They put down butter and pick up a margarine spread. They swap ice cream for frozen soy treats packed with fat and sugar. When they do eat vegetables, it is typically as a side dish glistening with "healthy" olive oil, the way most Americans eat them. Ignorant of the damage to their health, they give themselves a congratulatory pat on the back for saving animals from suffering. However, they are leaving one very important animal off their list of concerns: themselves.

Calorie for calorie, fake foods are not much better nutritionally than the animal foods they replace. In some cases, they are worse. Even though they may contribute less fat and more carbohydrate, the isolated soy protein in these foods increases calcium loss as much as animal protein does, hastening the path toward osteoporosis and kidney

Nutritional Comparison of Animal Foods and Their Vegan Substitutes

FOOD	FAT	PROTEIN	CARBOHYDRATE
Hamburger	65	35	0
Soy burger	28	62	10
Cheese	70	28	2
Soy cheese	60	10	30
Butter	100	0	0
Nondairy spread	100	0	0
Ice cream	55	7	38
Soy ice cream	20	13	67
Duck	75	25	0
Mock duck	0	65	35

Figures represent percent of total calories.

stones.[1–3] It also increases growth factors that promote cancer and aging more readily than does cow's milk.[4–6] Olive oil and nondairy butter replacements are just as high in fat and have exactly the same effect: fat stored on your thighs, hips, and buttocks. Vegetable oils often contribute even more than do animal fats to promoting cancer.[7–10]

A FAT IS A FAT IS A FAT

We all know that vegetable oils, like olive oil, protect us from heart disease . . . right? That may not be the case. In fact, the heart-healthy benefits of the widely promoted Mediterranean diet—an elusive concept considering that a wide range of diets is eaten throughout that part of the world—have been shown to accrue from the starches those populations eat, such as pasta and beans, accompanied by fruits and vegetables.[11–13] But what gets the credit? The olive oil. In fact, the Mediterranean diet promotes health *in spite* of olive oil, not because of it.

Do Vegetable Oils Prevent Heart Disease?
Many Studies Show They Do Not.

- Serial angiograms of human heart arteries over a year of study showed that all three types of fat—saturated (animal fat), monounsaturated (olive oil), and polyunsaturated (omega-3 and omega-6 oils)—were associated with significant increases in new atherosclerotic lesions.[14] Decreasing total fat intake was the only way to stop the lesions from growing.

- Both omega-3 and omega-6 polyunsaturated oils are found in human atherosclerotic plaques; thus they are involved in damaging the arteries and increasing the progression of atherosclerosis.[15]

- One of the most important predictors of heart attack risk is an elevated level of factor VII, a substance that enables blood clotting. The formation of blood clots inside the arteries causes most heart attacks and strokes. Olive oil increases blood clotting activity by increasing clotting factor VII as much as animal fats do.[16,17]

- Vegetable oils also impair circulation,[18,19] resulting in a 20 percent reduction in blood oxygen.[20] Reduced circulation can lead to angina (chest pain), impaired brain function, high blood pressure, fatigue, and compromised lung function.

In short, it doesn't matter what type of fat you eat; saturated animal fat and polyunsaturated vegetable oils all have adverse effects on your heart and health.

Nuts and Seeds Are Too Rich for Every Day

Growing up in a lower-income family in the suburbs of Detroit, I had the luxury of eating nuts just once a year. At Christmastime, my father would splurge on a 5-pound bag of mixed nuts still in their shells. Over the next 7 days, breaking through the hard shells with a nutcracker and a steel pick, we six McDougalls would feast on almonds, Brazil nuts, cashews, hazelnuts, pecans, and walnuts.

Nowadays, eating nuts is as easy as unscrewing a lid and pouring out handfuls of shelled, oil-roasted nuts. Eight chews and a swallow later—taking all of about 5 seconds—we've gulped down 170 calories of nearly solid fat with every ounce. Three hours later, our body has stored away that fat to help us through the next famine. The famine never arrives, but we keep storing up the fat, quite visibly, just in case. Our bodies were built to store fat to ensure our survival.

Trees produce nuts as a means of storing energy. Seeds, legumes, and grains serve the same botanical function. All of these storage organs can sprout into a seedling, which in turn can grow a new plant. One of the main differences among seeds, legumes, grains, and nuts is the amount of energy they store, either as fat or carbohydrate. Nuts and seeds store energy mostly as fat—approximately 80 percent of their calories are from fat, and 10 percent from carbohydrates. Grains and legumes (beans, peas, and lentils) store their fuel as carbohydrate—only about 5 to 10 percent of their calories come from fat, with carbohydrates supplying about 65 to 80 percent. In both cases, the remaining calories come from protein. Peanuts are the exception among legumes; like tree nuts, they are very high in fat (60 percent of calories), which is why we generally think of them as a nut. Soybeans are also high in fat (40 percent of calories).

All of these edible storage bins are also rich in proteins, vitamins, minerals, and thousands of other nutrients essential for the seedling's growth. The high nutrient density of these packages—especially their fat—has a major impact on human health. Overindulging in fat-filled nuts and seeds brings about oily skin and excess weight gain, at least.

(continued on page 140)

Star McDougaller:

Elizabeth TeSelle,
Office Worker and Former Overweight Vegan,
Nashville, Tennessee

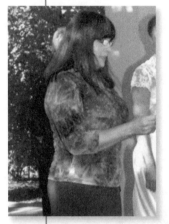

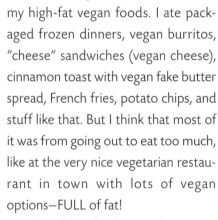

I admit it. I was a failed McDougaller before becoming a successful one.

My first time following the McDougall Diet, I lost the 70 pounds I had gained in my thirties. Afterward, I gradually slipped off the McDougall wagon, gaining back every pound I had lost plus a few more. It was not eating the Standard American Diet that put the pounds back on. I have been vegetarian since 1986 and vegan since 1992. Yet I still gained back the weight when I returned to my high-fat vegan foods. I ate packaged frozen dinners, vegan burritos, "cheese" sandwiches (vegan cheese), cinnamon toast with vegan fake butter spread, French fries, potato chips, and stuff like that. But I think that most of it was from going out to eat too much, like at the very nice vegetarian restaurant in town with lots of vegan options—FULL of fat!

I hit a low of 128 pounds in 1999 and, 10 years later, a high of 207. In June 2010, I fully recommitted myself to the McDougall Diet. This time I have lost almost 90 pounds, reaching a new low of 120. At my height of 5 foot 6 inches, this gives me a very healthy BMI of 19.4. Whereas I once wore a size 16, I now shop for size 4. My cholesterol has dropped from 181 to 123 milligrams per deciliter (mg/dL), and my blood pressure is down from 160/100 to 122/70 millimeters of mercury (mmHg). My fasting blood glucose has gone from 113 to 79 mg/dL. I am on no medication of any kind. At age 49, I am fit and healthy, and I look and feel great. Best of all, I'm riding my horses again!

I love what I am eating: green and yellow veggies, fruits, grains, legumes, potatoes, and other starchy veggies, and as little processed food as possible. As an all-or-nothing type, picking out the foods that are best and giving up the others has not been difficult. The biggest motivation, though, is that I feel my best when I stick with whole foods. I keep my kitchen stocked with basic ingredients: canned no-salt beans and tomatoes, plenty of frozen veggies and fruits, and lots of potatoes and brown rice, adding in fresh veggies and fruits that catch my eye at the market.

The most amazing part is that I can eat until my appetite is completely satisfied without worrying about wavering from my weight goal. That can mean second, third, or even fourth helpings at times. On the McDougall Diet, I never feel deprived.

When I made this commitment, weighing 207 pounds, I was certain that following the McDougall Diet would mean suffering. I have to smile when I think about that. I most certainly am not suffering; on the contrary, I enjoy my food a great deal and am immensely grateful to have been given a second chance at a healthy weight and an active life. The payoff doubles when I remember how I dodged the serious health problems that were lurking just around the corner. I can honestly promise that this time there will be no going back. Ever.

For many people, the resulting complications of obesity are type 2 diabetes and degenerative arthritis of the hips, knees, and ankles.

A casual review of the popular press and some of the scientific literature might convince you that nuts do not, in fact, cause weight gain. But how could eating so many concentrated fat calories be a part of any legitimate weight-loss plan? At 170 calories, a small handful—a single ounce—of nuts every day would add up to approximately 5,000 calories, or more than a pound and a half of body fat, over the course of a month. One trick lies in limiting the nuts you eat to about an ounce a day.[21]

Many explanations have been put forth for the perplexing phenomenon that an ounce of nuts a day *does* not appear to cause much weight gain.[21] One is that nuts are so satisfying they cause people to eat less of other foods; they replace cakes, pies, and other more fattening options. Or is it that their monounsaturated and polyunsaturated fatty acids are more easily burned? Or that they are not well digested, and the excess is eliminated?

Even if an ounce of nuts a day does not cause appreciable weight gain, the evidence shows that upping the quantities to more than an ounce daily, without restricting other sources of calories, will indeed increase your weight.[21] So I ask you, faced with a 24-ounce jar of roasted, salted, mixed nuts, how likely are you to stop at one small handful? You think: How could just one more cashew hurt me?

Soy Foods Can Be Fake Foods

As I was developing my first live-in program at St. Helena Hospital in the mid 1980s, I found myself looking for a good vegetarian meal around dinnertime. This particular corner of Northern California's wine country happens to be home to a large community of Seventh Day Adventists, known for eschewing tobacco, alcohol, illicit drugs, and often meat as well. I expected they would be a great source of vegetarian dining advice. So when my new friends suggested the

A&W west of town, I headed down for a veggie burger. My first bite told me they'd made a serious mistake. I leaned over the counter, beckoned to the cook, and complained he'd served me a real beef burger. He thanked me for the compliment, beaming with pride that their veggie burger had fooled me with the look, taste, and texture of the real thing. I walked out in disgust, leaving my dinner unfinished, scratching my head at how a burger made from soy could taste just as bad as the beef burgers I long ago left behind. For at least three decades, the sights and smells of the meat aisle at my local supermarket have nauseated me. I have no desire to replace those foods with fake meats made from soy that imitate the same unpleasant effects.

Nutritionists and health experts deliver conflicting news about soy foods. Those who recommend them point to the good health of populations that have included soy in their diets for more than 5,000 years, the Chinese and Japanese chief among them. Based on this observation alone, scientific research over the past three decades has tried to prove that soybeans can help reduce the risk of cancer and heart disease, lower blood pressure and cholesterol, relieve hot flashes, and build stronger bones.

But not all soy foods are the same. Populations following any traditional Asian diet are likely to include soy in the form of fresh soybeans boiled in their pods (edamame), soy milk, soybean sprouts, soy sauce, soy flour, tempeh, tofu; tofu by-products yuba and okara; and fermented soy pastes natto and miso. These foods are eaten fresh or are made using simple processes, like cooking, sprouting, grinding, and fermenting. A traditional family in Japan or China gets fewer than 5 percent of their daily calories from soy. That comes to about 2 ounces of soy foods daily, providing 7 to 8 grams of soy protein.

This small amount of soy food has little health impact, good or bad. The main reason those following a traditional Asian diet are healthy is that starch is at the center of every meal, supplemented generously with vegetables and fruits. Depending on regional differences and personal taste, that starch might be rice, sweet potatoes, or buckwheat.

Fake Soy Foods Cause Harm

While traditional soy foods provide no magic bullet, centering your diet around synthetic soy foods, or taking soy supplements, can cause real harm.[22] In fact, the manufactured soybean derivatives may actually *increase* your risk for cancer; impair thyroid, immune, and brain function; and cause bone damage and reproductive problems.[23-33]

Manufacturing begins with an extract known as isolated soy protein, also noted on ingredient lists as defatted soy flour, organic textured soy flour, textured vegetable protein, soy protein concentrates, or soy concentrates. These isolated, concentrated soy proteins are mixed with extracts of wheat protein, vegetable oils, and sometimes starch, sugar, salt, artificial sweeteners, and even dairy and egg proteins to create concoctions meant to satisfy the health seeker's meat and dairy cravings. The concentrated chemical cocktail often undergoes additional processing, using compression and heat, to form products that look and taste as much as possible like the foods they seek to replace: cheese, chicken, turkey, lunch meats, sausages, hot dogs, and hamburgers. Soy protein is often found in energy bars, candy bars, yogurt, ice cream, breads, pastries, and cookies.

Fake soy foods lack the vital elements found naturally in the bean's original design: fiber, carbohydrate, fat, vitamins, minerals, and hundreds of beneficial plant chemicals. Once these components are stripped away, the results on your health can be as far reaching as constipation from lack of fiber to a reduction in endurance due to carbohydrate deficiency.

More concerning than what is missing is the fact that the concentrated, isolated proteins burden the liver and kidneys, which play a key role in excreting surplus protein from the body. In time, protein overload wears out these organs, potentially contributing to outright liver or kidney failure, especially for people who already suffer from organ damage. Excess protein leaves in its wake an overly acidic environment that leaches calcium and other materials from the bones, over time leading to osteoporosis and kidney stones.[34,35] Adding just 40 grams of concentrated soy protein to experimental subjects' diets has been found to plunge the body into a negative calcium balance where more of the mineral is excreted through the urine and lost in the bowels than is absorbed by the intestines.[1] Many soy products also contain isolated wheat protein, which compounds the calcium loss.[35] (See Chapter 3 for a detailed discussion of the effects of excess protein on the body.)

Cancer is a real concern when it comes to isolated soy protein, which promotes tumor growth by increasing growth hormone levels. Resembling insulin in its chemical structure, the hormone insulin-like growth factor 1 (IGF1) accelerates the growth rate of normal tissue, like bone, as well as that of diseased tissues, like cancer.[36] Adding 40 grams of isolated soy protein to the human diet increases IGF1 almost twice as much as adding concentrated proteins isolated from cow's milk.[4] Cow's milk protein is itself notorious for stimulating an increase in growth hormones; consider that milk is responsible for growing a 60-pound calf into a 600-pound cow by the time it is weaned. Increased amounts of IGF1 have been strongly linked to the development and progression of cancers of the breast, prostate, lung, and colon.[36]

IGF1 also accelerates aging.[37–39] Big dogs, for example, such as Doberman pinschers and Rottweilers, live an average of 10 years, while Chihuahuas and small terriers have an average life of 13 years. The smaller dogs have lower levels of IGF1.[40] Humans exhibit the same inverse relationship between size and longevity: Taller and heavier people have shorter life spans than do shorter, thinner ones.[41] Researchers believe our best hope for increasing longevity is by taking actions that lower IGF1 activity.[39] Removing meat, poultry, fish, shellfish, eggs, and dairy are well recognized dietary changes that lower IGF1 levels. Isolated soy proteins should be added to the top of that list.

It doesn't take much to inadvertently add 40 grams of isolated soy protein a day to your diet—the amount used in the experiments to cause calcium loss and to raise growth hormones. Snacking on a couple

Soy Protein Isolates in Some Common Foods

ITEM	SERVING SIZE	SOY PROTEIN (g)
Clif Builder's Bar	1 bar	20
Revival Soy Shakes with Splenda	1 shake	20
Boca Burger Original	1 burger	13
MorningStar Farms Original Sausage Patties	1 patty	10
Smart Dogs	1 dog	9
Veggie Shreds cheese	2 oz	6

of soy energy bars will do it, or washing down a soy bar with a soy shake. So will eating one soy chicken patty for lunch and two soy burgers for dinner, or starting the day with four soy breakfast patties.

CONCERNS OVER SOY LEAD TO CHANGING RECOMMENDATIONS

Governments and health organizations worldwide have raised concerns about the effects of isolated soy proteins found in foods and infant formulas. After a year of study, a committee of experts from the Israeli Ministry of Health warned that babies should not be fed soy formula, and that children should eat no more than 1 ounce of soy per day, no more than three times per week. They suggested that adults should exercise caution because of adverse effects on fertility and increased breast cancer risk.[42] The French Agency for Food, Environmental and Occupational Health and Safety was the first government agency to require removal of isoflavones from infant formula, and to require warning labels on packages of soy foods and soy milk.[43,44] Child advocacy groups in New Zealand and Canada have taken this concern for soy's effects on the young a step further and are lobbying to have soy formulas removed from the general markets and made available only with a doctor's prescription.[45]

For Vegans, a Starch-Based Diet Furthers Their Causes

Vegans already have made a radical change based on their commitment to bettering the world. Yet, like the vast majority of Americans (and many others around the world) who follow a Western diet, most vegans continue to get the bulk of their calories from fat and protein. Going one step further, to base their diets on starch, would be far from a sacrifice. Instead, it would mean greater satisfaction and better health, while deepening their commitment to their own lives and that of our planet.

Even my Coke-and-potato chips intern back in Honolulu had alternatives during his 100-hours-a-week stint in the hospital. The dining room served oatmeal and cold grain cereals with fruit juice for breakfast. For lunch and dinner, he could have chosen salads with vinegar or salsa, rice, potatoes, sweet potatoes, corn, beans, low-fat vegetable soups, vegetables, and fruit. With just a little knowledge and minimal effort, he could have been a more effective doctor and a far more influential crusader with his peers and patients for a cause dear to his heart: saving animals' lives.

I admire vegans' character, self-sacrifice, and commitment to making a difference. Rather than harm the beautiful creatures with whom they share this earth, vegans are willing to risk not only accusations from family, friends, and physicians that they may become deficient in protein and calcium, but also social isolation. Vegans are industrious: They must shop and read menus carefully, sometimes turning down dinner invitations and social opportunities, as well as passing up tempting food in situations where they are hungry and the options are limited. It all requires a great deal more effort than the average person is willing to muster.

Vegans are duly rewarded for their deep sacrifice when they discover that, in fact, plants provide all of the protein, amino acids, essential fats, vitamins, and minerals they need, and that eliminating meat and dairy from their diet provides a great many health benefits. Turning away from the fatty, empty calories in harmful, processed soy foods and vegetable oils allows vegans to truly shine, inspiring a change in their public perception from being marginalized to being admired for being healthy, trim, active, strong, energetic, and committed to changing the world. Isn't it fortunate that the same choices that best serve the planet and its inhabitants also benefit our personal health?

Chapter 11

Just to Be on the Safe Side: Stay Away from Supplements

Nobody loves me more than my mother does. Still, there were times as a child when I wasn't convinced. The chemical aftertaste, the belching, and the nausea caused by the One A Day multivitamin capsule she forced on me with my orange juice every morning made me suspicious. She reassured me they were meant to taste bad so a little child like me wouldn't mistake them for candy. It turns out my hunch about vitamins was right.

What I have never understood is why we take these nasty-tasting pills when there is no apparent reason to do so. Medical achievements had long before cured the deadly diseases associated with vitamin deficiencies, such as scurvy, beriberi, and pellagra, with supplements. But that didn't stop the pharmaceutical industry from turning necessity into mythology. It has convinced many of us that if vitamins could cure these deadly illnesses, then supplementing our diets with vitamins and minerals must also be the answer to cancer, heart disease, and a host of other diseases. But is it?

With the hope of improving on Mother Nature, fueled by the desire for profit, scientists and entrepreneurs have developed thousands of products based on isolated, concentrated nutrients. To do this, they identify a pharmacologically active ingredient in a common food, then use science and manufacturing technology to purify it, replicate it in large quantities, and sell it to eager consumers as a "potent, natural remedy." Familiar examples include soy and whey protein isolates, omega-3 fish and flaxseed oils, and all manner of vitamins and minerals. They may be taken in the form of pills, powders, liquids, nutrition bars, "health" drinks, or fortified foods.

These concentrated nutrients are said to offset the effects of our destructive habits and to cure our ill health almost effortlessly, naturally, and with little or no side effects. Enormous profits motivate companies to keep these supplements on the market, whether or not they are effective. The consumer's desire for a quick fix to health problems guarantees steady sales. However, doctors, dietitians, nutritionists, and health food store clerks who prescribe supplements are practicing "faith-based medicine." They've got to believe, because they have no good evidence supporting their actions, no valid research to guide them, and no patient results to reward them.

Supplements can fix deficiencies, not excesses. How many friends and relatives do you know who have suffered from illnesses caused by a vitamin deficiency, such as scurvy from vitamin C deficiency, beriberi from insufficient vitamin B_1, or pellagra from a lack of niacin? How about protein or essential fatty acid deficiencies? Most likely *none*. Now, turn your vision 180 degrees. How many people do you know who suffer from diseases caused by nutritional *excess?* How many have health problems from consuming too much fat, cholesterol, sodium, protein, or just plain too many calories? I'm not going far out on a limb to guess you know more people who are overweight or who are suffering from heart disease, clogged arteries, high blood pressure, arthritis, and diabetes than those suffering from scurvy, beriberi, or pellagra.

Now, have any of those friends suffering from these excesses significantly reduced their weight by taking supplements? Have any cured

E-MAIL TO DR. McDOUGALL

A year ago I began your 10-day program. That
means I have not intentionally eaten meat, fish,
dairy, or added fat for a whole year now. I have
lost 55 pounds, and am off my blood pressure
pills as well as a host of supplements. I have
generally regained my health. I just got my
blood work back, the first since the end of the
10-day program. The prediabetic stuff was great—
normal insulin and blood glucose. I was a little
disappointed in my lipids. My cholesterol was
185, and even though that is perfectly normal,
my goal was 150. Considering that it started out
at 220, I know I am not doing bad. Still, I was
a bit surprised as I have not ingested a par-
ticle of cholesterol for a year. I guess it
doesn't really matter, though, since those are
just numbers and the proof is in the way I feel,
which is great.

Anne Sampson, MD

their arthritis, hypertension, colitis, or type 2 diabetes with vitamins
and minerals? I'm quite sure they have not.

I never hear about miraculous results from supplements, but what I
do hear every day, whether by telephone, e-mail, or in person, are
reports from those who have achieved amazing health improvements
by adopting a starch-based diet, along with a little exercise and some
sunshine.

What Are Vitamins and Minerals?

Vitamins are organic compounds that cannot be synthesized by the body. In order to remain healthy, we must take in these vitamins by eating food. Of the 13 known vitamins, there are only two that plants don't make: D and B_{12}. Vitamin D is not actually a vitamin at all, but rather a hormone that the body produces when we expose our skin to sunlight. Vitamin B_{12} is more complicated. Neither plants nor animals synthesize it; rather, it is produced by bacteria. B_{12} is then stored in animal tissue, so one way we can get it is by eating meat.

In addition to vitamins, we get all of our minerals by eating plants. These minerals are in the soil, and the plants draw them up into their stems, leaves, flowers, and fruits through their root systems. By eating plants and spending a little time in the sun, we get all the vitamins and minerals we need with the exception of vitamin B_{12}. If you eat no animal products at all, or foods that have been sufficiently fortified with B_{12}, then that's the one vitamin supplement you should seriously consider taking.

Please note: The word "supplement" encompasses many different kinds of products. The discussion in this chapter is focused on isolated, concentrated vitamins and minerals, rather than natural remedies such as St. John's wort, ginkgo biloba, glucosamine, ginger, and the like.

THE PERFECT HARMONY OF PLANTS

If I put a fruit plate in front of you, you could easily pick out the banana, the orange, the apple, and the cluster of grapes. Every fruit and vegetable comes with a precise molecular architecture that makes it easy to identify. This architecture gives fruits and vegetables more than their characteristic appearance; it also specifies the constellation of tens of thousands of proteins, fats, carbohydrates, fibers, vitamins, minerals, and other phytochemicals (plant chemicals) in each food. If one component of a fruit is especially healthy for us—say, the lycopene in a tomato—it is safe and beneficial because it comes packaged in nature with a bunch of other compounds that support its ability to promote health.

We take in nutrition from whole foods by breaking them apart with our teeth (and through preparing and cooking), then swallowing and digesting them. As we digest our food, its nutrients flow through our bloodstream to our 10 trillion cells. Components of this nutrient-rich blood pass through the cell membranes into the cell's inner fluid, or cytoplasm. If too few or too many of any of the nutrients of the digested and assimilated food are present within the cell, then imbalances occur. Scientists barely understand the orchestrations that take place between our foods and our bodies, but they do recognize that perfect harmony exists. If you add a little too much of this and not enough of that by manipulating the individual nutrients by taking vitamin pills, the cells' metabolisms become very unbalanced. Eventually, these imbalances can lead to heart disease, cancers, and early death.

Two highly respected Cochrane Reviews concluded that "beta-carotene, vitamin A, and vitamin E given singly or combined with other antioxidant supplements significantly increase mortality (death)."[1,2] There is no higher authority than a report from the Cochrane Collaboration. The harm from supplementing with isolated, concentrated nutrients like beta-carotene is in stark contrast to the benefit from eating beta-carotene-rich fruits and vegetables.

A Pill Is Not a Plant

It was well established three decades ago that people who consume more beta-carotene in their diets are less likely to develop many kinds of cancer, including lung cancer.[3,4] Following this observation, a

(continued on page 156)

Randomized, Controlled Trials Prove Supplements Are Useless or Dangerous

SUPPLEMENTS DO NOT REDUCE AND MAY INCREASE CANCER RISK

- *Alpha-Tocopherol, Beta-Carotene Cancer Prevention Study group:* 29,133 male smokers were assigned to one of four regimens: alpha-tocopherol (vitamin E) alone, beta-carotene alone, both alpha-tocopherol and beta-carotene, or a placebo.[5] *Findings:* There were both an 18 percent greater incidence of lung cancer and 8 percent more deaths in those from the two groups that took the beta-carotene.

- *Beta-Carotene and Retinol Efficacy Trial:* 18,314 smokers, former smokers, and workers who had been exposed to asbestos were assigned to take either beta-carotene and retinol (vitamin A) or a placebo.[6] *Findings:* There were increases of 17 percent for death, 46 percent for lung cancer, and 26 percent for cardiovascular disease in those who took the beta-carotene and retinol supplements.

- *Selenium and Vitamin E Cancer Prevention Trial (SELECT):* 35,533 men were assigned to one of four groups: selenium, vitamin E, selenium plus vitamin E, or a placebo.[11,12] *Findings:* There were both a 13 percent greater incidence of prostate cancer in the two groups taking vitamin E and no reduction in prostate cancer from any of the supplements.

SUPPLEMENTS DO NOT REDUCE AND MAY INCREASE HEART DISEASE

- *MRC/BHF Heart Protection Study:* 20,536 adults with coronary disease, other occlusive arterial disease, or diabetes were assigned to receive daily antioxidant vitamin supplementation from a combination of vitamin E, vitamin C, and beta-carotene or receive a placebo.[13] *Findings:* Those who took the vitamin supplements did have higher levels of the vitamins in their blood, but they did not reduce the incidence of vascular disease, cancer, or death.

- *Alpha-Tocopherol, Beta-Carotene Cancer Prevention Study:* 1,862 male smokers who had had previous heart attacks were assigned to groups that were given dietary supplements of beta-carotene, alpha-tocopherol, both, or a placebo.[14] *Findings:* There were 75 percent more deaths from coronary artery disease in the groups taking beta-carotene and a slight increase in deaths in the group taking only alpha-tocopherol compared with those taking the placebo.

- *Iowa Women's Health Study:* self-reported supplement use of 38,772 older women was reported between 1986 and 2008.[15] *Findings:* The use of multivitamins, magnesium, zinc, and copper was associated with increased risk of total mortality when compared with corresponding nonuse.

- *HOPE-TOO Trial:* 9,541 patients were assigned to receive either vitamin E or a placebo.[16] *Findings:* No difference was found between the two groups, either in cancer or cardiovascular deaths. Patients in the vitamin E group did, however, have a higher risk of heart failure.

- *Folate After Coronary Intervention Trial:* 636 patients with stents (a metal tube inserted into an artery to prop it open) in their heart arteries were assigned to receive either a combination of folic acid,

(continued)

Randomized, Controlled Trials Prove Supplements Are Useless or Dangerous (*cont.*)

vitamin B_6, and vitamin B_{12} or a placebo.[17] *Findings:* Those taking the combination experienced a greater degree of restenosis (closure of the artery) and more repeat heart surgeries.

- *NORVIT Trial:* 3,749 men and women who had experienced a heart attack in the past 7 days were assigned to one of four groups, receiving either folic acid, vitamin B_{12}, and vitamin B_6; folic acid and vitamin B_{12}; vitamin B_6 only; or a placebo.[18] *Findings:* In the two groups that took folic acid, the risk of heart attack, stroke, and cancer increased 20 to 30 percent, even though they showed a 27 percent decrease in homocysteine, an amino acid associated with blocked arteries, which should have predicted a lower rate of these diseases.

- *Women's Antioxidant and Folic Acid Cardiovascular Study:* 5,442 women who had either a history of cardiovascular disease or three or more coronary risk factors were assigned to receive either a combination of folic acid, vitamin B_6, and vitamin B_{12} or a placebo.[19] *Findings:* The risks of heart attack, stroke, heart surgery, and death were not reduced by taking the combination, although the disease indicator homocysteine decreased 19 percent.

- *Antioxidants for Atherosclerosis Study:* 819 older adults with elevated concentrations of plasma total homocysteine were assigned daily supplementation of 800 micrograms of folic acid for three years.[20] *Findings:* Supplementation raised folate and lowered homocysteine concentrations in the blood but did not slow the progression of atherosclerosis or reduce arterial stiffening.

- *SEARCH Trial:* 12,064 survivors of heart attacks were assigned to take either 2 milligrams of folic acid and 1 milligram of B_{12} or a placebo for an average of 6.7 years.[21] *Findings:* Even though homocysteine levels were reduced 28 percent in the supplement group, there was no beneficial effect of reducing the incidence of heart attack, stroke, or heart surgery.

SUPPLEMENTS INCREASE KIDNEY DAMAGE IN DIABETICS

- *Diabetic Intervention with Vitamins to Improve Nephropathy Trial:* 238 participants with clinical diagnosis of kidney disease and either type 1 or type 2 diabetes were assigned to one of two groups. One group received a combination of folic acid, vitamin B_6, and vitamin B_{12} and the other received a placebo.[22] *Findings:* The group taking the supplement had worse kidney function and twice as many vascular events as those taking the placebo.

SUPPLEMENTS CONTRIBUTE TO FRACTURES IN THE ELDERLY

- *Annual High-Dose Oral Vitamin D and Falls and Fractures in Older Women Trial:* 2,256 noninstitutionalized women age 70 years or older were assigned to receive either 500,000 IU of vitamin D or a placebo.[23] *Findings:* Those who took the vitamin D had more falls and fractures than those who did not.

SUPPLEMENTS MAKE RESPIRATORY INFECTIONS MORE SEVERE

- *Randomized Trial on Vitamin E and Infections:* 652 noninstitutionalized elderly subjects were assigned to one of these four groups: multivitamins-minerals, 200 milligrams of vitamin E, both, or placebo.[24] *Findings:* Taking vitamin E didn't alter the frequency of respiratory infections, but it did increase their severity.

hypothesis was developed that a single, plant-derived nutrient, beta-carotene, was the key to cancer prevention. Two well-designed trials published in 1994 and 1996 compared the effects of beta-carotene supplements to a placebo for people at high risk for developing lung cancer (smokers and those exposed to asbestos).[5,6]

Unexpectedly, during these two investigations more cancers were found in people taking the beta-carotene pills than those taking the placebo. However, these findings did not invalidate the original observation: People who eat more fruits and vegetables have a lower risk of cancer. Beta-carotene is found only in plants; thus it serves as a marker for the quantity of fruits and vegetables a person consumes. A diet high in plant foods protects against cancer. The same effect does not carry

The "Depleted Soils" Sales Pitch

The sales pitch goes like this: "You must take supplements because of the poor condition of soil these days. The crops you eat were grown in soil that has been drained of its nutrients from years of overfarming. Now the foods that grow in them are also deficient in vitamins and minerals. My brand of supplements will correct this problem for you by providing these missing nutrients."

This simply is not true. Plants synthesize vitamins; they are not in the soil. If a plant is going to bear roots, seeds, flowers, and/or fruits fit for sale in your market, then it is going to have to produce all of the organic chemicals that are necessary for its own survival. We call the plant-derived organic chemicals vital for human nutrition vitamins.

Mineral deficiency from depleted soil is theoretically possible, but highly unlikely to affect anyone living in a modern society. The classic example of a mineral deficiency is iodine deficiency, which caused the "goiter belts" of the Great Lakes region nearly a century ago and still causes goiters in underdeveloped parts of the world, such as Africa.

over to consuming a single nutrient, like beta-carotene. A pill is not a plant.[7–10]

Beta-carotene is one of about 50 similar naturally occurring active substances in our diet, classified as *carotenoids*, that are especially abundant in colorful fruits and vegetables. After nutrients move into the cytoplasm, they attach themselves to the cellular machinery through a specific receptor, the way a key fits into a lock. Beta-carotene, like all of the other biologically active carotenoids, must attach to these specific carotenoid receptors before it can function.

When a cell is flooded with one type of carotenoid, in this case beta-carotene from vitamin supplementation, there is overwhelming competition for the carotenoid receptor sites.[7] The other 49 functional

There are also some rare cases of selenium deficiency and possibly zinc deficiency in underdeveloped countries. These deficiencies occur because of the geographically restricted supply of foods available to these people. Their foods are grown locally, generally within about 25 miles of their village. The soil in their neighborhood may be deficient in one of these minerals, resulting in health problems among those who eat only those local foods.

Your risk of suffering from mineral deficiency caused by depleted soil is so incredibly small that a single case would make national headlines. That's because you eat foods grown in a wide variety of soil: corn grown in Nebraska, grapes from Chile, bananas from Panama, and so forth. In the unlikely chance that one food was low in a mineral due to depleted soil, your next bite would likely contain an abundant supply. People take supplements to protect against unfounded fears of developing deficiencies, and false hopes of preventing and curing illnesses that those deficiencies have never been known to cause (for example, heart disease and cancer).

carotenoids are displaced by the beta-carotene from their cellular connections, creating deadly nutritional imbalances.

People continue to put their faith in the latest supplement and its new, enticing marketing claim, regardless of what the preponderance of scientific evidence shows. The most careful studies on isolated, concentrated nutrients have focused on the effects of beta-carotene, vitamin E, and folic acid. Randomized, controlled trials involving more than 150,000 subjects have proven that taking these and other supplements actually increases your risk for heart disease, cancers, and premature death. Studies of supplement use have also reported more fractures in women at risk for osteoporosis, damage to the kidneys in diabetics, and an increase in the severity of respiratory infections.

Vitamin D: The Sunshine Vitamin

Vitamin D is unusual in two ways. First, it is actually a hormone and not a vitamin, even though we call it a vitamin. And second, we get it not from eating food, but rather through exposure to sunlight. Not everyone lives in sunny Florida or California, so depending on where you live, you might need to work a little harder to get enough sun to manufacture needed levels of this essential hormone.

If you take a calcium pill, or consume dairy foods, there's a good chance some vitamin D has been added. Cow's milk typically has both vitamins A and D added, and calcium pills often come combined with vitamin D, which is believed to help with the mineral's absorption into our system. The problem is that drinking milk and taking calcium pills are both harmful practices, as we learned in Chapter 8. I don't recommend doing either. So how will you get enough vitamin D?

The answer is easy: Go outside. Sunshine is the best way to get your vitamin D, which safely and effectively prevents weak bones. Sadly, instead of that easy and no-cost solution, your doctor is more likely to suggest a vitamin D supplement. The problem is that, while a pill will indeed increase the level of vitamin D in your blood, making it look as if you are benefiting from the vitamin, studies show that getting your D through pills or milk is not very effective at strengthening your bones. The benefits for bone fracture prevention are small and largely restricted to institutionalized elderly women, and to subjects who take a combination of vitamin D and calcium, not vitamin D alone.[25,26]

As your skin soaks up ultraviolet sunlight, it produces vitamin D with the help of the liver and kidneys. The average person living in the United States produces about 90 percent of his or her vitamin D from sunlight and gets only about 10 percent from food or supplements.[27–29]

Changes in vitamin D levels in the body are affected mostly by sun exposure rather than by diet.[30,31] Your body stores in your body fat the extra vitamin D you produce during the sunniest months of the year, then slowly releases it during the darker months.

For white people, exposing a large part of the skin to the summer sun for 20 to 30 minutes at one time provides about 10,000 international units (IU) of vitamin D.[32] The Scientific Advisory Committee on Nutrition and the National Institutes of Health recommend 200 IU daily, so you can see that 10,000 units is far more than enough. In spring, summer, and fall, exposing the hands, face, and arms to the noontime sun for 5 minutes two to three times a week is plenty for light-skinned people.[33] Because their skin is darker and does not absorb the sun as well, people of Asian or Indian descent may require three times as much sun under similar conditions, and those of African descent 10 times as much, compared with light-skinned people of European descent, in order to produce enough vitamin D.[34]

Ultraviolet radiation from the sun provides benefits beyond the production of vitamin D.[34] Sunlight directly alters the immune system, modulates other hormones, and changes the number and function of skin cells.[35,36] Sunlight also establishes circadian rhythms and resets your biological clock after jet lag. Increased sun exposure improves survival rates for those with cancers of the breast, colon, prostate, and lung, as well as melanoma and lymphoma.[37–40]

Exposure to sunlight for extended periods of time does not cause vitamin D toxicity, but overexposure to the sun or a tanning bed can cause skin damage.

The most dramatic consequence of sunlight deficiency is the bone-deforming childhood disease rickets, which can be corrected by increased sunshine and supplements. A similar softening of the bones in adulthood is called osteomalacia. In most cases, sunlight deficiency causes no symptoms, but it can contribute to diffuse muscle and bone pain and weakness, which may be misdiagnosed as fibromyalgia.[41]

CONFOUNDING FACTORS INFLATE THE BENEFITS OF VITAMIN D

Recently, lack of vitamin D has been associated with many other illnesses, such as heart disease, strokes, type 2 diabetes, common cancers (breast, prostate, and colon), and multiple sclerosis. People living farthest from the equator, whether north or south of it, are at greater risk for these common diseases, which is blamed on the lesser amount of sunshine they receive over the course of the year. But this assumption overlooks a crucial fact: As people move farther away from the equator, they eat fewer plant foods and more animal foods. Sunshine plays a big part in overall health, but a small part in the prevention of common Western diseases. Vitamin D supplements will not cure these diseases.

VITAMIN D: NORMAL VALUES ARE EXAGGERATED

Examining a patient's blood for vitamin D levels has become common practice, with many millions of tests performed annually in the United States. Based on the current standards of normal—30 or more nanograms per milliliter—between 50 and 90 percent of adults and children are considered deficient in vitamin D.[42-46]

Even people who get quite a lot of sun exposure cannot meet this standard. My wife, Mary, recently had her vitamin D level tested shortly after a spring and summer of abundant California sunshine and a July trip to Costa Rica, where she spent long hours sunbathing. Her vitamin D level was a hair short of the recommendation, at 29.6 nanograms per milliliter. Many well-meaning doctors would have told her to take a vitamin D supplement, perhaps for a lifetime.

Mary is not an unusual example. Similar results were found during a study of active young people living in Hawaii with average sun exposure of 29 hours per week. Even with all that vitamin D–promoting sunshine, 51 percent of the group failed to meet the minimum recommended level.[47] Another study of 495 women in Hawaii with an average age of 74 found 44 percent of subjects to have vitamin D values below this normal standard.[48]

Recent scientific literature suggests that the level for normal of 30 nanograms per milliliter is exaggerated and should be lowered.[46,49,50] I believe a level of 20 or more is adequate; most children and adults already meet this target. If your test comes back with a level below 20, I suggest the first thing you do is take a second test to rule out laboratory error. If it is still under 20, try spending more time in the sun and test again before considering something so drastic, and potentially dangerous, as taking vitamin D supplements.

Current Standards for Blood Vitamin D (ng/ml)

Definitely deficient: 10 or less

Deficient: 19 or less

Insufficient: 20 to 29 (although recent research says this level is sufficient)

Sufficient: 30 to 80

Excess: 81 to 199

Toxic: above 200

Note: To convert nanograms per milliliter (ng/ml) to nanomoles per milliliter (nmol/ml), multiply the nanogram figure by 2.496.

Why are so many doctors promoting vitamin D testing these days? Because with the inflated standards, your levels are inevitably found to be too low, and the business of medicine benefits by increasing your need for more medical visits and blood tests, while the pharmaceutical industry benefits by selling you supplements you don't need. I call this practice, where healthy people are turned into patients through unnecessary medical testing, *disease mongering*. Sadly, it is rampant.

Tanning Beds Are the Second Best Way to Boost Vitamin D

Indoor tanning devices for home or commercial use emit the same spectrum of ultraviolet radiation as sunlight. In areas of the world where sunlight hours are limited or when getting outdoors is impossible or impractical, artificial ultraviolet light is the preferred way to correct vitamin D deficiency.

Tanning beds have a bad reputation because they can cause skin damage when used improperly. After all, they can provide higher doses of ultraviolet rays than the midday Mediterranean sun. Tanning beds' reputation for being damaging is influenced by the fact that users, typically women age 17 to 30, tend to smoke more cigarettes, drink more alcohol, and eat a less healthy diet than do nonusers.[51] Just like sunshine, improper use of tanning beds can indeed increase risk for skin cancers, skin damage, and premature aging. However, when used appropriately, like sunshine, they can safely prevent or reverse vitamin D deficiency.[52,53]

Supplements Are the Choice of Last Resort

While sunshine promotes good health, taking vitamin D supplements may actually increase your risk for certain diseases. Unless you are unwilling or unable to get out in the sun and don't have access to a tanning bed, I hope you will avoid supplements, because the benefits are meager and the costs and risks substantial.

When consumed as isolated, concentrated nutrients, vitamin D supplements cause nutritional imbalances that can lead to illness. At what are considered "safe" dosages, they have been shown to contribute to increased LDL (bad) cholesterol, prostate cancer, pancreatic cancer, immune system suppression, autoimmune diseases, gastrointestinal symptoms, kidney disease, and kidney stones.[54–61] Supplements may actually hurt the bones. A major research article in the May 2010 *Journal of the American Medical Association* showed that a large dose of vitamin D given to elderly women resulted in more falls and 26 percent more fractures than in women taking a placebo.[23] In my opinion, the adverse effects of vitamin D therapy are understudied, underestimated, and underreported.

For those who must take vitamin D supplements, such as elderly people who are unable to get outdoors or use a tanning bed, 200 IU per day should be adequate. This is compared with the commonly recommended levels of 2,000 to 4,000 IU per day of over-the-counter vitamin D to correct low vitamin D blood levels. Vitamin D_2 is as effective as vitamin D_3 in maintaining circulating concentrations of 25-hydroxyvitamin D.[62] Taking 10,000 IU or more per day can cause vitamin D toxicity.

VITAMIN B_{12} DEFICIENCY— THE MEAT EATERS' LAST STAND

Defending eating habits seems to be a primal instinct. These days, Westerners are running out of excuses for their gluttony. Well-read people no longer believe meat is necessary to meet our protein needs, or that milk is the favored source of calcium. With the crumbling of these two time-honored battlefronts, the vitamin B_{12} issue has become the trendy argument against being vegan. Since the usual dietary

(continued on page 166)

Deb Tasic, Retired Administrator, University of Illinois Performing Arts Center, Champaign, Illinois

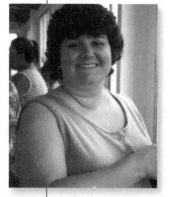

The attacks began when I was 41. Nausea and dizziness made the room spin so fast I couldn't lift my head from the pillow. Our family doctor diagnosed an inner ear infection by phone, but the medicine he prescribed didn't help. I remained incapacitated. Several days later, a friend drove my husband and me to the doctor. He referred me for an MRI and a visit with the neurologist, who delivered the decree as we sat in stunned silence: I had MS, multiple sclerosis.

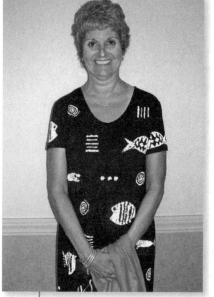

The doctor drew a big X in the upper left-hand corner of his white-board, and another X in the middle, with a downward line between them. He tapped the higher X: This is where you are now. He pointed to the middle X: This is you in 5 years, in a wheelchair. He placed a final X in the lower right corner: This is 10 years from now; you will be bedridden. He scheduled me for a spinal tap, and when I refused the risky and painful test he threatened to remove my name from consideration for clinical drug trials, our only hope for a possible future cure.

For the next 2 years I wallowed in self-pity as my condition worsened. I planned for my future care, made sure the house was fully accessible, and took out long-term disability insurance. I joined an MS support group, but it only depressed me more. I read everything I could find on the disease, but it was one short paragraph in a mountain of books that caught my eye: Dr. Roy Swank, doctor and neurology professor at the Oregon Health & Science University medical school, suggested a low-fat diet might help.

Seventy pounds overweight, I returned to Weight Watchers, where I'd once shed 50 pounds for a class reunion. I began walking with a friend; my first mile took 40 minutes. When I reached my goal weight 9 months later, I was walking 6 miles most days. I met Dr. John McDougall when he spoke at the North American Vegetarian Society Summerfest. I was semi-vegetarian at the time, eating just a little chicken and shrimp. He was committed to getting people out of the health care system and off medications and supplements, an appealing notion as I was spending over $100 a month on vitamins and supplements. I followed his suggestions.

I've lived beyond the decade that was expected to land me in a wheelchair, with some mild imbalance and slight memory loss to show for my MS. I take a low dose of thyroid medicine and no other drugs or supplements. I've dropped from 203 to 135 pounds and my cholesterol is down to 155 from 192 milligrams per deciliter (mg/dL). I look and feel great.

For the first 6 years of my disease, MRIs showed continued progression of MS activity and an increasing number of lesions. Things changed after I switched to a very low-fat diet. After that, my MRI report read, "Compared to two years earlier the multiple brain

(continued)

source of vitamin B_{12} for omnivores is meat, the obvious conclusion is
that those who choose to avoid eating it are destined to become
deficient in B_{12}. There is a grain of truth in this concern, but an otherwise healthy vegan's risk of developing *a disease* from B_{12} deficiency
is extremely rare—less than one chance in a million. Subclinical,
metabolic changes may be seen, but actual disease is exceedingly
uncommon.

The human body has evolved with highly efficient and unique
mechanisms to absorb, utilize, and conserve this vitamin. Our daily
requirement is less than 3 micrograms (a microgram is one-millionth
of a gram).[63] By design, we need be exposed to only minuscule amounts

of this essential nutrient. Typically, the liver stores 2 to 5 milligrams (or 2,000 to 5,000 micrograms) of B_{12}, at least a 3-year reserve. The body has many efficiency mechanisms, including reabsorbing the vitamin in the small intestine and recirculating it for future use. This means it could take you 20 to 30 years after adopting a vegan diet to become B_{12} deficient.[64] This assumes you take in no new vitamin B_{12}, which is all but impossible since, even on a vegan diet, you will take in some B_{12} through bacterial sources on your food, in your gut, and in the environment, even if you aren't trying.

There is evidence suggesting that during pregnancy and nursing, a mother is more dependent on B_{12} from her diet as her stored B_{12} is less available for the baby.[65] During these crucial times, a vegan woman should take a B_{12} supplement.

WHERE DOES B_{12} COME FROM?

Although vitamin B_{12} is found in animal foods, neither animals nor plants synthesize it. Bacteria make vitamin B_{12}. The intestines of animals, especially ruminants, such as cows, goats, and sheep, are populated with B_{12}-synthesizing bacteria. Animals store it in their tissues, and it gets passed up the food chain when one animal eats another. From the mouth to the anus, the human gut contains bacteria that synthesize vitamin B_{12}.[66] These bacteria are an important reason that disease from B_{12} deficiency occurs so rarely, even among lifelong, dedicated vegans. The colon contains the greatest number of bacteria and is where most of our intestinal B_{12} is produced. However, because B_{12} is absorbed in the ileum, upstream of the colon, this plentiful source of B_{12} is not immediately available for absorption.

Feces from cows, chickens, sheep, pigs, and people contain large amounts of active B_{12}. Until recently, most people lived in close contact with their farm animals, meaning that they consumed plenty of B_{12} left as bacterial residue, and also obtained B_{12} from their unsanitized vegetables.

The lack of vitamin B_{12} is the one blemish on an otherwise perfect diet that holds out hope for preventing or curing our most common chronic diseases. This blemish is not because a plant-based diet is somehow lacking, but rather because we have developed unnatural conditions by sanitizing our surroundings with fanatical washing, powerful cleansers, antiseptics, and antibiotics. The rare case of B_{12} deficiency may be one important consequence of too much cleanliness. Regardless, I recommend supplementation with vitamin B_{12}.

RISK OF VITAMIN B_{12} DEFICIENCY VERSUS RISK OF HEART DISEASE AND CANCER

The effects of B_{12} deficiency are observed first in the blood and then in the nervous system. In the blood, the deficiency shows up as megaloblastic anemia, characterized by very large blood cells. Even when the megaloblastic anemia is severe, the low red blood cell count doesn't typically cause problems for the patient, and the anemia is *always* cured with vitamin B_{12} supplementation.

The most common nervous system symptoms of B_{12} deficiency are numbness and tingling in the hands and feet. In the early stages of the deficiency, these neurological problems are entirely reversible. However, prolonged and severe deficiency can cause more serious and lasting nerve damage.

All in all, the risk of vitamin B_{12} deficiency is quite remote. On the other hand, eating lots of the foods that are highest in B_{12} means a diet rich in fatty animal foods, which hands you a 50 percent chance of dying prematurely from a heart attack or stroke, a one in six chance of developing prostate cancer (if you are male), and a one in seven chance of getting breast cancer (if you are female). In addition, this same diet increases your chances of obesity, diabetes, osteoporosis, constipation, indigestion, and arthritis. You can see these consequences of a rich, typically American, B_{12}-sufficient diet every day. You probably also know some vegetarians and vegans, but have you ever met one who has suffered from anemia or nervous system damage as a result of his or her diet? I doubt it.

Recommendation for Supplementing B_{12}

Regardless of the minimal risk of vitamin B_{12} deficiency, I recommend taking a vitamin B_{12} supplement. In fact, it is the *only* supplement I recommend. I make this recommendation largely to plug the one hole critics might focus on in the otherwise exceptional diet I recommend, as well as protect against the minuscule risk of harm.

Here's my specific recommendation: If you strictly follow the McDougall Diet in *The Starch Solution* or another vegan diet for more than 3 years, or if you are pregnant or nursing, I suggest you take a daily supplement of 5 micrograms of vitamin B_{12}.

When you go to purchase a supplement, you will find that the pills sold in stores typically contain not 5 micrograms but 500 to 5,000 micrograms (0.5 to 5 milligrams). These high concentrations are meant to correct B_{12} deficiency in people who may be unable to absorb it normally.[67,68] Fortunately for the rest of us, these excessive quantities of B_{12} appear to be safe and nontoxic. If you are an otherwise healthy vegan and are using typical dosages of B_{12} (500 micrograms or more per pill), a weekly, rather than daily, dose of this vitamin will be more than sufficient.

Please check the bottle: B_{12} is often sold as cyanocobalamin, which some researchers have questioned for treating vitamin B_{12} deficiency, especially neurological problems. The methylcobalamin and hydroxycobalamin forms of B_{12} are better choices.[69] Also note that B_{12}-like substances found in food supplements such as spirulina and other algae are ineffective and not a reliable substitute for vitamin B_{12}.[70]

Fermented foods, such as tempeh and miso, are also unreliable sources.[71] Fortified foods, including some nutritional yeasts, may be reliable sources of B_{12}. The seaweed nori, used to wrap maki (sushi rolls, which can be made with vegetables and brown rice rather than fish), has been found to contain substantial amounts of active vitamin

B_{12} thanks to symbiotic organisms that live on it, making nori a "most excellent source of vitamin B_{12} among edible seaweeds, especially for strict vegetarians."[71-73] If you have any question about your B_{12} status, I suggest that you check your B_{12} levels through blood testing; if they are adequate, recheck every 3 years.

OBTAIN NUTRIENTS NATURALLY

In order to maximize your health and minimize the risk of any health problems, I recommend that you and your family follow a diet based on starches, vegetables, and fruits. Expose yourself to adequate sunshine and get a little exercise. To avoid the extremely rare chance of becoming a national headline, add a reliable B_{12} supplement. Failure to follow the starch-based diet that is the natural one for humans is the reason that more than a billion people are overweight and sick today. Trying to fix modern-day health problems with supplements adds to the injury at great financial costs. Scientific facts and reasoning call for the blind and misguided faith placed in supplements to stop.

Chapter 12

Salt and Sugar: The Scapegoats of the Western Diet

The shift to a starch-based diet requires a little discipline at first. In the beginning, you may fear that leaving behind your favorite foods will cause hunger pangs and profound feelings of loss. I promise it won't be long before you prefer to fill your plate with healthy, satisfying starches, and turn your nose up at the overly rich, fatty, chemical-infused foods you may now love. Until you reach that point, it is essential that you stick with this new way of eating, because sticking with it is the only way you are going to become and stay healthy.

I have good news: I'm going to make this adjustment easier by inviting you to add two flavor-enhancing ingredients to the food you eat—ones you probably assumed were off limits on a healthy diet: salt and sugar. Are they nutritious? No, but they cause no real harm for most people.

You may recall from high school biology class that the tip of your tongue finds salt and sugar pleasurable. In fact, you are physiologically designed to seek out these two substances essential to providing for your energy and mineral needs. Most critical is that they will help you to adopt and stick with a plan that leads to shedding excess pounds and

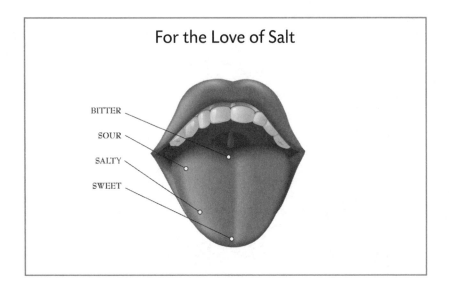

For the Love of Salt

BITTER

SOUR

SALTY

SWEET

improving your lifelong health. This makes these two ingredients well worth including.

The reason you may believe these two added ingredients represent the core of culinary evil has more to do with marketing than with science. Scapegoating salt and sugar deflects attention from the real problems: meat, dairy, fats, oils, and processed foods.

FOR THE LOVE OF SALT, SHOULD I DIE?

Sodium restriction is the most widely publicized, nonmedicinal recommendation for preventing heart disease and stroke. This advice is based mostly on older research and largely reflects studies involving extreme changes in sodium intake, such as reducing sodium to less than 500 milligrams per day in order to lower blood pressure.[1]

Has this recommendation made any difference in the average person's health? Not according to recent research and careful analysis of the data. Why? First, almost no one has been able to follow this advice because a low-salt diet simply is not palatable. People would rather risk illness and death than make this kind of sacrifice. If handfuls of costly blood pressure–lowering pills will allow them to get their salt back and avoid a bland-tasting diet, swallow them they will. The second reason is that reducing salt consumption is of little medical benefit and may even be hazardous to your health.[2]

The major medical concern about salt is that it raises blood pressure, and high blood pressure—more than 140/90 millimeters of mercury (mmHg)—is a risk factor for heart attack, stroke, and kidney disease. Randomized clinical trials, however, show that reducing high sodium intake by an average of 1,725 milligrams (a teaspoon and a half of salt) to 2,300 milligrams per day, the current USDA recommendation, lowers the systolic blood pressure (the top number in your blood pressure reading) by 1 to 5 points and the diastolic (bottom number) by 0.6 to 3 points.[3,4] On the McDougall Diet, with no limitation of the amount

---

Salt Is Synonymous with Value

- Roman soldiers were paid a *salarium* of salt, the derivation of the modern "salary."

- Greek slave-traders often bartered salt for slaves, giving rise to the expression that someone was "not worth his salt."

- Covenants in both the Old and New Testaments of the Bible were often sealed with salt, the origin of "salvation."

- Jesus referred to his disciples as "the salt of the earth." We still use this term to speak well of good, honest, hard-working people.

- The French greeting *salut* is derived from the word for salt.

- The Romans called a man in love *salax,* or in a salted state, from which is derived the word *salacious.*

- "Sitting above the salt" refers to the place of aristocracy above the common folk.

of salt added to foods at the table, the average reduction for people starting out with this level of blood pressure (140/90 mmHg or greater) is 15 points systolic and 13 points diastolic in just 7 days. This is especially remarkable considering that in almost all cases, blood pressure medications are stopped on the first day of my 10-day live-in program. This profound change in blood pressure is due to the overall impact of a healthy diet that is low in fat, animal protein, and calories, and high in potassium, dietary fiber, and carbohydrates.[5] These healthy dietary components improve the health of the blood vessels and overall circulation, significantly lowering elevated blood pressure as a result.

What I observe in my patients can also be seen in society as a whole. Hypertension is rare in indigenous communities with diets that are based on starches, even when the diet is quite high in sodium.[6] When these healthy indigenous people move to urban settings and adopt a Western diet rich in animal products and processed foods, they develop hypertension, type 2 diabetes, heart disease, and obesity. The importance of the overall diet, rather than any single component (sodium), is the fundamental reason that vegetarians tend to have low blood pressure regardless of how much salt they consume.[7]

Reducing Salt May *Increase* Your Risk of Death and Disease

In 2007, the Third National Health and Nutrition Examination Survey (NHANES III), studying nearly 100 million US adults, reported "a robust, significant, and consistent inverse association between dietary sodium and cardiovascular mortality."[8] In other words, people who ate *more* salt had *less* risk of dying from heart disease and strokes.

In a population study published in 2011 in the *Journal of the American Medical Association* involving 3,681 participants without cardiovascular disease, investigators found that the less sodium a person consumed, the higher his or her risk of death from strokes and heart attacks.[9] The authors' conclusion: "The associations between systolic pressure and sodium excretion did not translate into less morbidity or improved survival. On the contrary, low sodium excretion predicted higher cardiovascular mortality. Taken together, our current findings . . . do not support the current recommendations of a generalized and indiscriminate reduction of salt intake at the population level."

The Cochrane Collaboration, an international, independent, not-for-profit health care research organization funded in part by the US Department of Health and Human Services, reported in 2011 in the *American Journal of Hypertension* its review of seven major studies.[10] It concluded that there was no strong evidence of benefit from salt restriction, and that this restriction increased the risk of death in people with congestive heart failure.

Why would cutting back on salt harm your cardiovascular system and increase your risk of dying? We are physiologically designed to seek out and eat salt. When we do not eat enough of it, the body changes in ways that include increasing its production of adrenal hormones, reducing salt losses from the kidneys and skin, and many other adjustments that help us to retain salt. Furthermore, salt restriction raises cholesterol and triglyceride levels.[11] Over the long term, stresses caused by these physiological adaptations for survival may injure our blood vessels and lead to more heart attacks and strokes.

WE LOVE SALT

The desire for salt leads us to consume minerals essential to life, sodium being just one of them. Attempting to deny this innate drive could be harmful and, more importantly, prevents many people from adopting a healthy diet because they simply won't tolerate food that doesn't taste right.

Thirty-five years ago, as an internal medicine resident in training at The Queen's Medical Center in Honolulu, I had the job of convincing my patients with severe kidney disease to eat salt-free butter and cheese. The most common response was, "You must be kidding,

Doc—this tastes like a glob of grease." People who eat steak also rely on salt to bring out its flavor. Without the salt, that slab of beef tastes pretty disgusting (think of boiled beef).

The natural instinct to eat salt in balance with all of the other healthy components of food was well and good until the food industry found clever ways to turn our drives against us. Nearly all of the salt we now eat—80 percent of it—is processed into our foods rather than added at the table. That leaves most people following a Western diet with no choice but to eat loads of salt, with the highest levels found in the unhealthiest foods: processed meats, cheeses, and packaged foods.

Don't Blame the Sodium

It's not the sodium that's to blame, but rather the foods it is mixed up with. Consider these common foods, with sodium expressed in milligrams per 100 calories.

American cheese: 404	Parmesan cheese: 409
Bacon: 415	Pepperoni: 406
Blue cheese: 396	Salami: 510
Cottage cheese: 560	Sour cream dip: 350
Ham: 830	Turkey pastrami: 745

If you were to eat 2,000 calories of these foods, you would take in 10,000 milligrams of sodium, or 435 percent of the USDA recommendation of less than 2,300 milligrams of sodium per day. If you ate 3,000 calories of them, it would total 15,000 milligrams of sodium. Note that corn, peas, potatoes, and rice have about 10 milligrams each of sodium per 100 calories.

When we blame salt, we are colluding with the food companies that have fooled us into focusing our attention on an innocent bystander when the real culprit is the foods that have been overly salted. Salt also tricks us into eating animal-derived foods, which, without excessive amounts of it, would be altogether unappealing. It's not the salt, but the bacon that makes us fat and sick.

How Much Salt Do You Need?

You need only as little as 50 milligrams of sodium per day to meet your baseline metabolic requirements.[12] A diet based on starches, vegetables, and fruits, with no added sodium, contributes about 200 to 500 milligrams, so there is no reason for concern that you won't get enough, even without adding salt.

Adding a half teaspoon of salt at the table to your starch-based meals over the course of a day adds about 1,100 milligrams of sodium, for a daily total of about 1,600 milligrams, 700 milligrams below the 2010 USDA Dietary Guidelines of less than 2,300 milligrams daily, and 400 milligrams below the 2,000-milligram low-sodium diet fed to hospital patients following a massive heart attack.

With these naturally low levels, I have no concerns about inviting people following my starch-based diet to sprinkle a little salt on their food. Assuming the food was not prepared with sodium, you could add up to three-quarters of a teaspoon of salt per day and still stay within the USDA's Dietary Guidelines. I suggest adding salt at the table rather than in cooking because salt added during cooking largely dissipates into the mix of other ingredients, losing the pleasurable flavor. Your big payoff is when you add salt to the surface of your food; it contacts your tongue directly.

Some people are, however, sensitive to salt and must follow a very restricted diet. These people can develop swollen feet from just a couple of glasses of salty tomato juice on a long airplane ride, or swollen fingers after eating Chinese food. For people with severely damaged hearts and kidneys, avoiding salt can be lifesaving. Obviously, these are good reasons to restrict salt for certain people, but not for the general population.

LIFE SHOULD BE SWEET

Along with salt, a little sweetness goes a long way toward making foods taste great. At least at first, you may find corn, beans, potatoes, and rice a little bland compared to what you're used to eating. So what if you enhance these healthy starches with familiar sauces you have enjoyed your whole life? If adding barbecue, blueberry, curry, ketchup, marinade, pasta, raspberry, salsa, steak, or a sweet and sour sauce keeps you eating plenty of healthy starches, I'm all for it.

Sugar is an energy source and taste pleaser with no fat, cholesterol, or sodium and very few chemical contaminants. It is inexpensive, costing about 40 cents per pound, or about a penny for every 45 calories of energy. The environmental footprint associated with sugar production is small, and no animals need be harmed in its production. Used appropriately, it is a helpful addition to your kitchen arsenal. Like salt, sugars add to the deliciousness of your food, ensuring enjoyment as you eat the best foods nature has to offer.

Sugar is clearly a better choice for enhancing flavor than fats and oils, which contribute two and a quarter times more calories per gram than pure white sugar and cause a host of health problems. Feel free to sprinkle a little brown sugar over your oatmeal, drizzle maple syrup over your pancakes, add a bit of refined sugar to a fruit dessert, or dress up your starches and vegetables with sweetened sauces. The shift from animal foods, processed foods, and fats to plant foods is already a giant leap forward for your health. A little sugar won't diminish the powerful effects of this dietary change for most people.

As with salt, you'll get the most flavor by putting the sweet stuff on your food at the table rather than cooking with it. A teaspoon of brown sugar on your bowl of oatmeal adds just 16 calories. These few extra calories will not cause you to put on weight, but they will make the difference in whether or not you look forward to your breakfast.

SUGAR WILL NOT MAKE YOU FAT OR DIABETIC

The misconception that carbohydrates are bad is at the root of your avoidance of some of nature's most perfect foods. Remember that there are three sources of calories—proteins, fats, and carbohydrates—that can be obtained from foods. Sugar, a carbohydrate, is the primary source of energy for cells throughout your body. If you avoid carbohydrates, you are left to fill your calorie void with fat and protein, most likely in the form of meat, poultry, fish, eggs, dairy products, and vegetable oils.

Studies show that people who eat more simple sugar tend to take in fewer calories altogether, which means less chance of becoming overweight.[13] One reason for this is that people who eat more simple and complex sugars generally eat less fat, the real culprit in weight gain and illness. This is because sugar and fat act as a sort of seesaw: When one goes up in a person's diet, the other goes down, naturally.

Type 2 diabetes is a direct result of obesity. Worldwide, the populations with the lowest rates of diabetes are those that eat the most carbohydrate; type 2 diabetes is all but unknown in rural Asia, Africa, Mexico, and Peru, where a high-carbohydrate diet is the cultural norm.[14-16] Some of the highest rates of obesity and diabetes are, however, found among people of Hispanic, Native American, Polynesian, and African descent living in prosperous countries, but not because of their genetic makeup or the starch-based diets of their distant ancestors. These ethnic groups became fat and sick when they adopted a high-fat, high-protein Western diet.[17]

Scientists understand that sugar does not cause type 2 diabetes; the American Diabetic Association recommends that diabetics consume 55 to 65 percent of their calories from carbohydrate, which may include sugary foods.[18] High-carbohydrate diets based on starches have been shown to help diabetics cure their underlying disease, get off their medications, and improve their overall health.[19-21]

That the role of sugar in common diseases has been overrated does not mean that sugar and white flour hold the keys to good health. As carbohydrates become increasingly refined, they become less efficient in inhibiting weight gain and increasing weight loss.[22,23] Refined sugars and flours are referred to as "empty calories" because most essential nutrients have been removed in their manufacturing. Complex carbohydrates in the form of whole starches, like brown rice, whole oats, corn, white potatoes, and sweet potatoes, are the best route to weight loss and good health.

THE GLYCEMIC INDEX: NOT READY FOR PRIME TIME

You've probably heard a lot recently about the glycemic index (GI), which measures the rise in blood sugar over 2 to 3 hours after we eat. Your blood sugar is *supposed* to rise after you eat. It's a *good* thing, not the sign of a problem. Why do we eat in the first place? Aside from the pure pleasure of it, we eat to get the energy needed to carry out our daily activities. GI measures the effectiveness of a particular food as a source of life-sustaining fuel.

This perfectly normal increase has become associated by the public with diabetes, the disease characterized by abnormally high blood sugar. As a result, consumers and medical professionals alike assume that foods with a higher GI, such as potatoes and rice, that cause some of the higher increases in blood sugar seen after a meal, are harmful and should be avoided.

This is far from true, and the mistake is leaving enormous health problems in its wake, including higher rates of diabetes itself. In the United States, Australia, and Western Europe, obesity and type 2 diabetes have reached epidemic proportions as people shun healthy carbohydrates, in part, because of their GI ratings and replace them with

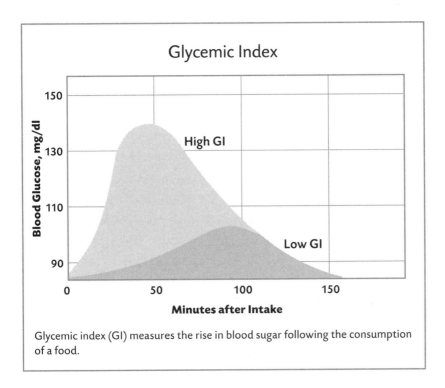

Glycemic index (GI) measures the rise in blood sugar following the consumption of a food.

unhealthy but very low-GI foods like vegetable oils, meats, and cheeses.

Starches high on the GI actually *prevent* weight gain in people who tend to be obese.[24,25] Rising blood sugar triggers satiety, telling you it's time to stop eating.[26] Rather than causing you to eat too much and gain weight, high-GI foods help you to feel satisfied, and thus to stop eating. Potatoes have a high GI, and for this reason they have been shown, based on the same number of calories, to satisfy the appetite twice as well as meat or cheese.[27]

Carbo-loading is practiced by all winning endurance athletes. Carbohydrates, stored as glycogen in the muscles and liver and later released into the bloodstream, provide immediate energy for the whole body during a race. Athletes have learned that the most efficient way to replenish their spent glycogen reserves is to choose foods high on the

GI.[28,29] Selecting foods with a high GI is sound advice not only for athletes, but for anyone yearning to be strong and energetic throughout the day.

Taking the GI out of context leads to some unfounded and dangerous conclusions. Think about a slice of pizza dripping with oily cheese and a nice, big slice of chocolate cake piled high with rich frosting versus a bag of raw carrots and some plain boiled potatoes. Which of these foods are healthier? You won't have any trouble picking the carrots and potatoes. Which have the lower GI? The pizza and cake. Will choosing what to eat based on its GI help you to avoid obesity and diabetes and a multitude of other illnesses? No.

SIMPLE SUGARS CAN CAUSE PROBLEMS

As a practicing physician, I mostly see elevated triglycerides and dental cavities as the primary problems resulting from people eating too much

When High GI Means Quality

JUNK FOODS WITH GI LESS THAN 40	HEALTHY FOODS WITH GI GREATER THAN 80
Fructose (a pure sugar) (19)	Corn meal porridge (109)
Pizza supreme (30)	Jasmine rice (109)
Egg fettuccine (32)	Boiled potato (101)
Peanut M&Ms (33)	Parsnips (97)
Sugar-sweetened chocolate milk (34)	Carrots (92)
No-bake egg custard (35)	Brown rice (87)
Nestle Nesquik Strawberry Drink (35)	Corn thins (87)
Sara Lee Premium Ice Cream (37)	Baked potato (85)
Chocolate cake (38)	Nabisco Shredded Wheat (83)

The glycemic index (GI) of a food is in parentheses.

simple sugar. Carbohydrates are commonly implicated in increased triglycerides, the elevated blood fat levels associated with risk for heart disease and strokes. But in order to demonstrate a rise in triglycerides from eating carbohydrates in experimental studies, subjects must eat a great deal of simple sugars and refined flours and/or must continue to eat after they feel full to the point of discomfort.[30,31] Under these special conditions, the liver will turn some of the excess dietary sugars to triglycerides.[32,33] On the other hand, when subjects are fed starches such as whole grains, beans, and potatoes, along with green and yellow vegetables, and when they are asked to eat only as much as they wish (not to overeat), their triglyceride levels do not increase.[31,34,35]

Only in a very few cases where a starch-based diet is ineffective in bringing cholesterol and triglyceride levels back to normal do I suggest my patients completely eliminate foods made with refined flours and simple sugars, including fruits and fruit juices, both of which contain large amounts of fructose, the type of sugar that causes the greatest increase in triglycerides (and cholesterol).[36] Otherwise, most people can enjoy small amounts of both refined flours and simple sugars without adverse effects.

Studies of ancient skeletons show that widespread tooth decay is largely a modern phenomenon, beginning with the production of refined foods and the widespread use of sugars in food.[37,38] Bacteria in your mouth convert simple sugars into strong acids, and these acids can eat through the protective enamel coating on your teeth to cause decay. It doesn't seem to matter what type of sugar you eat; they all produce enamel-eating acids. Rinsing out your mouth after eating sugars and brushing your teeth will help remove most of these sugars and acids.

DON'T DENY YOUR NATURAL CRAVINGS

Our biological cravings for salt and sugar have made limiting them an unachievable goal for most of us. Focusing on an impossible target—eat little salt and no added sugar—ensures that our health will not improve, consumers will continue their same buying habits, food companies will remain highly profitable, people will remain sick, and drug companies will enjoy record profits. In contrast, a meaningful message, like "stop eating meat and cheese, and instead focus your diet on rice and potatoes," would revolutionize the world—but those now in control of governments and "health" organizations representing profitable businesses don't want to see that day come any time soon. The status quo will indeed continue until the truth about salt and sugar becomes accepted.

The goals of a starch-based diet are to improve your happiness and health and to simultaneously help heal our troubled environment. A diet only works to the extent that you stay on it. The Starch Solution is not a religion based on perfection, but rather a practical means to solve many everyday problems. These two highly pleasurable ingredients, salt and sugar, along with a variety of spices, will increase your enjoyment of your foods and help you to stick with the Starch Solution for a lifetime.

Part III

LIVING THE SOLUTION

CHAPTER 13

Practicing the Starch Solution

Ready to get started? Your friends are going to be mighty envious. First they'll notice you've lost weight; then that you're looking great. Next they'll hear you've gotten your blood pressure down so far that your doctor was incredulous—especially because you gave up the meds you were prescribed to control it. They may also hear that your type 2 diabetes is under control for the first time, also without medication, and that you're eating all the starches *their* doctors (and yours) told them to avoid. They'll also hear that your cholesterol is down to 150 from 270, and that you're off those muscle-damaging statins. Your friends will do a double take when they see you slamming balls on the tennis court, or when you zoom past them on foot heading up a steep hill, overtaking them effortlessly while they stop, bend over, and strain to fill their lungs with air. Oh, no—they are not going to be happy about this at all.

Why won't your friends be happy for you? You've done something you say is very simple—you've only changed the way you eat. Yet, for them, the task seems next to impossible. Give up bacon and eggs for breakfast? They'd rather lie down and die, right now. Don't worry. It's not your job to tell them they're already headed down that path. That, in fact, if they want to ensure more time with friends and family, to enjoy their favorite music and even their favorite foods, a very straight-forward change can help.

What you *will* need to have in your back pocket are some snappy responses for when your family and friends tell you how worried they are about you. How you can't possibly be getting enough protein. Enough calcium. Enough vitamins B_{12} or D. Having read the appropriate chapters in this book, I know you are well prepared for that.

But first, let's get down to the practical advice you need to begin dropping excess weight and reclaiming your health, right here and now. You'll find everything you need to know in this chapter: which foods to seek out and which to avoid; tips for replacing meat and processed foods with real foods; healthy substitutions for your favorite products; a guide to setting up and stocking your kitchen and pantry; how to find healthy food if you don't like to cook; what to order in a restaurant; how a starch-based diet can help you keep costs down; and those few final tips on responding to your well-meaning family members and friends.

What to Eat, What to Avoid

One of the most exciting things about the Starch Solution is that it is not a diet in the traditional sense of restricting how much you can eat. So long as you choose the right foods, you can always eat until you feel comfortably full and satisfied. If you are hungry again an hour later, eat some more. This is one of the key benefits of the Starch Solution and part of what makes it so successful: You need never again feel hungry or deprived.

The Starch Solution does not require you to purchase special pre-pared foods, count calories or starch equivalents, keep a food journal or exercise log, or eat only specified menus or dishes at particular times. So long as you eat only the permitted ingredients, you can combine them in any way you like, in any preparation, to suit your own taste. You can eat a wide variety or limit your choices to a few simple dishes repeated over and over again.

If you prefer the guidance of a specific menu as you get started, you will find a 7-day plan in Chapter 14. Whether you choose to follow a menu or create your own meals depending on your mood, Chapter 15 includes nearly 100 easy-to-prepare recipes for tempting, delicious foods to keep you and your family healthy and satisfied.

The cardinal rule of the Starch Solution is that you must *center the food on your plate around starches, adding color and flavor with nonstarchy vegetables and fruits.* Use fat-free seasonings and sauces generously to add variety to your meals and make them more interesting. The sidebar beginning on page 190 explains which foods are starches and should make up the greatest portion of your meals, and which are the nonstarchy vegetables and fruits that should surround them.

In addition to knowing which foods you should eat, you need to know which to avoid. The following foods are never part of a healthy diet, and should be meticulously avoided if you are to benefit from the Starch Solution.

- Meat, such as beef, pork, lamb
- Poultry, such as chicken, turkey, duck
- Fish and shellfish
- Dairy foods, such as milk, cheese, yogurt, sour cream
- Eggs
- Animal fats, such as lard and butter
- Vegetable oils, including olive, corn, flaxseed, canola, and safflower
- Processed and packaged foods, except for ones containing *only* permitted ingredients

If you have a "slip" and eat one of these foods, the best way to protect your health is to immediately return to following the Starch Solution. Although diverging from the plan once or twice a year will not undo all of its benefits, it can be a slippery slope. If you indulge too often, you may find it difficult to get back on track. For most people, eliminating a food altogether is far easier than figuring out when it is

(continued on page 192)

Starch, Vegetable, or Fruit?

STARCHES

Most starches can be classified as whole grains, legumes, or starchy vegetables. Some commonly available whole grains are barley, brown rice, bulgur wheat, corn, farro, millet, oats, rye, spelt, triticale, and wheat berries. Products made with these grains include breads, tortillas, flatbreads, pasta, couscous, and whole grain cereals.

Legumes include dried beans, peas, and lentils. There are a great variety of beans to choose from: adzuki, cranberry, black, cannellini, fava, chickpeas, great northern, kidney, lima, mung, navy, pinto, soy, and white beans. Common pea varieties include black-eyed peas and split or whole yellow and green peas. Small, flat lentils can be found in green, red, or brown, each with its own flavor and texture. Pea and bean pods that must be shelled before eating are generally the starchy ones, such as cranberry beans, fava beans, and soybeans.

Peanuts are also a legume, although like tree nuts, they are high in fat and should be minimized or avoided altogether, especially if you are trying to lose weight.

Starchy vegetables include most tubers and root vegetables, including burdock, cassava, potatoes, sweet potatoes, taro, and yams. Winter squashes are also high in starch; some examples are acorn, buttercup, butternut, Hubbard, and kabocha, as well as pumpkins.

GREEN, YELLOW, AND ORANGE (NONSTARCHY) VEGETABLES

Nonstarchy vegetables are a plentiful source of vitamins and minerals, fiber, and water. On their own, these vegetables don't provide enough calories to make them a filling meal, but they do add flavor, aroma, texture, color, and variety to the plate.

Nonstarchy vegetables are the green, yellow, orange, and more multicolored ones, and they come in many forms. The summer squash family includes zucchini, straight and crookneck squash, chayote, cocozelle, and pattypans in colors ranging from white to yellow to green, and sometimes striped varieties. Some root vegetables, lower in starch, are carrots, beets, jicama, and radishes. Edible bulbs include fennel, garlic, and onions. Related to roots are rhizomes like ginger, turmeric, and lotus root.

Some vegetables grow in pods, with the more delicate varieties housing immature, nonstarchy beans such as green beans, sugar snap peas, and snow peas. These are the ones you can pop in your mouth, pod and all.

Among mushrooms, white button, cremini, portobello, oyster, enoki, and shiitake varieties are cultivated, while lobster, porcini, and black trumpet varieties grow wild.

Some of the vegetables we eat are actually the plant's unopened or partially opened flower. Broccoli, cauliflower, artichokes, and Brussels sprouts are examples. With others, like asparagus, celery, and rhubarb (it's not a fruit), we eat the stalk. Leafy vegetables include lettuce, arugula, radicchio, spinach, cabbage, chard, kale, collards, and mustard greens.

Some things we know as vegetables are classified botanically as fruits. Fruits are the plant parts used for reproduction, namely seeds and the plant parts that contain the seeds. (Think of seed-covered strawberries.) Common vegetables that are classified botanically as fruits include eggplant, tomato (actually a berry), cucumber, and avocado. Bean pods and squashes are fruits as well. For our purposes, we talk about these as vegetables if they are more often eaten for dinner than dessert.

(continued)

okay to eat it, how much is safe to eat and remain on the plan, and when it's time to stop. For that reason, I recommend staying away from these foods altogether, all of the time, for the rest of your life. It may seem inconceivable now, but once you make the commitment and experience the profound effects, you will not miss the foods you give up.

There are a few foods that won't spoil your success with the Starch Solution, but will slow your progress. If you seek to accelerate your weight loss, or if you suffer from a chronic disease or are on the cusp of developing one, I recommend avoiding these foods altogether. If, on the other hand, you are already happy with your weight or not in a hurry to lose, and you do not suffer from a chronic illness, you might wish to consider including small quantities of these higher calorie foods in your starch-based meals.

- Avocados
- Dried fruits
- Flours (whole grain, white, all-purpose)

mons, dates, figs, and grapes. Tropical fruits include banana, pine-apple, guava, mango, lychee nut, passion fruit, kiwifruit, and melons such as cantaloupe, honeydew, crenshaw, watermelon, and others.

In parts of Asia and the Philippines, avocados are enjoyed as fruit. Avocado and olives, also a fruit, are notable for their high fat content compared with other fruits and vegetables. Like peanuts, tree nuts like almonds and walnuts are comparatively high in fat and thus should be limited or avoided altogether if weight loss is a primary goal. In dried fruits, sugars are concentrated as moisture evaporates in the drying process, leaving a highly concentrated food that is supersweet and high in calories.

- Fruit and vegetable juices
- Nuts
- Peanuts and peanut butter
- Seeds
- Simple sugars (i.e., table sugar, maple syrup, molasses, agave)

How to Prepare Your Food

There are endless ways to prepare starchy grains, legumes, and vegetables. As you are getting started, you might like to choose familiar foods, the ones you grew up with. I was raised in the Midwest on potatoes. If you were raised in a family of Asian ancestry, rice may well be your favorite starch. If your *nonna* and *nonno* called Italy home, you might turn to pasta (without eggs) for sustenance and comfort.

Spices and other seasonings can help to keep your food varied and interesting. They can also help you to make familiar-tasting foods from less familiar ingredients. Try adding curry powder as you cook if you enjoy Indian foods, rice wine vinegar and soy sauce for Asian-style food, and chili powder, cilantro, or salsa for a Latin flavor.

Most any supermarket offers a broad array of both fresh and dried herbs and spices. Natural food stores often have even more. Stores that sell the most spices have the greatest turnover and therefore the freshest, most flavorful ones. Store spices in a cabinet away from heat and light to keep them tasting fresh. Buy in small quantities and use liberally. For the freshest flavor, replace older herbs and spices every 6 months.

Salt and sweeteners used in reasonably small quantities also help to enhance taste and make adjusting to a new eating plan a little easier (see Chapter 12). When you purchase prepared sauces, or any prepared product, read the label carefully to avoid oils and other fats. Choose products with the fewest artificial ingredients.

Mary and I recommend making the recipes in this book in large quantities and packaging them in individual or family-sized servings in the refrigerator and freezer. That way there is always something good to eat on hand when you get hungry.

Healthy Substitutions for Your Favorite Foods

The suggestions that follow can help you find foods that are healthy and part of the Starch Solution to substitute for your favorite familiar foods.

Setting Up Your Kitchen and Pantry

The best way to ensure that you stick with the Starch Solution is to keep an assortment of healthy ingredients on hand in your kitchen. A well-stocked pantry and refrigerator will make the difference between success and failure. These ingredients can be used to prepare a wide variety of quick and easy meals.

AVOID	ENJOY
Butter and margarine	Bean spreads, jellies and jams, tofu mayonnaise
Cereals, refined and sugar coated	Hot or cold whole grain cereal without refined ingredients
Cheese	Tofu ricotta (page 296)
Cookies, cakes, and other desserts	Fresh fruit or a McDougall dessert
Chocolate, in recipes	Fat-free cocoa powder
Coffee, decaf coffee, and black teas	Noncaffeinated herbal teas, cereal beverage, hot water with lemon
Colas and other sodas	Mineral water, club soda, or unsweetened seltzer (flavored or plain)
Eggs, to eat	Tofu scramble, Eggless Egg Salad (page 241)
Eggs, in recipes	Ener-G Egg Replacer
Fats, in baking	Prune puree, fat replacers, or applesauce
Flour, white	Whole wheat, white whole wheat, or other whole grain flours
Ice cream	Banana ice cream, pure fruit sorbet, frozen juice bars
Meat, poultry, fish	Starchy vegetables, whole grains, pastas, and beans
Oils, vegetable, for pans	Use nonstick pots and pans
Oils, vegetable, for sautéing and in recipes	Omit oil, or replace with water, vegetable broth, or other liquids; sauté in water or broth
Mayonnaise	Tofu Mayonnaise (page 243)
Milk, as a beverage	Water, juice, or herbal tea
Milk, on cereal and in cooking	Soy milk, rice milk, nut milk, fruit juice, or water
Rice, white	Brown rice or other whole grains
Salad dressing	Squirt of fresh lemon or lime juice, or a low-fat dressing
Sour cream	Tofu Sour Cream (page 242)
Yogurt	Soy or nut-based yogurt

Which Soy Foods Are Healthiest?

The following guidelines will help you choose soy foods that fit with the Starch Solution (see Chapter 10).

Enjoy traditional soy foods, like soy milk and tofu, as a small part of your diet—no more than 5 percent of your calories, or about 2 ounces per day. These foods aren't necessary for good health, but they do add richness and variety without the hazards of vegetable oils and animal foods.

Avoid synthetic and highly processed soy products, like soy burgers, soy sausage, soy bacon, soy cheese, and soy-based protein powders and energy bars.

Instead of commonly consumed soy meats and dairy:

- Replace soy burgers with low-fat bean and grain burgers.

- Add rice to your bean chili instead of fake sausage.

- Pass up the soy margarine on your baked potatoes and vegetables.

- Use recommended dips, sauces, and spreads.

- Skip the soy cheese on your whole wheat pizza. (Eat it topped with tomato sauce and vegetables.)

- Finish dinner with fruit or sorbet rather than soy ice cream or cheesecake.

To enjoy soy in healthy ways:

- Splash a little soy milk on your morning cereal.

- Add a few ounces of tofu to a stir-fry.

- Season grains with a small dollop of miso paste or a squirt of soy sauce.

- Occasionally whip up a tofu pudding or pie filling for dessert.

Shelf-stable foods

Keep the following shelf-stable foods in your pantry and you will always be prepared with the components to make a quick meal or snack, and the flavorings and condiments to give your foods flavor and variety.

Agave nectar

Apple juice

Applesauce

Baking powder (aluminum free)

Baking soda

Barbecue sauces (oil free)

Beans (canned, all kinds, including fat-free refried; dried)

Brown sugar or Sucanat

Canned chopped tomatoes (with herbs or plain)

Canned green chiles

Canned vegetables (artichokes, roasted red peppers, pumpkin)

Cereals (made from whole grains with minimal ingredients and no added fat)

Coffee substitutes (Teeccino, Roma, etc.)

Cornstarch

Dip and dressing mixes

Dr. McDougall's Right Foods soups, cereals, and cup meals

Dried fruits (prunes, raisins, currants, figs, dates, apricots, etc.)

Ener-G Egg Replacer

Flours (unbleached, all-purpose white flour; whole wheat flour; whole wheat pastry flour; white whole wheat flour)

Grains (brown rice, barley, rolled oats, steel-cut oats, other grains as desired)

Herbal teas

Hot sauce (Tabasco, hot chili sauce, etc.)

Kabuli pizza crust

Ketchup

Molasses

Mustard (prepared)

Pasta (egg free, and made from whole wheat, corn, quinoa, spelt, or rice)

Pasta sauces (fat free)

Peanut butter

Pimiento (chopped, bottled)

(continued)

Pure maple syrup

Salad dressings (fat free)

Salsa (bottled)

Soy or rice milk

Soy sauce (regular or low sodium; no MSG)

Sunsweet Lighter Bake (butter and oil replacement)

Tomato sauce and tomato paste

Vegetable broth

Vegetarian Worcestershire sauce

Vinegars (balsamic, rice, wine)

Wonderslim Wondercocoa Fat-Free Cocoa Powder

Fresh foods to keep on hand

Bread (from a local bakery: 100 percent whole grain flour, low fat, low sodium)

Garlic

Onions

Potatoes

Tomatoes

In the refrigerator

Garlic (minced, bottled)

Ginger (minced, bottled)

Jellies and jams

Lemons or lemon juice

Limes or lime juice

Milk (nondairy soy, nut, or rice)

Miso paste

Salsa ("salsa fresca" on page 319)

Tofu, silken or regular

Variety of fresh vegetables and fruits

Frozen foods at your fingertips

Brown rice (precooked)

Burgers (made from beans and grains; free of meat or soy products)

Corn tortillas (no added fat)

Fruit

Fruit sorbet

Hash brown potatoes (no added fat)

Vegetables (without sauces)

Whole wheat buns

Whole wheat tortillas

Herbs and spices

To keep your food tasty and appealing, in addition to the condiments, sauces, and seasonings previously mentioned, McDougallers following the Starch Solution do best when they keep a well-stocked spice cabinet. Stock up on whatever herbs and spices you like best. Here are some suggestions:

Allspice	Mustard (dry)
Basil	Nutmeg
Bay leaf	Onion powder
Celery seed	Oregano
Chili powder	Paprika (smoked and/or sweet)
Cinnamon	Parsley flakes
Cloves	Pepper (black, red, or smoked)
Coriander	Rosemary
Crushed red pepper	Sage
Cumin	Tarragon
Curry powder	Thyme
Dill seed and dill weed	Turmeric
Garlic powder	Vanilla beans or pure vanilla extract
Ground red pepper	
Marjoram	Vegetable seasoning mixture

The two most popular seasonings are salt and sugar, and they add the most value when they are sprinkled on the surface of your food before eating, rather than lost in the mixture as it cooks. (See Chapter 12 for more information about salt and sugar.)

To add familiar flavorings of meat or fish, look for vegetarian products that mimic these flavors, such as beef and poultry seasoning mixes made from spices, and seaweeds that provide a fishy taste.

Snack foods

Keep the following foods on hand to feed a midday or late night snack attack:

Corn thins

Crackers (rice or wheat; fat free)

Hummus or other spreads
(fat free)

Popcorn (just corn; avoid instant popcorn with added fat)

Cookware

Having the right cookware can help you turn out delicious foods without added fats. We recommend cookware made from cast iron, stainless steel, glass, or ceramic. Nonstick cookware is helpful, but please avoid any that puts aluminum in direct contact with your foods. (Aluminum is associated with Alzheimer's disease.) You can find baking pans in a variety of shapes and sizes made from silicone, which releases foods easily without coating them with fat or oil. They clean up quickly and easily.

The following items make a good cookware starter kit:

Baking pans (square, round, and rectangular)

Baking sheets (nonstick or lined with silicone baking mats)

Cake pans (nonstick, silicone, or lined with parchment paper)

Casserole dishes

Colanders and strainers

Frying pans (nonstick)

Griddle (nonstick)

Kitchen tools (cutting board, forks, knives, slotted spoons, spatulas)

Loaf pans (nonstick, silicone, or lined with parchment paper)

Muffin cups (nonstick, silicone, or lined with cupcake liners)

Pasta pot with strainer insert

Pressure cooker

Rice cooker

Saucepans in various sizes

Slow cooker

Soup pots

Teakettle

When You Don't Feel Like Cooking

There will be times when you just don't feel like cooking, or don't have time. It is for these occasions that we've suggested keeping your pantry shelves, refrigerator, and freezer well stocked. Preparing, portioning, and refrigerating or freezing foods in advance when you do have time to cook leaves you with easy meals for later. In fact, many soups, stews, and casseroles taste even better the second day.

Remember, if your favorite dinner is a plate of beans and rice with salsa and corn tortillas, or a big bowl of soup with whole grain bread, or a sweet potato with steamed broccoli, there is absolutely no reason not to enjoy that same food, day after day and night after night. These foods are healthy. There is no reason to eat them only occasionally or in moderation. Variety is good if you *like* variety, but some people find comfort in eating the foods they know and love on a regular basis.

Frozen cooked brown rice and frozen vegetables make quick and easy work of preparing a meal when there is no time to cook. Microwave the rice, bake a potato, or boil some pasta, then throw in some cooked frozen vegetables and add some sauces you have purchased or made earlier. Fresh or bottled salsa or even soups make great toppings for potatoes, rice, and vegetables.

You might also wish to take advantage of the packaged Dr. McDougall's Right Foods soups, cereals, and cup meals. Keeping these foods on hand ensures that you always have something good to eat.

Some supermarkets and restaurants sell foods that can be brought home for a quick meal. Also look in natural food stores for prewashed, precut, packaged salad greens and other salad ingredients. At the salad bar, you can easily make up a satisfying salad of leafy greens, carrots, radishes, onions, cucumbers, celery, corn, peas, and beans, or purchase ingredients that are all ready to cook, although at a premium compared with unprepared raw ingredients. Some stores also sell precut carrots, onions, and celery to use in soups; peeled, cubed squash; and other prepared ingredients that make cooking quick and easy.

Low-fat dressings and seasoned or balsamic vinegars are a great way to quickly and easily dress up tossed salads or steamed vegetables.

If you can afford it, you might consider hiring someone to prepare your meals. Private chefs are available to cook in your home—often making a week's worth of meals for you in just a day—or deliver prepared meals. Just be sure that they fully understand the requirements of your diet. Try www.hireachef.com or the bulletin board at your local natural foods store as useful resources for finding a personal chef.

DINING OUT

When you go out to eat with friends or family, as a break from cooking at home or to celebrate a special occasion, you will have to put some thought into it. You will also need to be prepared to politely stick to your plan when dining in a friend's home.

Ethnic restaurants like Mexican, Chinese, or Thai tend to offer the best options. (Remember that these populations have traditionally followed a starch-based diet.) Speak directly with the chef if you are able, making it clear that you wish to eat mostly starches such as rice, beans, and potatoes, with a few added vegetables, and that your food must be prepared without any oil or animal products. You cannot rely on vegetarian and vegan restaurants or options as they are listed in the menu, as typically they are loaded with vegetable oils. Don't be bashful about sending your meal back if it doesn't match the starch-based, low-fat meal you asked for.

At other types of restaurants, look for side dishes that can be put together into a plate, such as potatoes, pasta, and/or rice with some plain steamed vegetables. For breakfast, you can often get oatmeal prepared without milk or butter (be sure to specify this), cold whole grain cereals with fruit juice, dry whole grain toast with jam, or hash browns cooked "dry," and a cup of fruit. For lunch, if the soups, sandwiches, and salads on the menu don't meet the requirements of your plan, ask for whole grain bread, some mustard, lettuce, tomatoes, pickles, and the like. You can always put these together into your own sandwich.

KEEPING COSTS DOWN ON A STARCH-BASED DIET

For many families, food is one of the greatest monthly expenditures. Luckily, grains, legumes, and starchy vegetables are some of the least expensive foods you can buy. Other vegetables and fruits may be more costly, especially if you purchase organic. You won't be eating as much of these as you will the starchier foods, and it will be worth the extra cost to get fresh fruits and vegetables, especially those in season.

You can easily figure the cost savings of a starch-based diet. On average, moderately active women consume about 2,000 calories per day and men 2,500 calories. The cost of a typical home-cooked meal featuring animal foods could easily be $10 per person or more per day.

People often underestimate the cost of eating at fast-food or other restaurants. Roughly half of US food dollars are spent eating out—about 40 percent in full-service restaurants and 40 percent in fast-food establishments. At least one in three Americans (adults and children) eats at a fast-food restaurant daily, although this expensive habit has been declining with increasing economic pressures; more than half of restaurant operators reported a decline in sales in January 2010.

Food Costs of a Diet Based on Animal Foods

FOOD	COST PER ITEM	COST PER 2,500 CALORIES
Beef rib eye (1 lb)	$9.99	$24.29
Ground beef (1 lb)	$2.99	$6.55
Chicken breast (1 lb)	$3.99	$13.72
Salmon (1 lb)	$9.99	$30.60
Cheddar cheese (1 lb)	$11.99	$15.48
Milk (½ gal)	$2.49	$10.37

Based on northern California prices.

Many consumers turn to fast-food restaurants to reduce their dining-out costs. But if you compare the "bargain" of a fast-food meal to the cost of a starch-based diet, you will quickly see the outrageous cost of eating in fast-food outlets: from $9 to $21 per person for a full day's worth of fast-food meals (2,500 calories). About $14 per person per day is the average cost.

FOOD	COST PER ITEM	COST PER 2,500 CALORIES
Burger King Whopper	$2.99	$11.12
Burger King Triple Whopper	$4.99	$11.03
Burger King Chicken Sandwich	$3.99	$12.62
Burger King BK Big Fish Sandwich	$3.39	$13.24
KFC Snacker	$1.19	$9.30
KFC Oven Roasted Twister	$3.59	$19.10
McDonald's Big Mac	$3.19	$14.77
McDonald's Large Fries	$2.00	$8.77
McDonald's Chicken Sandwich	$3.49	$20.77
McDonald's Filet-O-Fish Sandwich	$3.19	$20.98
Round Table Gourmet Veggie Pizza	$21.35	$19.34
Round Table Ulti-Meat Pizza	$21.35	$14.83
Taco Bell Taco	$0.99	$14.56
Taco Bell Steak Burrito	$3.19	$12.65
Taco Bell Chicken Salad	$5.39	$17.06
Based on northern California prices.		

In comparison, a starch-based diet with added fruits, vegetables, and condiments will cost you about $3 per person per day. Starches are among the least expensive foods in the supermarket. Getting your full daily supply of calories from starches alone would cost you less than $1.50 (for 2,500 calories). Perishable fruits and vegetables cost a little more, but you will not be eating them in as large quantities as the starches. Choosing fruits and vegetables in season will also help keep your food bill affordable. (Add another $1.50 daily for fruits and vegetables, for a total of $3.00 a day for your starch-based diet.)

FOOD	COST PER ITEM	COST PER 2,500 CALORIES
White potatoes (20 lbs)	$6.99	$1.75
Sweet potatoes (10 lbs)	$5.99	$3.00
Pinto beans (25 lbs)	$13.79	$1.05
Brown rice (25 lbs)	$24.75	$1.52
White rice (50 lbs)	$14.99	$0.44
Corn tortillas (120 pieces)	$2.79	$1.00
Corn grits (50 lbs)	$41.99	$1.28
Oats (9 lbs)	$6.99	$1.09
Based on northern California prices.		

Keeping grains, potatoes, and legumes on hand at home cuts your transportation costs by requiring fewer trips to the market, especially compared to eating at restaurants and fast-food outlets, which requires a trip for each and every meal.

Dry goods (beans, rice, grains) are easily stored for long periods without refrigeration, cutting another hidden food cost: the energy associated with refrigeration. Since these foods do not easily spoil, there is little waste. Potatoes, sweet potatoes, and winter squashes may also be stored at cool room temperature away from light for up to several months.

Cleaning up after a plant-based, low-fat meal is relatively easy and cheap. What takes the most soap and elbow grease to scrub? Fats and oils.

The net savings from switching your 2,500 calories per day from fast foods to starch-based meals is $11 per person, per day ($14 minus $3). Over the course of a year, this puts savings in your pocket of more than $4,000. If you are feeding a family of four, this means an additional $16,000 saved annually on food costs alone that you could save for other expenses. Of course, these savings do not take into consideration the indirect financial benefits: reduced medical expenses, reduced medication costs, decreased need for supplements, increased productivity, and more. Nor do they reflect your contribution to creating a healthier environment and alleviating senseless suffering of animals.

You can further bring down costs on a starch-based diet by following these tips:

- Purchase products with a long shelf life in large quantities.
- Select unprocessed foods.
- Buy in bulk at natural food stores, co-ops, and grocery stores.
- Shop warehouse clubs and stores for bulk prices and specials.
- Purchase local fruits and vegetables in season.
- Patronize farmers' markets; you can sometimes get deals from producers at the end of the day.
- Grow fruit trees, plant a vegetable garden, and buy herbs in pots for an ongoing supply rather than purchasing cut herbs.
- Shop when you're not so hungry, to avoid impulse buys.
- Plan your grocery list before you shop and cluster your errands to reduce gasoline use and wasted time.
- Walk or bicycle to the store and leave the car at home.
- Look for deals online or by mail order.
- Prepare as many of your meals as possible at home.

CHAPTER 14

The 7-Day
Sure-Start Plan

A re you ready for a challenge? Try the starch-based diet I recommend for 7 days. In a week you will know whether the Starch Solution is right for you. When I suggest that returning to a historically validated diet rich in starch and vegetables, low in fat, and without meat, fish, or dairy is simple, I don't mean to suggest that it's an easy change to make. For most people, this change is a big deal.

The good news is that with big changes come big results. Experience tells me that you will come to love it, and surprisingly quickly. I also know that you will be relieved to eat as much as you wish, be completely satisfied afterward, and lose excess weight as you improve your health more than you ever could from any pill or surgery prescribed by your well-meaning doctors.

This is not an all-or-nothing program. However, change is usually easier when you draw clear boundaries for yourself, like: Today I am a smoker and tomorrow I will not be. My recommendation is to go at this with your full will and intention to become different. Today I am a meat, dairy, and junk-food eater and tomorrow I will not be. Tomorrow, and from now on, I will be a starch eater, the way nature always intended me to be.

Get Ready

It is always best to consult your physician before making any major change to your diet; it is essential to do so if you are ill or on medication. While you're there, why not take the opportunity to get a little more data by having your blood pressure, blood sugar, cholesterol, and triglycerides measured along with your weight before you begin? I also suggest checking your thyroid function, as low thyroid can influence your weight and health. Measured before you begin following this plan and again after you have followed it faithfully for a week (and at reasonable intervals as you continue), these test results will provide some of the best evidence that the Starch Solution is helping you not only drop those excess pounds but improve your overall health. They will also help get your doctor on board so that he or she can support your ongoing commitment to this change. You may even end up helping others as your doctor passes along this secret to good health.

On the opposite page is a lab slip you can hand your doctor to ask for the simple tests that will show you whether this diet is effective for you.

Copy the page, fill out the information about yourself in the first two boxes, and bring it to your doctor. Tell your doctor that you will be following a starch-based diet for 7 days. Ask whether there is any reason you should not try this 7-day challenge. I cannot think of a valid reason your doctor could give you not to try the Starch Solution; nonetheless, it is important that he or she knows what you are doing, especially if you are on medications or have any serious health problems. Most commonly, medications for high blood pressure and type 2 diabetes need to be reduced or stopped when you begin your new diet. Antacids, laxatives, and pain medications are reduced or stopped by most people when they begin. All of these changes in medication need to be made under the supervision and with the recommendations of a competent health care provider. Also let your doctor know that you will be returning in 7 days to repeat these tests.

Ask your doctor or nurse to record the information in the bottom box for you:

DATE: _____

WEIGHT: _____

HEIGHT: _____

BLOOD PRESSURE: _____

General Medical Laboratory Request

PATIENT

NAME: _____

ADDRESS: _____

DATE OF BIRTH: _____

E-MAIL ADDRESS: _____

PHONE NUMBER: _____

FAX NUMBER: _____

MEDICAL RECORD NUMBER: _____

MEDICAL INSURANCE INFORMATION: _____

PHYSICIAN

NAME: _____

ADDRESS: _____

PHONE NUMBER: _____

Please obtain the following laboratory tests and send one copy of the results to the patient and one copy to the requesting physician.

GLUCOSE (BLOOD SUGAR): _____

TOTAL CHOLESTEROL: _____

HDL CHOLESTEROL: _____

LDL CHOLESTEROL: _____

TRIGLYCERIDES: _____

THYROID FUNCTION (TSH): _____

GET SET

Before you get started, weigh yourself and write down your weight. Store it someplace you will remember. This may be the biggest clue as to how effective this new way of eating is for you.

The rules of the 7-Day Sure-Start Plan are easy to follow:

1. Eat more starch. Eat as much starch as you like. Don't go hungry.

2. Choose the least processed starches and other foods you can find. (For example, brown rice is better than white; cooked whole grains are better than products made with white flour.)

3. Eat plenty of vegetables and fruits.

4. Eliminate animal food from your diet, including meat, poultry, fish, eggs, cheese, and milk.

5. Keep your fat intake as low as possible, enjoying avocado, coconut, other nuts, and seeds only as occasional treats.

6. Avoid any added fat in your food, including butter, margarine, and all vegetable oils, even olive oil.

7. When eating soy foods, skip those that are highly processed (e.g., soy burgers) and enjoy minimally processed soy foods like tofu, edamame (soybeans), and soy milk as infrequent additions in small quantities; they're richer than you think.

8. Go easy on sugar and salt, but don't sweat the unimportant stuff. They're usually the scapegoat, not the problem. Whenever possible, add them to the surface of the foods.

Over many years of working with patients making the transition to a starch-based diet, I have heard over and over again that two tips helped them above all others to get comfortable with this new style of eating:

- Avoid temptation by keeping unhealthy foods you crave out of your home and workplace. If a food feels like an addictive drug when you eat it—you have a hard time stopping—it's not a good food to keep around.

- Prepare or purchase healthy foods you enjoy so there is always something you can feel good about eating, especially when you are in a hurry. Keep your refrigerator and cupboards filled with good foods you can grab on the go and bring along with you to work or on the road.

That's everything you need to get started. Easy, right? But to make things even easier, I've provided you with a 7-day menu plan.

GO! THE STARCH SOLUTION 7-DAY SURE-START MENU PLAN

The menus that follow are meant to offer variety; they are not set in stone. This is an endlessly flexible way of eating. You can swap any dish on the menu for any of the recipes in Chapter 15 or those included in other McDougall books or in the McDougall Cookbook app. For a quick fix, you can purchase a variety of Dr. McDougall's Right Foods cups in many supermarkets. If on Day 5 you are in the mood for the menu on Day 3, no problem, swap them. If you really enjoyed the lunch on Day 2, follow that menu twice, or three times, or seven. In fact, if you simply adore sweet potatoes and broccoli, you can eat them for breakfast, lunch, dinner, and between-meal snacks—every day of the week for many years. As you have learned in this book, starches along with vegetables and fruits provide complete nutrition.

Although the menus are based on three meals per day, the number of times you eat is not important. You can eat once a day or 14 times. Eat when you are hungry and stop when you are satisfied. If you do that, it makes no difference how often you eat.

In Chapter 13 you will find practical advice about how to stock your refrigerator and kitchen cabinets, substitutions for the foods you are accustomed to eating, cooking techniques, and more. You might wish to scan that chapter and the recipes in Chapter 15 for ideas as you get started.

As long as you follow the basic rules on page 210, you are taking part in the Starch Solution and can expect to achieve results. The only imperatives are that you eat plenty of starch, supplemented with fruits and vegetables, avoid vegetable oils and animal-based foods, and eat rich foods like nuts, seeds, minimally processed soy products, and dried fruits and juices in moderation, if at all. The less of these richer foods you eat, the more dramatic your weight loss and health improvement will be. If you are already at your desired weight, or are underweight, you can use these richer plant foods to keep your weight in check.

DAY 1

Breakfast: Super Simple Overnight Cereal (page 221) with fresh blueberries

Lunch: Eggless Egg Salad (page 241) on whole wheat bread with lettuce and sliced tomatoes

Dinner: Bean and Corn Enchiladas (page 287), tossed green salad with low-fat dressing or seasoned vinegar, Decadent Chocolate Pudding (page 318)

DAY 2

Breakfast: Hash Brown Potatoes (page 227) with barbecue sauce, ketchup, or fresh salsa; sliced fresh fruit

Lunch: McDougall Veggie Burger (page 250) on a whole wheat bun with lettuce, sliced tomatoes, and ketchup and/or mustard

Dinner: Tunisian Sweet Potato Stew (page 277), brown rice, steamed broccoli, Peach-Oatmeal Crisp (page 317)

DAY 3

Breakfast: Fluffy Pancakes (page 222) with pure maple syrup and sliced bananas

Lunch: Festive Dal Soup (page 269) with whole wheat bread

Dinner: Baked Penne Florentine (page 303), steamed green beans and carrots, Carrot Cake (page 315)

DAY 4

Breakfast: French Toast (page 223) sprinkled with cinnamon; sliced cantaloupe

Lunch: Fresh Tomato Wraps (page 257), steamed kale

Dinner: Polenta with Black Beans and Mango Salsa (page 286), tossed green salad with low-fat dressing or seasoned vinegar, Banana Ice Cream (page 312)

DAY 5

Breakfast: East-West Breakfast (page 231) with warm corn tortillas and salsa

Lunch: Split Pea Vegetable Soup (page 268), baked potato

Dinner: Tofu Lasagna (page 296), steamed Swiss chard, Chocolate Brownies (page 313)

DAY 6

Breakfast: No-Huevos Rancheros (page 228), papaya with lime wedges

Lunch: Quinoa Chowder (page 270), whole wheat bread or dinner rolls

Dinner: Spicy Lima Beans and Cabbage (page 290), corn tortillas, tossed green salad with low-fat dressing or seasoned vinegar, Apple Crisp (page 316)

DAY 7

Breakfast: Veggies Benedict (page 230), fresh strawberries

Lunch: Ventana Lentil Stew (page 275), brown rice

(continued on page 217)

Mike Teehan,
Retired from the US Postal Service, Honolulu, Hawaii

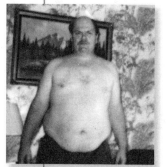

My whole life has been centered around food. When things with my alcoholic father got bad, Mom would pack up me and my sister and we'd go on an eating binge of candy, hot dogs, and potato chips. By the sixth grade I weighed nearly 200 pounds.

In high school I brought my weight down so I could enlist in the US Marine Corps. After I

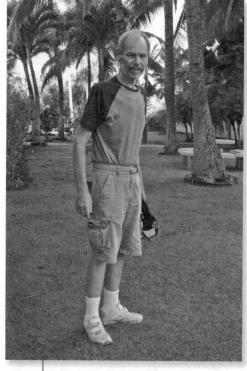

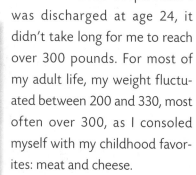

was discharged at age 24, it didn't take long for me to reach over 300 pounds. For most of my adult life, my weight fluctuated between 200 and 330, most often over 300, as I consoled myself with my childhood favorites: meat and cheese.

At age 28 I came across one of Dr. McDougall's books and, after reading that you could eat all you want, I took it home. I bought 10 pounds of potatoes thinking, "I'll show him!" The next morning my scale showed a 2-pound loss. This was Nirvana! It wasn't long before I began adding sour cream and butter to those potatoes, and the weight loss came to a standstill.

Fourteen years later, I managed to lose 99 pounds, dropping from 331 to 232. I had the idea that I could capitalize on this by going on the Atkins diet, which I understood was deadly but also quick and effective. Once I got below 200, I figured, I'd use McDougall to regain my health. Five years later I'd bounced back to 300 pounds, where I stayed for several years.

At age 50, in January 2005, I decided to give the McDougall plan another try. By August I weighed 288 pounds and by early December, 229. A combination of holiday treats and cockiness from my success led me to stray and my weight shot right back up to 270. I tried Medifast and lost 34 pounds in 30 days, but also developed kidney stones. I have never known such pain.

When I finally committed myself 100 percent to the McDougall Maximum Weight-Loss Plan (see page 216), I stopped counting calories, ate only when I was hungry, and ate exclusively from the approved list of foods. I set a goal of 175 pounds, though I honestly could not remember ever weighing that little. Today, weighing 159 pounds at age 55, I have exceeded that goal. My blood pressure is 100/70 millimeters of mercury, my BMI is normal at 22.9, my cholesterol is 117 milligrams per deciliter (mg/dL), and my glucose is under 100 mg/dL. I wake up in the morning excited about the day ahead and I feel better than I have in years. Food has gone from a way to stuff my feelings to the pleasure of truly tasting it for the first time. The most fun is telling people I eat 85 to 90 percent carbohydrates—some accuse me of lying!

Achieving Maximum Weight Loss

Follow this more restricted version of the Starch Solution to lose more weight more rapidly.

- Increase the amount of nonstarchy green, yellow, and orange vegetables you eat to about one-third to one-half of the food on your plate.
- Fill the remainder of your plate with starch.
- Avoid all simple sugars, including dried fruits and juices.
- Keep fresh fruits to one or two a day.
- Avoid flours and flour products, including breads, bagels, and pastas.
- Steer clear of all high-fat plant foods, such as nuts, seeds, avocados, olives, and soy-based foods.
- Eat many small meals a day rather than one or two large ones.
- Eat a simple meal plan, like sweet potatoes and broccoli or beans and rice with a nonstarchy vegetable. Greater variety results in more food consumed.
- Don't eat out at restaurants.
- Exercise more frequently to burn more calories and to tame an overactive appetite.

A word of caution: Enjoyment and satisfaction are the keys to successful diet change and weight loss. Avoid becoming too overzealous about eating very low-calorie green, yellow, and orange vegetables and reducing the starches you eat so much that you feel hungry all the time. It will make the program difficult to follow and increase your risk of giving it up. If you feel hungry, eat more starches.

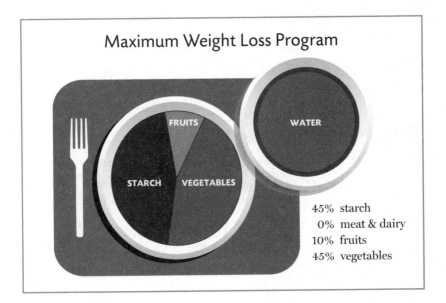

Maximum Weight Loss Program

45% starch
0% meat & dairy
10% fruits
45% vegetables

(continued from page 213)

Dinner: Thai-Style Noodles (page 295), steamed cauliflower, Banana Bread (page 311)

Enjoy hot or iced herb tea and still or sparkling water with and between meals. If you are hungry between meals, snack freely on:

- Raw or steamed green, yellow, and orange vegetables, including carrots, pea pods, peppers, celery, cucumbers, and broccoli
- Fresh fruits, including apples, bananas, berries, peaches, grapes, and melons
- Sliced, cooked potatoes, sweet potatoes, or yams, hot or chilled
- Corn thins, rice crackers, and whole grain crackers, all with no added fats or oils
- Whole wheat bread
- Corn tortillas with salsa
- Air-popped corn seasoned with soy sauce or nutritional yeast

- Seasoned nori seaweed

- Dr. McDougall's Right Foods cups (available in grocery stores)

- Any leftovers from meals on the plan or from the recipes in Chapter 15

McDougall Weekly Menu Planner

On the next page is a weekly menu planner that I recommend you copy and fill in with several weeks' worth of meals. The recipes you choose can be as simple or varied as you like. Start by filling in the daily breakfast sections. This should be easy, because people tend to eat the same items for breakfast every day. In our home we eat oatmeal with fruit almost every morning because it's simple, tasty, satisfying, inexpensive, and easy to prepare.

Next, choose your favorite recipes to fill in the dinner sections. When doing this, remember to plan your meal around a starch (potatoes, rice, etc.) and keep it simple. Lunches can simply be leftovers from the previous night's dinner or a sandwich made with one of the spreads from Chapter 15 and layered with lettuce, tomatoes, onions, and other vegetables.

Complete three or four different weekly menus so that you will be able to alternate them from week to week. This way you will avoid the panic that hits when you realize you haven't planned ahead. Make a weekly shopping list on the back of your menu planners so you will be prepared to buy all of the ingredients when you shop.

McDougall Weekly Menu Planner

	SUNDAY	MONDAY	TUESDAY	WEDNESDAY	THURSDAY	FRIDAY	SATURDAY
Breakfast							
Lunch							
Dinner							

CHAPTER 15

Our Favorite Recipes

BY MARY MCDOUGALL

Starting the Day

These breakfast favorites will get your day off to a strong start. Many of these recipes also work well for supper or snacking.

SUPER SIMPLE OVERNIGHT CEREAL

Prepared the night before in almost no time, this breakfast makes mornings deliciously easy.

PREP: 5 MINUTES • SERVES 1

1 cup rolled oats

1 cup soy milk or rice milk, apple juice, or water

1 tablespoon currants or raisins

$\frac{1}{2}$ teaspoon ground cinnamon

Sliced bananas, fresh berries, or other fruits (optional)

Stir together the oats, milk or juice or water, currants, and cinnamon in a bowl or airtight container until everything is well coated. Cover and refrigerate overnight.

In the morning, enjoy the cereal cold or heat in a microwave oven until hot. Top with fruit before serving, if you wish.

FLUFFY PANCAKES

Sparkling water keeps these easy pancakes light and fluffy. Use all whole wheat pastry flour for heartier cakes—you'll be surprised at how light they remain. My grandson, Jaysen, and I prefer these plain, but a little pure maple syrup or applesauce on top is good, too.

> To make the pancakes ahead of time, prepare the batter and refrigerate overnight. When you are ready to cook the pancakes, add a bit more soy milk, rice milk, or sparkling water until the consistency of the batter is similar to when it was first prepared. The cooked pancakes can be refrigerated overnight or frozen for up to a week in individual zip-top bags. Thaw frozen pancakes in their packaging overnight in the refrigerator. Enjoy the refrigerated or thawed pancakes cold as a snack, or microwave on high power for about 30 seconds, until they are warm.

PREP: 10 MINUTES | COOK: 10 MINUTES • MAKES 10 TO 12

$3/4$ cup whole wheat pastry flour

$3/4$ cup unbleached all-purpose flour or whole wheat pastry flour

2 teaspoons baking powder

Dash of salt

1 tablespoon Ener-G Egg Replacer

1 cup mashed ripe bananas (2 to 3 bananas)

1 cup soy milk or rice milk

$1/2$ cup sparkling water

1 tablespoon Sunsweet Lighter Bake

1 tablespoon fresh lemon juice

$1/3$ cup fresh blueberries (optional)

Mix together the whole wheat and all-purpose flours, baking powder, and salt in a medium bowl.

In another medium bowl, whisk the Egg Replacer with $\frac{1}{4}$ cup warm water until frothy. Add the bananas, mixing well. Add the milk, sparkling water, Lighter Bake, and lemon juice until well mixed. Stir the banana mixture into the dry ingredients just until combined. Gently stir in the blueberries, if you are using them.

Heat a nonstick griddle over medium heat. When it is hot, ladle pancakes onto the griddle, using $\frac{1}{4}$ cup per pancake, allowing space for them to spread. When bubbles form on the surface, use a spatula to flip them over. Cook until lightly browned. Repeat with the remaining batter.

Serve immediately.

FRENCH TOAST

I like to cook up a batch, then refrigerate or freeze individual slices in zip-top bags. A quick heating in the toaster or microwave oven and breakfast is ready. Substitute a tablespoon of brown sugar for the dates if you wish. The turmeric is for color; if you don't have it, just leave it out.

PREP: 10 MINUTES | COOK: 15 MINUTES • MAKES 12 SLICES

2 cups Cashew Milk (page 249)

3 tablespoons chopped, pitted dates

$\frac{1}{8}$ teaspoon ground cinnamon

Dash of ground turmeric

12 slices whole wheat bread

Pure maple syrup, fruit sauce, or fruit spread, for serving

Process 1 cup of the Cashew Milk and the dates, cinnamon, and turmeric in a blender until smooth. Add the remaining 1 cup Cashew Milk and blend a few more moments.

Pour the mixture into a bowl and dip slices of bread in it, one at a time, coating them well.

Heat a nonstick griddle or skillet over medium heat. Cook as many slices as your pan will handle at a time, turning until both sides are evenly browned.

Serve warm with toppings of your choice.

Pumpkin-Walnut Muffins

When I make these mildly spiced muffins for my grandchildren Jaysen, Ben, and Ryan, they are all standing around the kitchen counter eagerly waiting to get a warm one from the first batch. We bake the muffins in standard-size silicone muffin cups, available online and at most cookware stores. After cooling for about 10 minutes, the muffins pop right out of the cups; no liners needed.

PREP: 20 MINUTES | BAKE: 30 MINUTES • MAKES 12

2 teaspoons Ener-G Egg Replacer

1 cup whole wheat pastry flour

$^3/_4$ cup unbleached all-purpose flour

$^1/_2$ cup dark brown sugar

$1^1/_2$ teaspoons ground cinnamon

1 teaspoon baking soda

1 teaspoon ground nutmeg

$^1/_2$ teaspoon baking powder

$^1/_8$ teaspoon salt

$^1/_2$ cup coarsely chopped walnuts

$^1/_4$ cup raisins

1 cup canned pumpkin

$^1/_2$ cup Sunsweet Lighter Bake

$^1/_4$ cup molasses

$^1/_4$ cup soy milk

Have ready a 12-cup standard-size silicone muffin pan or line a muffin pan with liners.

Preheat the oven to 375°F with a rack in the lower third of the oven. Whisk the Egg Replacer with $^1/_4$ cup warm water in a small bowl until frothy, then set aside.

In a large bowl, whisk together the whole wheat and all-purpose flours, brown sugar, cinnamon, baking soda, nutmeg, baking powder, and salt. Stir in the walnuts and raisins.

In a separate bowl, stir together the pumpkin, Lighter Bake, molasses, and soy milk until no lumps remain. Add the reserved Egg Replacer. Stir this mixture into the flour mixture just until combined.

Spoon the batter into the prepared muffin cups and bake for 30 minutes, or until they are golden and a wooden pick inserted in the center comes out clean. Set the pan on a rack to cool completely before removing the muffins from the pans.

Blueberry Muffins

Use fresh or frozen blueberries to enjoy these muffins all year round. To use frozen berries, thaw them in the bag, drain in a large sieve, then gently toss with about a tablespoon of flour in the sieve, shaking out any excess.

PREP: 20 MINUTES | BAKE: 25 MINUTES • MAKES 12

1 tablespoon Ener-G Egg Replacer

1 cup whole wheat pastry flour

1 cup white whole wheat flour or whole wheat pastry flour

2 teaspoons baking powder

$\frac{1}{8}$ teaspoon sea salt

$\frac{1}{2}$ cup applesauce

$\frac{1}{2}$ cup agave nectar

$\frac{1}{2}$ cup soy milk or rice milk

1 teaspoon pure vanilla extract

1 teaspoon fresh lemon juice

1 cup blueberries

Have ready a 12-cup standard-size silicone muffin pan or line a muffin pan with liners.

Preheat the oven to 350°F. Whisk the Egg Replacer with $\frac{1}{4}$ cup warm water in a small bowl until frothy, then set aside.

Stir together the whole wheat pastry and white whole wheat flours, baking powder, and salt in a large bowl.

In another bowl, stir together the applesauce, agave nectar, milk, vanilla, and lemon juice. Add the reserved Egg Replacer. Stir this mixture into the flour mixture just enough to combine. Use a spatula to gently fold in the berries.

Spoon the batter into the prepared muffin cups and bake for

25 minutes, or until they are golden and a wooden pick inserted in the center comes out clean. Set the pan on a rack to cool completely before removing the muffins from the pans.

Whole Wheat Biscuits

Serve these biscuits warm from the oven, either plain or with fruit spread. Fold in blueberries for a breakfast biscuit, or leave them out to serve with salads and soups. These are best the day they are made, but you can store leftover biscuits at room temperature in a tightly sealed bag for up to 2 days.

PREP: 15 MINUTES | BAKE: 16 TO 18 MINUTES • MAKES 12

2 cups white whole wheat flour or 1 cup each all-purpose and whole wheat flour

$\frac{2}{3}$ cup rolled oats

$\frac{1}{4}$ cup granulated sugar

2 teaspoons baking powder

$\frac{1}{4}$ teaspoon salt

$\frac{2}{3}$ cup soy milk or rice milk

$\frac{1}{2}$ cup sparkling water

$\frac{1}{4}$ cup Sunsweet Lighter Bake

1 teaspoon fresh lemon juice

$\frac{2}{3}$ cup fresh blueberries (optional)

Preheat the oven to 400°F.

Stir together the flour, oats, sugar, baking powder, and salt in a medium bowl.

In a small bowl, whisk together the milk, sparkling water, Lighter Bake, and lemon juice. Add this mixture to the flour mixture, stirring just until combined. Gently fold in the blueberries, if you are using them.

Use a scoop or spoon to scoop out 12 even mounds of the batter onto a nonstick or lined baking sheet, spacing them evenly to allow for spreading. Bake 16 to 18 minutes, until the tops are golden.

Cool the biscuits on a wire rack and serve warm.

Hash Brown Potatoes

Use fresh or frozen potatoes in this McDougall breakfast staple. If using frozen potatoes, there's no need to thaw them first, though they will take a little longer to cook. You can easily shred your own potatoes in a food processor—skins on, or off for a more pristine look. To vary, mix some chopped onion and bell peppers into the potatoes before cooking.

PREP: 2 MINUTES | COOK: 15 TO 20 MINUTES • SERVES 2

4–5 cups fresh or frozen shredded potatoes

Heat a nonstick skillet over medium-high heat for 30 seconds. Add all of the potatoes to the dry pan, flattening them slightly with the back of a spatula or a fork. Cover the pan with a lid and cook until they begin to brown, 5 to 8 minutes. Use a spatula to turn the potatoes in one large round or break into pieces while flipping. Cook the potatoes until they are heated through and evenly browned, 7 to 10 minutes, turning as often as you wish.

Serve immediately.

Potato Pancakes

A food processor makes easy work of grating the potatoes and onion. Grate the potatoes right before making these to prevent browning. (It's your choice whether to include the skins or not.) Depending on your mood and what you are eating them with, these are good topped with applesauce, ketchup, barbecue sauce, gravy, or fresh salsa.

PREP: 20 MINUTES | COOK: 30 MINUTES • MAKES 6

4 or 5 russet potatoes, grated

$\frac{1}{2}$ onion, peeled and grated

5 tablespoons white whole wheat flour

3 tablespoons parsley, chopped

Preheat the oven to 200°F.

Mix the potatoes, onion, flour, parsley, and 3 tablespoons of water in a medium bowl until everything is well combined.

Ladle about ¼ cup of the mixture for each pancake onto a hot, non-stick griddle, flattening slightly with a metal spatula. Cook 5 to 8 minutes on one side, until golden, then turn and cook 5 to 8 minutes on the other side. Continue making the pancakes in batches until you have used all of the batter.

As you finish each batch, transfer the pancakes to a plate and hold in the warm oven until you have cooked all of them.

Serve warm.

No-Huevos Rancheros

This vegan version of a Mexican breakfast uses scrambled tofu in place of eggs. The scramble is good on its own, or tuck it into tortillas with a spoonful of salsa. For a creamy finish, top with a dollop of Tofu Sour Cream (page 242). For the beans, smash some warm, cooked beans with a fork or use the Smashed Slow-Cooked Beans on page 306.

PREP: 10 MINUTES | COOK: 8 MINUTES • SERVES 4

¼ cup vegetable broth

½ cup chopped scallions (green and white parts)

1 pound firm tofu, drained well and mashed with a fork

1 teaspoon regular or reduced-sodium soy sauce

¼ teaspoon ground turmeric

1 tablespoon chopped green chile peppers (optional)

Chopped fresh cilantro (optional)

Dash of salt

Freshly ground black pepper

8 small soft corn tortillas

2 cups cooked pinto beans, warmed and smashed

Salsa fresca, for serving

Pour the vegetable broth into a large nonstick skillet. Add the scallions and cook, stirring frequently, for about 3 minutes, until they soften. Add the tofu, soy sauce, turmeric, and the peppers, if using. Cook and stir for about 5 minutes, until the mixture is hot. Stir in the cilantro, if using, and salt and pepper to taste. Set the skillet aside, off the heat.

To serve, warm and soften the tortillas briefly on a dry nonstick griddle. Center a tortilla on a plate, spread with warm beans, then top with another tortilla and more beans. Spoon some of the tofu scramble over the tortilla stack. Top with salsa, or serve the salsa in a bowl at the table. Repeat to make the remaining servings. Serve immediately.

STELLA BLUES TOFU SCRAMBLE

My daughter, Heather, and I love the tofu scramble at Stella Blues Cafe on Maui, where they serve it with country-style potatoes and onions. This is my rendition of the dish, and I like it even better than the original. We serve it on its own, over Potato Pancakes (page 227), or with a side of Hash Brown Potatoes (page 227) for breakfast, lunch, or dinner.

PREP: 15 MINUTES | COOK: 12 MINUTES • SERVES 4

4 cups small broccoli florets

1 bunch scallions (green and white parts), chopped

1 pound fresh mushrooms, sliced

1 pound firm tofu, drained and cut into $\frac{1}{2}$" cubes

$\frac{3}{4}$ cup Tahini Sauce (page 247)

2 teaspoons regular or reduced-sodium soy sauce

Sriracha hot sauce (optional)

Steam the broccoli over boiling water just until it is tender, about 5 minutes. Remove from the heat, drain, and set aside.

Put the scallions and mushrooms in a large nonstick skillet with 2 tablespoons of water. Cook over medium-high heat, stirring frequently, for 5 minutes, until they begin to soften. Add the tofu and cook for 3 minutes. Add the Tahini Sauce, soy sauce, the reserved broccoli, and a few squirts of Sriracha, if you wish. Mix and cook 2 to 3 minutes, until everything is heated through and the sauce has thickened slightly.

Serve immediately.

Veggies Benedict

Use your creativity to come up with endless variations of this dish using steamed broccoli, spinach, sautéed mushrooms, or other vegetables in place of or in addition to the tomato and avocado. The sauce is also very good served over steamed asparagus, other vegetables, or thick-sliced, cooked potatoes. It can be prepared up to a day ahead; cover tightly and refrigerate, then reheat gently over low heat, whisking steadily to prevent scorching.

PREP: 15 MINUTES | COOK: 5 MINUTES • SERVES 2 TO 4

1 tablespoon cornstarch

1 cup Cashew Milk (page 249)

2 tablespoons fresh lemon juice

1 teaspoon nutritional yeast

$\frac{1}{2}$ teaspoon onion powder

$\frac{1}{8}$ teaspoon garlic powder

$\frac{1}{8}$ teaspoon salt

$\frac{1}{16}$ teaspoon ground turmeric

Pinch of paprika

2 fat-free English muffins, split

1 vine-ripened tomato, cut into 4 slices

$\frac{1}{2}$ avocado, sliced

Stir the cornstarch with 2 tablespoons of cold water in a small bowl until it is completely dissolved. Set aside.

In a saucepan, whisk together the Cashew Milk, lemon juice, nutritional yeast, onion and garlic powders, salt, turmeric, and paprika. Add the cornstarch mixture, mixing well. Bring to a boil over low heat, stirring constantly, then continue to cook and stir until the mixture is smooth and thick. Set aside.

Toast the English muffin halves and place 1 or 2 halves per serving onto plates. Top each muffin half with a tomato slice and some of the avocado. Ladle the sauce over the muffin halves and serve immediately.

East-West Breakfast

This breakfast is a great way to use leftover cooked potatoes and rice. It's great served plain, spiced up with salsa, or rolled into tortillas. Store leftovers in the refrigerator, tightly covered, for up to 4 days; reheat in a saucepan over medium heat or in a microwave oven.

PREP: 15 MINUTES | COOK: 10 MINUTES • SERVES 4

1 cup vegetable broth

$\frac{1}{2}$ cup chopped onion

$\frac{1}{2}$ cup chopped red bell pepper

$\frac{1}{2}$ cup chopped celery

2 large red potatoes, boiled and cut into large chunks

1 cup cooked brown rice

1 cup chopped fresh spinach

1 tablespoon regular or reduced-sodium soy sauce

$\frac{1}{2}$ teaspoon ground cumin

Dash of Tabasco sauce (optional)

Put $\frac{1}{2}$ cup of the broth in a large nonstick skillet along with the onion, bell pepper, and celery. Cook, stirring occasionally, for 5 minutes, until the vegetables soften. Add the potatoes and the remaining $\frac{1}{2}$ cup broth and cook for 5 minutes.

Stir in the rice, spinach, soy sauce, and cumin. Cook and stir until everything is heated through and the spinach has softened slightly. Season with a dash or two of Tabasco sauce, if desired.

Serve immediately.

Salads

Salad doesn't always have to mean a bowl of leafy greens. Most of the time we skip those light, unsatisfying versions in favor of heartier combinations of potatoes, grains, and vegetables.

Many of these salads make a complete meal, perhaps accompanied by a slab of whole grain bread. Others are perfect on the side with your favorite sandwiches, soups, or main dishes.

See Dressings, Sauces, and Condiments (page 242) for more recipes you can use to season and dress your own creations.

YUKON POTATO SALAD

This is our family's favorite potato salad. Tossing the potatoes with a bit of vinegar after cooking gives them a burst of flavor. We enjoy this best served slightly warm.

> Yukon Gold potatoes have a naturally buttery color and flavor—there's no need to add fat. Yellow Finns or red- or white-skinned new potatoes also work well in this salad.

PREP: 20 MINUTES | COOK: 10 TO 12 MINUTES | REST: 30 MINUTES • SERVES 6

2 pounds Yukon Gold potatoes, peeled and cut into large chunks

3 tablespoons white wine vinegar

$\frac{1}{2}$ cup Tofu Mayonnaise (page 243)

1 tablespoon soy milk or almond milk

1 tablespoon prepared mustard

1 tablespoon chopped parsley

$\frac{1}{4}$ teaspoon chopped fresh dill fronds or dried dill weed

$\frac{1}{4}$ teaspoon salt

Freshly ground black pepper

$^1\!/_2$ cup finely chopped celery

$^1\!/_2$ cup chopped scallions (green and white parts)

$^1\!/_2$ cup shredded carrots (optional)

Put the potatoes in a large pot and cover them with cold water. Bring to a boil, then reduce the heat to cook the potatoes at a slow boil just until they are tender, 10 to 12 minutes. Drain the potatoes well, then put them in a large bowl, toss with the vinegar, and let sit for 30 minutes.

To make the dressing: In a small bowl, whisk together the Tofu Mayonnaise, milk, mustard, parsley, dill, salt, and pepper to taste. Set aside.

After the potatoes have cooled for 30 minutes, add the celery, scallions, carrots (if you are using them), and the dressing. Stir gently to mix.

Serve immediately or refrigerate, covered, for up to 24 hours and serve cold.

VEGETABLE TABBOULEH

This tabbouleh is fresh and delicious on its own. For a heartier meal, add 2 cups of cooked or canned chickpeas or kidney, black, or white beans. If using canned beans, be sure to rinse and drain them well before adding.

PREP: 15 MINUTES | HYDRATE: 30 MINUTES | CHILL: 2 TO 3 HOURS • SERVES 8

1 cup bulgur wheat

2 cups boiling water

3 tomatoes, chopped

1 cucumber, chopped

1 green bell pepper, chopped

6 scallions (green and white parts), chopped

1 cup chopped parsley

$^1\!/_2$ cup chopped fresh mint

$^1\!/_2$ cup fresh lemon juice

Freshly ground black pepper

Put the bulgur in a medium bowl and pour the boiling water over it. Cover the bowl and set the bulgur aside for 30 minutes to hydrate. Transfer the bulgur to a colander to drain.

While the bulgur hydrates, combine the tomatoes, cucumber, bell pepper, scallions, parsley, and mint in a large bowl. Stir in the drained bulgur, the lemon juice, and pepper to taste.

Stir well, then cover and refrigerate until cold, 2 to 3 hours. Serve cold.

Macaroni Salad

Make this summertime salad a day ahead to allow the flavors to develop. Feel free to substitute or add any vegetables you like. We often add bite-size broccoli florets.

PREP: 30 MINUTES | CHILL: AT LEAST 4 HOURS • SERVES 6 TO 8

12 ounces elbow macaroni

1 cup Tofu Mayonnaise (page 243) or Nasoya Fat-Free Nayonaise

1 teaspoon prepared mustard

2 tablespoons chopped parsley

$1/2$ teaspoon dried dill weed

1 cup finely chopped celery

1 cup finely chopped green bell pepper

1 cup finely chopped red bell pepper

$1/4$ cup chopped scallions (green and white parts)

$1/4$ cup shredded carrots

Salt

Freshly ground black pepper

Cook the macaroni according to package directions or in plenty of boiling water until it is just tender, about 8 minutes. Drain and set aside to cool.

In a large bowl, whisk together the Tofu Mayonnaise, mustard, parsley, and dill. Stir in the celery, green and red bell peppers, scallions, and carrots. Add the macaroni and stir gently until everything is evenly coated. Add salt and pepper to taste.

Cover and refrigerate at least 4 hours or up to 1 day before serving.

Summer Tomato Panzanella

My daughter, Heather, returned home from a trip craving a bread salad she'd enjoyed while away. She created this one, which is best when it's made with vine-ripened tomatoes from the garden or farmers' market.

PREP: 20 MINUTES | REST: 15 MINUTES • SERVES 4

1 loaf fat-free French or Italian-style bread, crusts on, cut into 1" cubes

1 cucumber, cut into $\frac{1}{2}$" cubes

1 green bell pepper, seeded and cut into $\frac{1}{2}$" cubes

3 ripe tomatoes, cut into $\frac{1}{2}$" cubes

$\frac{1}{2}$ cup chopped fresh basil

$\frac{1}{4}$ cup kalamata olives, pitted and cut into quarters

1 cup Fat-Free Balsamic Vinaigrette (page 244) or bottled vinaigrette

3 cloves garlic, crushed or minced

2 tablespoons hot water

2 tablespoons vegetable broth

2 teaspoons balsamic vinegar

Preheat the oven to 300°F.

Spread out the bread cubes on a baking sheet and bake for 15 minutes to dry. Let cool on the sheet.

Put the cucumber, bell pepper, tomatoes, basil, and olives in a large bowl.

In a small bowl, whisk together the Fat-Free Balsamic Vinaigrette, garlic, water, vegetable broth, and vinegar.

About 15 minutes before serving, add the toasted bread cubes to the vegetable mixture and mix to distribute the ingredients evenly. Add the dressing and toss again. Let the salad stand for 15 minutes before serving to allow the bread cubes to soak up some of the dressing.

Pasta Salad with Avocado and Tomatoes

This simple summer salad should be made using the nicest avocados and tomatoes you can find. You can let the teenagers loose on this one—it's easy enough for them to make and enjoy on their own. This salad is best served the day it is made.

PREP: 10 MINUTES | COOK: 10 MINUTES • SERVES 4

3 cups medium pasta shells or other shapes

3 ripe tomatoes, chopped

2 avocados, peeled, seeded, and chopped

2 or 3 cloves garlic, crushed or minced

2 tablespoons fresh lime juice

Salt

Freshly ground pepper

Cook the pasta in plenty of boiling water until it is al dente, about 8 minutes. Drain and rinse under cool running water.

Combine the tomatoes, avocado, garlic, and lime in a large bowl. Add the pasta and stir gently to coat it evenly. Add salt and pepper to taste.

Serve immediately, or cover and refrigerate for several hours and serve chilled.

Picnic Lentil Salad

I began making this salad 25 years ago, when we lived in Hawaii. We would take it along on our beach excursions.

> If you can't find sweet onions, soak chopped yellow or white onions in cold water for 5 minutes and drain before adding them to the salad.

PREP: 15 MINUTES | COOK: 30 MINUTES | CHILL: 3 HOURS • SERVES 6

1 cup dried lentils

2 tablespoons red wine vinegar

$\frac{1}{2}$ cup chopped parsley

1 clove garlic, crushed or minced

1 tablespoon regular or reduced-sodium soy sauce

2 teaspoons Dijon mustard

1 teaspoon vegetarian Worcestershire sauce

$\frac{1}{2}$ teaspoon dried oregano

1 cup grated carrots

$\frac{1}{2}$ cup chopped sweet onion

Freshly ground black pepper

Put the lentils in a medium saucepan with 4 cups of water. Bring to a boil, reduce the heat, cover, and cook for about 30 minutes, until the lentils are tender but still firm. Drain well.

In a large bowl, whisk together the vinegar, parsley, garlic, soy sauce, mustard, Worcestershire sauce, oregano, and 1 tablespoon of water. Add the carrots, onion, lentils, and pepper to taste, stirring gently to coat everything evenly with the dressing.

Cover and refrigerate at least 3 hours or up to 2 days before serving.

Fiesta Mexican Salad

For variety, substitute kidney or pinto beans for the black beans in this hearty dish that provides starch in three forms: rice, beans, and corn. Consider this one for a picnic or potluck—it holds well in a cooler.

PREP: 10 MINUTES • SERVES 4 TO 6

$2\frac{1}{2}$ cups cooked brown rice

1 can (15 ounces) black beans, drained and rinsed

1 cup fresh or frozen and thawed corn kernels

1 tomato, chopped

4 scallions (green and white parts), chopped

$\frac{1}{2}$ cup salsa fresca

$\frac{1}{4}$ cup Tofu Mayonnaise (page 243) or Nasoya Fat-Free Nayonaise

Gently stir together the rice, beans, corn, tomatoes, and scallions in a large bowl.

In a small bowl, mix the salsa and Tofu Mayonnaise until well combined. Pour over the rice and bean mixture and stir to coat everything well.

Serve immediately, or cover and refrigerate up to 24 hours.

RAINBOW SALAD

This salad is fantastic with fresh peas and corn when they are in season. If they're not in season, frozen corn and peas work perfectly well; simply thaw at room temperature before adding them.

PREP: 15 MINUTES | CHILL: 2 HOURS • SERVES 6 TO 8

3 cups cooked brown rice

1 can (15 ounces) kidney beans, drained and rinsed

1 can (15 ounces) chickpeas, drained and rinsed

1 can (15 ounces) black beans, drained and rinsed

1 cup fresh or frozen and thawed corn kernels

1 cup peas

$\frac{1}{4}$ cup finely chopped red onion

$\frac{1}{4}$ cup finely chopped pimiento

2 tablespoons chopped black olives

2 tablespoons chopped fresh cilantro

$\frac{3}{4}$ cup bottled or homemade fat-free salad dressing

1 tablespoon regular or reduced-sodium soy sauce

$\frac{1}{2}$ teaspoon Tabasco sauce

Put the rice and all of the beans and the chickpeas in a large bowl; stir to combine. Add the corn, peas, onion, pimiento, olives, and cilantro and mix again.

In a small bowl, whisk together the salad dressing, soy sauce, and Tabasco until smooth. Pour the dressing over the salad and mix to coat everything well.

Cover the salad and refrigerate at least 2 hours or up to 2 days before serving. Taste and adjust the seasonings right before serving.

Quinoa Market Salad

Quinoa provided strength and endurance to the ancient Incas as they prepared for battle. You can purchase this grain—which is actually a seed—in bulk at many natural food stores, or in packages where you find pasta and rice in your grocery store.

> Before cooking, always rinse quinoa in a strainer under cool running water for several minutes, agitating it with your fingers, to remove its natural bitter coating.

PREP: 15 MINUTES | COOK: 15 MINUTES | CHILL: 2 HOURS • SERVES 6 TO 8

1 cup quinoa, rinsed well in a strainer under cool running water

$\frac{1}{2}$ red bell pepper, chopped

$\frac{1}{2}$ green bell pepper, chopped

$\frac{1}{2}$ yellow bell pepper, chopped

$\frac{1}{2}$ orange bell pepper, chopped

1 small zucchini, chopped

2 tomatoes, chopped

1 bunch scallions (green and white parts), coarsely chopped

1 can (15 ounces) chickpeas, drained and rinsed

$\frac{1}{2}$ cup parsley, coarsely chopped

$\frac{1}{4}$ cup fresh cilantro, coarsely chopped

$\frac{1}{8}$ cup fresh mint, coarsely chopped

$\frac{1}{2}$ cup fresh lemon juice

1 tablespoon regular or reduced-sodium soy sauce

Several dashes of Tabasco sauce

Freshly ground black pepper

Stir the drained quinoa with 2 cups of water in a medium saucepan. Bring the mixture to a boil, reduce the heat, cover, and simmer for 15 minutes, or until the quinoa is tender and the water is absorbed. Remove from the heat, cover, and set aside.

While the quinoa cooks, combine the bell peppers (all colors), zucchini, tomatoes, scallions, chickpeas, parsley, cilantro, and mint in a bowl. Add to the cooked quinoa and stir to combine. Add the lemon juice, soy sauce, Tabasco, and pepper to taste; mix well.

Cover and refrigerate for at least 2 hours or up to 8 hours.

My Caesar Salad

The versatile dressing for this salad can be made several hours in advance and refrigerated in a jar until serving time; shake well before adding it to the salad. Store any leftover dressing tightly covered in the refrigerator for up to 1 week to use on any green salad. For a more traditional Caesar salad, toss in some dry toasted bread cubes just before serving. Miyoko Schinner, cookbook author and one of our McDougall Program cooking instructors, taught me how to make this dressing about 8 years ago and it has become my family's favorite salad dressing!

Almond meal is made by grinding the nuts until they are almost the texture of flour. You can find almond meal at Trader Joe's, Bob's Red Mill, or natural food stores. To make your own, grind unsalted, blanched or skin-on, raw almonds in a food processor until very fine, taking care not to go so far that you make almond butter. (Using cold nuts helps to prevent this.) Store almond meal in the freezer for up to 6 months.

PREP: 15 MINUTES • SERVES 4

2 tablespoons almond meal

3 tablespoons Dijon mustard

3 tablespoons nutritional yeast

3 cloves garlic, crushed or minced

3 tablespoons fresh lemon juice

2 tablespoons regular or reduced-sodium soy sauce

2 heads romaine lettuce, washed, spun dry, and torn into pieces

Put the almond meal, mustard, nutritional yeast, and garlic into a 12-ounce jar. Stir with a fork to make a paste. Add the lemon juice, soy sauce, and 1 tablespoon of water. Close the jar tightly and shake vigorously to mix.

Put the lettuce in a large bowl. Shake the dressing well, then pour about half of it over the lettuce. Toss, taste, and continue to toss in dressing until the salad is dressed the way you like.

Eggless Egg Salad

This salad has morphed more than a few times over the 20-plus years I have been making it. The only ingredients that have stayed the same are the tofu that serves as the base of the salad and the turmeric that gives it the yellow color of egg salad. If there is something you have always liked in egg salad, feel free to try it here. A little pickle relish, perhaps?

Serve the salad on a bed of greens or spread it on bread or bagels, adding lettuce, tomatoes, pickles, or other toppings of your choice.

PREP: 10 MINUTES | CHILL: 2 HOURS • MAKES 1¾ CUPS

1 package (14 ounces) firm tofu, drained well and mashed with a
    fork

¼ cup Tofu Mayonnaise (page 243) or Nasoya Fat-Free Nayonaise

¼ cup finely chopped celery

2 tablespoons finely chopped onion

2 teaspoons vinegar

½ teaspoon ground turmeric

¼ teaspoon onion powder

¼ teaspoon garlic powder

¼ teaspoon dried dill weed

¼ teaspoon salt

Put the tofu in a bowl and add the rest of the ingredients. Mix well.

Cover tightly and refrigerate for at least 2 hours or up to 2 days before serving.

Dressings, Sauces, and Condiments

These dressings and sauces will not only dress up the recipes in this book but also help you get started creating new dishes of your own.

In a pinch, turn to the oil-free dressings, salsas, and other condiments at your local supermarket or natural food store. You will also find our quick and easy No-Parmesan Cheese recipe, as well as Cashew Milk, a terrific base for creating creamy sauces.

Tofu Taco Topping

We use this quick topping on our Tex-Mex Potatoes (page 289). It also makes a very good dip for cooked, chilled potato chunks or raw vegetables.

PREP: 5 MINUTES | CHILL: 3 HOURS

1 package (12.3 ounces) silken tofu, drained in a fine-mesh strainer

$\frac{1}{2}$–1 packet taco seasoning mix

Combine the tofu and seasoning mix in a food processor until very smooth. Taste, and add more of the taco seasoning for a spicier flavor, if desired. Transfer to a bowl.

For best flavor, cover and chill for several hours before serving.

Tofu Sour Cream

This makes a great substitute for sour cream. Refrigerating the mixture for a few hours before using it allows it to thicken and the flavors to develop.

PREP: 5 MINUTES | CHILL: 2 HOURS • MAKES 1½ CUPS

1 package (12.3 ounces) silken tofu, drained in a fine-mesh strainer

$2\frac{1}{2}$ tablespoons fresh lemon juice

$2\frac{1}{2}$ teaspoons granulated sugar

Dash of salt

Combine the drained tofu, lemon juice, sugar, and salt in a food processor and process until the mixture is completely smooth.

Transfer to an airtight container, cover, and refrigerate for at least 2 hours or up to 2 weeks.

Tofu Mayonnaise

This is my go-to creamy mayonnaise for dressings and sandwiches.

PREP: 5 MINUTES • MAKES 1½ CUPS

1 package (12.3 ounces) silken tofu, drained in a fine-mesh strainer

1½ tablespoons fresh lemon juice

1 teaspoon granulated sugar

½ teaspoon salt

¼ teaspoon mustard powder

⅛ teaspoon ground white pepper

Combine the drained tofu, lemon juice, sugar, salt, mustard, and pepper in a food processor and process until the mixture is completely smooth. Transfer to an airtight container, cover, and refrigerate for at least 2 hours or up to 1 week.

Tofu Island Dressing

This thick, flavorful dressing with bits of vegetables can be used in salads and on sandwiches in place of Thousand Island.

PREP: 5 MINUTES | CHILL: 2 HOURS • MAKES ABOUT 2 CUPS

1 package (12.3 ounces) silken tofu, drained in a fine-mesh strainer

3 tablespoons ketchup

1 teaspoon regular or reduced-sodium soy sauce

1 tablespoon fresh lemon juice

2 tablespoons sweet pickle relish

1 tablespoon finely chopped red onion

1 tablespoon finely chopped parsley

Freshly ground black pepper

Combine the tofu, ketchup, soy sauce, lemon juice, and ⅓ cup water in a blender or food processor and process until smooth. Transfer to a bowl and stir in the relish, onion, parsley, and pepper to taste. Transfer to an airtight container, cover, and refrigerate for at least 2 hours or up to 1 week.

Fat-Free Balsamic Vinaigrette

A tasty oil-free bottled salad dressing is difficult to come by, and getting it right at home isn't easy, either. This dressing solves the problem of both taste and texture. It's worth splurging on top-quality vinegars to create a dressing with great flavor.

The secret to this creamy vinaigrette is a bit of xanthan or guar gum (often available in natural food stores), which gives it enough viscosity to coat salad greens without running off. These gums can be used to thicken other uncooked sauces and dressings, as well.

PREP: 10 MINUTES | CHILL: 2 HOURS • MAKES 2½ CUPS

¼ cup balsamic vinegar

¼ cup apple cider vinegar

¼ cup red wine vinegar

¼ cup unseasoned rice wine vinegar

3–4 cloves garlic

¼ cup ketchup

1 tablespoon Dijon mustard

1–2 tablespoons agave nectar

½ teaspoon xanthan gum or guar gum

Pour the balsamic, cider, wine, and rice vinegars into a blender. Add the garlic, ketchup, mustard, 1 tablespoon of the agave, and 1 cup of water. Blend until the mixture is very smooth. With the blender running, slowly add the xanthan or guar gum through the top to avoid forming clumps. Continue to blend until the dressing is smooth and thickened. (The dressing will thicken further as it chills.) Taste, and add more agave if you like.

Refrigerate the dressing in a tightly covered container for at least 2 hours or up to 2 weeks before serving.

CREAMY CILANTRO-GARLIC DRESSING

Include some cilantro stems along with the leaves for the boldest flavor. Or improvise by substituting other fresh herbs for the cilantro: basil, parsley, or mint all make a lively dressing.

PREP: 5 MINUTES | CHILL: 1 HOUR • MAKES ABOUT 2 CUPS

1 package (12.3 ounces) silken tofu, drained in a fine-mesh strainer

$\frac{1}{2}$ cup rice wine vinegar

$\frac{1}{4}$ cup regular or reduced-sodium soy sauce

2–3 cloves garlic, crushed or minced

$\frac{1}{2}$ bunch fresh cilantro

Combine the tofu, vinegar, soy sauce, and garlic in a blender or food processor and blend or process until smooth. Add the cilantro and process again just until the cilantro is chopped.

Pour the dressing into a jar, cover, and refrigerate for at least 1 hour or up to 5 days.

CITRUS-CHILI DRESSING

To make a thicker dressing that clings better to salad greens, add up to $\frac{1}{2}$ teaspoon of xanthan gum or guar gum to the blender through the feed tube while it is running, then chill the dressing for 20 to 30 minutes to let it thicken.

PREP: 5 MINUTES • MAKES ABOUT 1½ CUPS

1 cup orange juice

$\frac{1}{4}$ cup Dijon mustard

$\frac{1}{2}$ cup rice wine vinegar

2 cloves garlic

1 tablespoon chili powder

1 tablespoon sweet Thai chili sauce, such as Mae Ploy

Combine the juice, mustard, vinegar, garlic, chili powder, and chili sauce in a blender and blend until smooth.

Refrigerate leftover dressing in an airtight container for up to 1 week.

Red Pepper Aioli

We use this aioli as a dip for raw veggies, a spread for crackers or bread, and as a change of pace from ketchup on our burgers.

PREP: 10 MINUTES | CHILL: AT LEAST 1 HOUR • MAKES 2 CUPS

1 package (12.3 ounces) silken tofu, drained in a fine-mesh strainer

1/2 cup jarred roasted red peppers, drained

2 tablespoons fresh lemon juice

1 tablespoon apple cider vinegar

Dash of salt

Process the tofu in a food processor until smooth. Add the peppers, lemon juice, vinegar, and salt and continue to blend for several minutes until very smooth.

Refrigerate in an airtight container for at least 1 hour or up to 4 days.

Enchilada Sauce

This versatile red sauce is the one I use in our Tamale Pie (page 285) and Potato Enchiladas (page 293). Keep some on hand in the fridge and I am certain you will find many other uses for it as well.

PREP: 5 MINUTES | COOK: 5 MINUTES • MAKES ABOUT 2½ CUPS

1 can (8 ounces) tomato sauce

1–1½ tablespoons chili powder

2 tablespoons cornstarch

1/4 teaspoon onion powder

1/8 teaspoon garlic powder

Whisk together the tomato sauce, chili powder, cornstarch, onion and garlic powders, and 1½ cups of cold water in a saucepan. Cook and stir over medium heat until the sauce thickens, about 5 minutes.

Serve warm. Refrigerate leftover sauce in an airtight container and refrigerate for up to 1 week. Reheat in a saucepan over low heat, stirring with a whisk, until warm.

Spicy Peanut Sauce

Used sparingly, just a small amount of this higher-fat dressing adds lots of flavor. We use the sauce to dress lettuce, sweet potatoes, raw or steamed vegetables, or brown rice.

PREP: 5 MINUTES • MAKES 2 CUPS

$\frac{3}{4}$ cup natural peanut butter

$\frac{3}{4}$ cup rice wine vinegar

$\frac{1}{4}$ cup regular or reduced-sodium soy sauce

1–2 tablespoons sambal oelek (Indonesian chili paste)

$\frac{1}{4}$ cup warm water

$\frac{1}{8}$ cup cilantro leaves

Combine the peanut butter, vinegar, soy sauce, and chili paste in a blender and blend until smooth and creamy. Add the warm water and cilantro leaves and process until well mixed.

Use immediately, or transfer to an airtight container and refrigerate for up to 1 week.

Tahini Sauce

We use this sauce in our Stella Blues Tofu Scramble (page 229) and Falafel Wraps (page 255). This is a higher-fat sauce because of the tahini, so use it sparingly. For a spicier taste, stir in a squirt or two of Sriracha or other hot sauce.

PREP: 5 MINUTES • MAKES 2 CUPS

$\frac{3}{4}$ cup raw or toasted tahini (sesame paste)

$\frac{1}{4}$ cup fresh lemon juice

2 cloves garlic, crushed or minced

Combine the tahini, lemon juice, garlic, and 1 cup of water in a food processor or blender and process or blend until smooth. Use immediately, or transfer to an airtight container and refrigerate for up to 3 days.

Marsala Mushroom Sauce

We use this sauce in our Yukon Stuffed Peppers (page 292), but it also works as a topping for grains, potatoes, pasta, or vegetables.

PREP: 15 MINUTES | COOK: 15 MINUTES • MAKES 3½ CUPS

2 leeks, white and light green parts only, thinly sliced

¾ pound fresh mushrooms, wiped clean, thinly sliced

½ teaspoon chopped fresh oregano (leaves only)

½ teaspoon chopped fresh sage (leaves only)

¼ cup regular or reduced-sodium soy sauce

⅛ cup Marsala wine (may be omitted)

3½ tablespoons cornstarch

Put the leeks and mushrooms in a saucepan with ½ cup of water. Cook over medium heat, stirring occasionally, for 5 minutes to soften the vegetables. Add the oregano, sage, soy sauce, wine, and 3 cups of water. Bring to a boil, reduce to a simmer and cook, uncovered and stirring occasionally, for 8 minutes.

In a small bowl, stir the cornstarch with ¼ cup of cold water to dissolve it. Add the cornstarch mixture to the sauce, stirring constantly. Continue to stir the sauce over medium heat until it boils and thickens slightly.

Golden Gravy

We use this comforting gravy on our New Old-Fashioned Tofu Loaf (page 282) but it is also very good over hash browns or mashed potatoes. I use brown rice flour, which is so forgiving that you can even whisk it into a smooth, lump-free sauce at the end of the cooking time.

PREP: 5 MINUTES | COOK: 10 MINUTES • MAKES ABOUT 2 CUPS

1½ cups vegetable broth

3 tablespoons regular or reduced-sodium soy sauce

2 tablespoons tahini (sesame paste)

¼ cup brown rice flour

Freshly ground black pepper

Pour the broth into a saucepan and stir in ½ cup of water. Whisk together the soy sauce and tahini in a small bowl, then whisk the mixture into the saucepan. Stir the mixture as you bring it to a boil.

Reduce the heat to a simmer and continue to stir as you sprinkle the brown rice flour slowly over the top, about a tablespoon at a time, until it is completely incorporated and begins to thicken. When it is the consistency of gravy, add pepper to taste, and serve immediately.

Refrigerate leftover gravy in an airtight container for up to 4 days. (The gravy will be very thick when it is cold.) Reheat in a saucepan over medium heat, adding a bit of water to thin if needed.

No-Parmesan Cheese

Our vegan substitute for Parmesan cheese contains no processed ingredients. It's perfect for shaking over soups, stews, and pastas.

PREP: 5 MINUTES • MAKES 2 CUPS

1 cup almond meal (page 240)

1 cup nutritional yeast

Dash of onion powder

Dash of salt (optional)

Put the almond meal, nutritional yeast, and onion powder in a jar. Cover and shake well. Taste and add a little salt if you wish; shake again.

Cover the jar and refrigerate for up to 1 month.

Cashew Milk

For 28 years, this has remained my favorite base for sauces and French toast. Be sure to use raw cashews (or blanched almonds).

PREP: 5 MINUTES • MAKES 2 CUPS

½ cup raw cashews

Combine the cashews with 1 cup of water in a blender and blend until smooth. Add another cup of water and continue to blend 1 to 2 minutes. Pour the mixture through a fine-mesh strainer into a bowl and discard the solids.

Refrigerate in a tightly covered container for 2 to 3 days.

Burgers and Wraps

The chance to roll up your favorite fillings in a tortilla or flatbread, just the way you like, makes wraps more fun than sandwiches. They're easy to make, and many of the recipes provide great leftovers.

Be sure to choose tortillas with no added fat, preferably made from corn or whole wheat, water, and few if any other ingredients. Just before serving, soften the tortillas one at a time on a dry nonstick griddle, or wrap them in a tea towel and warm them in the microwave oven just until they are soft and pliable.

Burgers can do double duty as lunch or supper. We avoid the supermarket type made from processed soy—they are no more healthful than the fast foods they're meant to mimic. Instead, we make our own hearty, satisfying burgers from beans and whole grains. You know exactly what you are eating, and you'll be surprised at how much better they taste.

Serve any of the burgers on whole wheat buns with lettuce, tomato, onions, and your favorite condiments, such as pickles or pickle relish, ketchup, mustard, or a dab of the Tofu Mayonnaise on page 243. Red Pepper Aioli (page 246) also makes a terrific burger topping.

Do I hear the lunch bell?

McDougall Veggie Burgers

Our McDougall Veggie (McVeggie) burgers have withstood the test of time: My family still requests them 30 years after I first served them. For authentic barbecue flavor, finish the baked burgers for a few minutes on the grill.

To prepare ahead, shape and bake the burgers, then refrigerate for up to 2 days, or freeze for up to 3 months in a zip-top bag or airtight container. Reheat the frozen burgers on a plate in a microwave oven for about 2 minutes, or on a dry griddle for about 5 minutes.

PREP: 30 MINUTES | BAKE: 40 MINUTES • MAKES 16

20 ounces firm tofu, well drained

1 package (12.3 ounces) silken tofu, drained in a fine-mesh strainer

3 cups quick-cooking oats

1 package (10 ounces) frozen chopped spinach, thawed, drained, and squeezed dry

1 large onion, chopped

$\frac{1}{2}$ pound mushrooms, chopped

3 cloves garlic, crushed or minced

2 tablespoons regular or reduced-sodium soy sauce

2 tablespoons vegetarian Worcestershire sauce

2 tablespoons Dijon mustard

1 teaspoon paprika

1 teaspoon fresh lemon juice

$\frac{1}{2}$ teaspoon freshly ground black pepper

Whole wheat buns and condiments, for serving

Preheat the oven to 350°F. Have ready two nonstick or parchment-lined baking sheets.

Combine the drained firm and silken tofu in a food processor and process until smooth, stopping several times to scrape down the bowl. Transfer the tofu to a large bowl and mix in the oats and spinach.

Put the onion, mushrooms, and garlic in a large nonstick skillet with $\frac{1}{2}$ cup of water. Cook over medium heat, stirring frequently, until the onion softens and all of the liquid has evaporated, 10 to 12 minutes. Add the onion-mushroom mixture to the tofu mixture, along with the soy sauce, Worcestershire sauce, mustard, paprika, lemon juice, and pepper. Mix very well, using your hands if you wish.

Use moistened hands to shape the mixture into 16 $\frac{1}{4}$"-thick patties, arranging them on the prepared baking sheets. Bake for 20 minutes, flip the burgers, then bake them for 20 minutes on the other side.

Serve the burgers warm on buns with the usual condiments.

LENTIL-POTATO BURGERS

These healthful, flavorful burgers are a great convenience. Freeze any remaining baked burgers in an airtight container or zip-top bag for up to 3 months. Reheat the frozen burgers on a plate in a microwave oven for about 2 minutes, or on a dry griddle for about 5 minutes.

PREP: 50 MINUTES | BAKE: 40 MINUTES • MAKES 12

1 cup dried lentils

2 cups frozen chopped hash brown potatoes

$\frac{1}{4}$ cup chopped onion

$\frac{1}{2}$ cup quick-cooking oats

$\frac{1}{2}$ teaspoon ground sage

$\frac{1}{2}$ teaspoon ground thyme

$\frac{1}{2}$ teaspoon ground marjoram

$\frac{1}{4}$ teaspoon poultry seasoning

Freshly ground black pepper

Whole wheat buns and condiments, for serving

Put the lentils in a saucepan with 2 cups of water. Cook over medium heat, covered, until the lentils are very soft and the water has been absorbed, about 40 minutes. Remove from the heat and set aside.

While the lentils cook, put the frozen potatoes into another saucepan with 2 cups of water. Cook over medium heat, uncovered, until the potatoes are soft and all of the water has evaporated, about 20 minutes. Remove from the heat and set aside.

Preheat the oven to 350°F. Have ready two nonstick or parchment-lined baking sheets.

Place the chopped onion in a small saucepan with $\frac{1}{4}$ cup of water. Cook over medium heat, stirring occasionally, until the onion softens, about 5 minutes. Remove from the heat and set aside.

Stir together the cooked lentils, potatoes, and onion in a large bowl until they are well mixed. Add the oats, sage, thyme, marjoram, and poultry seasoning, and pepper to taste. Mix well.

Use moistened hands to shape the mixture into 12 patties, arranging them on the prepared baking sheets. Bake for 20 minutes, flip the burgers, and bake for 20 minutes on the other side.

Serve the burgers warm on buns with the usual condiments.

TAMALE BURGERS

We tuck these burgers into tortillas, but you could also form them into patties and serve them on buns. Either way, Mexican toppings are the perfect condiments. Freeze any remaining baked burgers in an airtight container or zip-top bag for up to 3 months and reheat on a plate in a microwave oven for about 2 minutes, or on a dry griddle for about 5 minutes.

PREP: 30 MINUTES | REST: 20 MINUTES | CHILL: 30 MINUTES | GRILL: 15 MINUTES •
MAKES 8 TO 10

$\frac{1}{3}$ cup masa harina (see page 307)

2 tablespoons vegetable broth

1 onion, finely chopped

1 small red bell pepper, seeded and finely chopped

$\frac{3}{4}$ cup fresh or frozen and thawed corn kernels

1 chipotle chile pepper in adobo sauce, finely chopped

2 teaspoons adobo sauce, from can

2 cloves garlic, crushed or minced

1 teaspoon ground cumin

3 cups cooked brown rice, warmed

$\frac{1}{2}$ cup chopped fresh cilantro

$\frac{3}{4}$ teaspoon lime peel

$1\frac{1}{2}$ tablespoons fresh lime juice

8 to 10 corn tortillas

Lettuce, tomatoes, avocado, and taco sauce, for serving

Mix the masa harina with $\frac{1}{2}$ cup water in a small bowl; set aside.

Pour the vegetable broth into a medium nonstick saucepan and add the onion, bell pepper, corn, chile, adobo sauce, garlic, and cumin. Cook, stirring occasionally, until the vegetables soften, about 10 minutes. Add the masa harina and mix well (mixture will be very thick). Cover the saucepan and cook over low heat, stirring once or twice, for 5 minutes.

Put the warmed rice in a large bowl and add the masa-vegetable mixture, along with the cilantro, lime peel, and lime juice. Mix very well. Set aside for 20 minutes.

Line two baking sheets with parchment paper. Fill a small bowl with water and place it by a work surface, along with the baking sheets.

Moisten your hands with the water, then pinch off and shape the mixture into 8 to 10 oblong, flattened burgers that fit across the middle of a tortilla. Arrange the shaped burgers on the baking sheets. Refrigerate the burgers on the baking sheets for 30 minutes.

Prepare a charcoal or gas grill, or heat a stovetop grill or griddle. Grill the burgers over medium heat until crusty, about 7 minutes per side.

To serve, place a burger on a tortilla, add toppings, fold up, and eat.

SLOPPY LENTIL JOES

These quick and easy sloppy joes reheat well. Refrigerate in an airtight container up to 4 days; reheat in a saucepan over low heat, stirring, until hot.

PREP: 15 MINUTES | COOK: 1 HOUR • SERVES 8 TO 10

1 onion, chopped

1 green bell pepper, chopped

1 tablespoon chili powder

1½ cups dried brown lentils

1 can (15 ounces) crushed tomatoes

2 tablespoons regular or reduced-sodium soy sauce

2 tablespoons prepared mustard

2 tablespoons brown sugar

1 teaspoon rice wine vinegar

1 teaspoon vegetarian Worcestershire sauce

Freshly ground black pepper

Whole wheat buns and condiments, for serving

Put ⅓ cup of water into a large saucepan and add the onion and bell pepper. Cook over medium heat, stirring occasionally, until the onion softens, about 5 minutes. Stir in the chili powder.

Add the lentils, tomatoes, soy sauce, mustard, brown sugar, vinegar, Worcestershire sauce, pepper to taste, and 3 cups of water; mix well. Bring the mixture to a boil, reduce the heat to low, cover, and simmer slowly for 55 minutes, stirring occasionally.

To serve, ladle the mixture over split whole wheat buns.

FALAFEL WRAPS

The traditional bread for falafel is pita, and the traditional way to serve it is with all the toppings on the table in bowls so that guests can make their own the way they like it best. But when I watched my daughter, Heather, mix all the toppings together in a bowl, then wrap them in a whole wheat tortilla, I realized this was even easier. I don't expect I will ever look back. Of course, you can still use the stuffing to fill a split pita. If you wish to further reduce the fat, substitute a no-fat hummus for the tahini.

> To make oil-free falafels, purchase bulk or boxed falafel mix and follow the instructions to mix. Instead of frying, bake the falafels on a nonstick baking sheet at 375°F until they are nicely browned, about 10 minutes per side, or brown them on a nonstick griddle with no oil.

PREP: 20 MINUTES (USING PREPARED FALAFEL) • SERVES 6 TO 8

Tahini Sauce (page 247)

¼ cup fresh lemon juice

1 tomato, chopped

1 cup chopped cucumber

3 scallions (green and white parts), chopped

Sriracha hot sauce

1 cup chopped lettuce

3 cups baked falafel, cut into large chunks

Whole wheat pita breads or tortillas

Put the Tahini Sauce in a medium bowl and mix in the lemon juice, tomato, cucumber, scallions, and Sriracha to taste. Mix in the lettuce and the baked falafel chunks.

To serve, tuck the falafel mixture into pita halves or roll up in tortillas.

Spicy Tofu Tacos with Shredded Cabbage and Cilantro-Garlic Aioli

Cabbage adds crunch and aioli punch to these colorful tacos. The elements all come together quickly enough for an impromptu lunch or dinner.

PREP: 30 MINUTES | COOK: 10 MINUTES • SERVES 6 TO 8

TOFU

¼ cup regular or reduced-sodium soy sauce

2 tablespoons fresh lime juice

2 tablespoons chili powder

2 teaspoons ground cumin

2 teaspoons garlic powder

½ teaspoon ground red pepper

24 ounces extra-firm tofu, drained and cut into ½" cubes

CABBAGE

4 cups finely shredded cabbage

3 tablespoons seasoned rice wine vinegar

½ tablespoon fresh lime juice

AIOLI

1½ cups Tofu Sour Cream (page 242)

⅓ cup cilantro leaves, coarsely chopped

2 large cloves garlic, crushed or minced

2 tablespoons fresh lime juice

Pinch of salt

12 small corn or whole wheat tortillas, warmed

Hot sauce (optional)

To make the tofu: Stir together the soy sauce, lime juice, chili powder, cumin, garlic powder, and pepper in a large bowl. Add the tofu, mix gently to coat, then let stand for 10 minutes to absorb the flavors.

Set a large nonstick skillet over medium heat. Add the tofu and all of the marinade. Cook, stirring occasionally, until the tofu begins to brown and crisp, about 10 minutes. Set aside.

To make the cabbage: Stir together the cabbage, vinegar, and lime juice in a medium bowl.

To make the aioli: Stir together the Tofu Sour Cream, cilantro, garlic, lime juice, and salt in a small bowl.

To serve, spoon some of the warm tofu mixture down the center of a tortilla and top with cabbage, aioli, and hot sauce, if desired. Roll up the tacos and serve.

FRESH TOMATO WRAPS

In August, when our garden is overflowing with fresh tomatoes, this is one of my favorite ways to use them. Perfect for those hot northern California late summer nights.

PREP: 15 MINUTES | CHILL: 30 MINUTES • SERVES 4 TO 6

2 cups chopped fresh tomatoes

1 can (15 ounces) black or pinto beans, drained and rinsed

1 cup chopped avocado

½ cup chopped scallions (green and white parts)

2 tablespoons chopped cilantro

2 tablespoons fresh lime juice

1 tablespoon chopped jalapeño pepper (optional)

Tabasco, Sriracha, or other hot sauce

Salt

4–6 corn or whole wheat tortillas, warmed

Chopped romaine lettuce, for serving

In a medium bowl, gently stir together the tomatoes, beans, avocado, scallions, cilantro, lime juice, and jalapeño, if using (wear plastic gloves when handling). Add a bit of hot sauce and salt, to taste. Cover and refrigerate for 30 minutes or up to 2 hours.

To serve, place a tortilla on a plate and lay down a line of the tomato mixture across the center. Top with lettuce and more hot sauce if you wish. Roll up and enjoy.

Baja Vegetable Wraps

Make the filling for these wraps once for a week of quick-fix lunches. Simply refrigerate in a covered container for up to 1 week and warm before serving, either in a saucepan over medium heat, stirring, or in a microwave oven. Set aside some of the cilantro to stir in just before serving. For variety, serve the filling over baked potatoes or cooked whole grains.

PREP: 20 MINUTES | COOK: 20 MINUTES • SERVES 6 TO 8

1 onion, chopped

1 green bell pepper, chopped

1 carrot, halved lengthwise, then sliced

1 clove garlic, crushed or minced

$\frac{1}{2}$ cup vegetable broth

1 bunch scallions (green and white parts), cut into 1" pieces

$1\frac{1}{2}$ cups sliced napa cabbage

1 tablespoon regular or reduced-sodium soy sauce

1 teaspoon chili powder

1 teaspoon oregano leaves

2 cups chopped fresh tomatoes

2 cups (packed) chopped fresh spinach

2 cans (15 ounces each) black beans, drained and rinsed

$\frac{1}{2}$ cup salsa fresca

1–2 tablespoons chopped fresh cilantro

Tabasco or other hot sauce

6 to 8 whole wheat tortillas, warmed

Put the onion, bell pepper, carrot, and garlic in a large saucepan. Add the vegetable broth and cook over medium heat, stirring occasionally, until the vegetables begin to soften, about 5 minutes. Add the scallions, napa cabbage, soy sauce, chili powder, and oregano and cook, stirring occasionally, for 10 minutes. Add the tomatoes, spinach, beans, and salsa and cook 5 minutes longer. Remove the saucepan from the heat and stir in the cilantro and hot sauce to taste.

Put a tortilla on a plate, spoon the filling across the center, roll up, and eat.

Barbecue Tofu Wraps

Feel free to substitute your favorite type of beans for the black beans in these roll-ups.

PREP: 20 MINUTES | COOK: 10 MINUTES • SERVES 6 TO 8

1 package (14 ounces) firm tofu, drained and cut into 1/2" cubes

3 teaspoons white wine vinegar

1 1/2 teaspoons ground cumin

1 1/2 teaspoons chili powder

1/2 cup vegetable broth

1 onion, chopped

1 red bell pepper, chopped

1 can (15 ounces) black beans, drained and rinsed

1 cup cooked brown rice

1 cup fresh or frozen and thawed corn kernels

3/4 cup barbecue sauce

6–8 whole wheat tortillas, warmed

Shredded lettuce, chopped tomatoes, chopped onion, and/or salsa, for topping (optional)

Put the tofu in a shallow bowl and add the vinegar, cumin, and chili powder. Stir gently to coat the tofu. Set aside.

Put the vegetable broth in a nonstick skillet and add the onion and bell pepper. Cook, stirring occasionally, until the vegetables soften, about 5 minutes. Stir in the beans, rice, corn, and barbecue sauce and cook, stirring occasionally, for 2 minutes. Add the reserved tofu and cook 3 minutes, giving it an occasional gentle stir.

To serve, lay a tortilla on a plate and spoon the mixture down the middle. Top with any of the optional toppings, roll up, and eat.

Hoisin-Tofu Lettuce Wraps

These wraps are fun to eat, but be prepared with the napkins—they can get messy. To reduce the fat, leave out the pine nuts and add ½ cup of chopped water chestnuts to the tofu as it cooks, and add an extra tablespoon of hoisin sauce.

PREP: 15 MINUTES | COOK: 10 MINUTES • SERVES 2

12 ounces firm tofu, drained and cut into ¼" cubes

3 tablespoons rice wine vinegar

2 tablespoons regular or reduced-sodium soy sauce

1 tablespoon granulated sugar

¼ teaspoon sambal oelek (Indonesian chili paste)

Drizzle of sesame oil

1 tablespoon hoisin sauce, plus more for serving

1 cup chopped fresh cilantro or Italian parsley

½ cup toasted pine nuts

8 iceberg or butter lettuce leaves

Put the tofu in a bowl and add the vinegar, soy sauce, sugar, sambal, and sesame oil. Stir gently to coat.

Heat a nonstick skillet over medium-high heat and add the tofu and all of the sauce in the bowl. Cook, stirring constantly, until the pan is dry, 3 to 4 minutes. Stir in the hoisin sauce, then the cilantro or parsley, continuing to heat and stir for 1 minute. Remove the pan from the heat and stir in the pine nuts.

To serve, put a lettuce leaf on a plate, spread with a little hoisin if desired, put some of the tofu across the middle, roll up, and eat.

Spreads for Wraps

ARTICHOKE SPREAD

This is delicious as a spread for sandwiches, as a dip for crackers or veggies, or stuffed into pita bread and topped with chopped tomatoes, cucumbers, and sprouts.

PREP: 10 MINUTES • MAKES 3 CUPS

2 cans (14 ounces) artichoke hearts in water, drained and rinsed

1 can (15 ounces) white beans, drained and rinsed

4 tablespoons lemon juice

2 cloves garlic, crushed

4 scallions, chopped

1 tablespoon soy sauce or low-sodium soy sauce

$\frac{1}{2}$ teaspoon ground red pepper

Combine all ingredients in a food processor and process until smooth.

NOT-TUNA SPREAD

This is a McDougall Program favorite, wonderful for spreading on a thick, hearty sandwich with lettuce, tomatoes, and onions.

PREP: 10 MINUTES | CHILL: 1 HOUR • MAKES 2 CUPS

1 can (15 ounces) chickpeas, drained and rinsed

$\frac{1}{4}$ cup Tofu Mayonnaise (page 243) or Nasoya Fat-Free Nayonaise

$\frac{1}{4}$ cup finely chopped onion

$\frac{1}{4}$ cup finely chopped celery

$\frac{1}{4}$ cup finely chopped scallions

1 tablespoon lemon juice

Place the chickpeas in a food processor and process until coarsely chopped, or mash with a bean masher. Do not overprocess to a smooth consistency. Place in a bowl, add the remaining ingredients, and mix well. Chill for at least 1 hour or up to 4 days.

Soups and Stews

These hearty soups and stews will quell any concern you may have had that following the Starch Solution would leave you hungry. Far from it—these dishes provide ample sustenance to keep your belly satisfied.

Soups and stews are also great for making ahead and reheating. In fact, many taste even better on the second day, after the flavors have had some time to develop. Add a salad and a slab of whole grain bread and you have yourself a satisfying meal.

Miso Soup

This simple, flavorful soup is light enough to enjoy on a hot summer night or at the start of a more substantial dinner. To turn the soup into a meal, add cooked soba or udon noodles when you add the miso.

PREP: 10 MINUTES | COOK: 5 MINUTES | REST: 2 MINUTES • SERVES 4

1 ounce wakame seaweed

$\frac{1}{4}$ cup mellow white miso

1 package (12.3 ounces) silken tofu, cut into small cubes

$\frac{1}{8}$ cup regular or reduced-sodium soy sauce

4 scallions (green and white parts), chopped

Put the wakame in a bowl and cover it with water. Soak for 5 minutes. Drain, squeeze out all the water with your hands, then cut the seaweed into bite-size pieces. Set aside.

Bring 4 cups of water to a boil in a saucepan. Put the miso in a small bowl and stir in $\frac{1}{2}$ cup of the boiling water until it forms a smooth paste. Return the miso mixture to the pan, stir, and cook 1 minute. Stir in the tofu, soy sauce, and the reserved seaweed. Stir gently, turn off the heat, and add the scallions. Let rest 2 minutes before serving.

CHUNKY GAZPACHO

I serve versions of this refreshing, cold tomato soup throughout the summer months, especially on those Santa Rosa nights when it is too hot to think of lighting a burner. To cut down on prep time, use a food processor instead of chopping the vegetables by hand. Beyond that, it is simple to make. Refrigerate any leftover soup, tightly covered, for up to 3 days.

PREP: 20 TO 40 MINUTES | CHILL: ABOUT 3 HOURS • SERVES 10

2 large ripe tomatoes

4 cups tomato juice

1 cup chopped cucumber

$\frac{1}{2}$ cup chopped red onion

$\frac{1}{2}$ cup chopped celery

$\frac{1}{2}$ cup fresh or frozen and thawed corn kernels

$\frac{1}{2}$ cup chopped green bell pepper

$\frac{1}{4}$ cup chopped scallions (green and white parts)

$\frac{1}{4}$ cup chopped zucchini

$\frac{1}{4}$ cup chopped canned green chiles

$\frac{1}{4}$ cup chopped parsley

$\frac{1}{4}$ cup chopped cilantro

1–2 cloves garlic, crushed or minced

2 tablespoons red wine vinegar

2 tablespoons lime juice

1 tablespoon Tabasco or other hot sauce (optional)

Peel the tomatoes using a serrated peeler, or dip them briefly into a pot of boiling water, then quickly transfer them to a bowl of ice water to keep them from cooking. The skins should easily slip off.

Seed and chop the peeled tomatoes and place them in a large bowl. Stir in the tomato juice, cucumber, red onion, celery, corn, green pepper, scallions, zucchini, chiles, parsley, cilantro, garlic, vinegar, and lime juice.

Cover and refrigerate until very cold, about 3 hours. Add the hot sauce, if desired, or allow guests to add it at the table.

Serve cold.

Minestrone Soup

I have many varieties of minestrone that I make throughout the fall and winter months, but this one is our favorite. You may use any type of uncooked pasta that you prefer; we like spaghetti broken into 2" pieces.

PREP: 30 MINUTES | COOK: 3 HOURS • SERVES 8

1¼ cups dried red kidney beans

1 onion, chopped

1 teaspoon minced garlic

1 rib celery, chopped

1 carrot, sliced into rounds

6–8 fingerling potatoes, cut into chunks

½ cup fresh green beans, cut into 1" pieces

1 cup tomato sauce

¼ cup parsley

1½ teaspoons dried basil

1½ teaspoons dried oregano

½ teaspoon dried marjoram

¼ teaspoon celery seed

¼ teaspoon ground black pepper

1 can (15 ounces) chickpeas, drained and rinsed

1 can (15 ounces) chopped tomatoes

1 zucchini, chopped

1½ cups shredded cabbage

½ cup uncooked whole wheat elbow pasta

Place the beans in a large pot with water to cover. Bring to a boil, cook for 2 minutes, turn off the heat, and let rest for 1 hour. (To eliminate this step, soak beans overnight.) Drain off water. Add onion, garlic, and 8 cups of fresh water. Bring to a boil, reduce heat, cover, and cook for 1 hour. Add celery, carrot, potatoes, green beans, tomato sauce, and all the seasonings. Return to a boil, reduce heat, and cook for 45 minutes. Add the chickpeas, canned tomatoes, and zucchini. Cook for another 30 minutes. Then add the cabbage and pasta and cook for an additional 30 minutes.

Quick Black Bean Soup

This is great to make ahead of time and then heat just before serving. Make a double batch so you can enjoy a quick bowl of soup when you are hungry.

PREP: 5 MINUTES | COOK: 10 MINUTES • SERVES 2 TO 4

3 cans (15 ounces) black beans, drained and rinsed

$1\frac{3}{4}$ cups vegetable broth

1 cup salsa fresca

$\frac{1}{4}$–$\frac{1}{2}$ teaspoon ground oregano

$\frac{1}{4}$ teaspoon chili powder (or more, to taste)

$\frac{1}{8}$ teaspoon smoked chipotle chili powder

Several dashes hot sauce (optional)

Reserve 1 cup of the beans in a separate bowl. Place the remaining beans, the vegetable broth, and the salsa in a blender jar. Process until fairly smooth and pour into a saucepan. Mash the reserved beans slightly with a fork or bean masher. Add to the saucepan with the remaining ingredients. Cook over medium heat for 10 minutes to blend flavors. Adjust seasoning to taste before serving.

Tortilla Soup

Make this with canned tomatoes when fresh tomatoes are not available or not very desirable (during the winter months). Use 1 can (15 ounces) of chopped tomatoes and add tomatoes with the beans and corn.

PREP: 15 MINUTES | COOK: 30 MINUTES • SERVES 6

4 cups vegetable broth

1 onion, chopped

$\frac{1}{2}$ cup chopped green bell pepper

$1\frac{1}{2}$ cups fresh chopped tomatoes

1 can (15 ounces) black beans, drained and rinsed

1 cup frozen corn kernels

¼–½ cup salsa (mild, medium, or hot)

1–2 tablespoons chopped green chiles

½–¾ cup chopped avocado

¾ cup broken fat-free tortilla chips

Place ½ cup of the broth in a medium saucepan. Add the onion, bell pepper, and tomatoes. Cook, stirring occasionally, for 15 minutes over low heat. Add the remaining broth, bring to a boil, reduce heat, and add the beans and corn. Add salsa and green chiles to taste. Cook over low heat for 10 minutes. Add the avocado and adjust seasonings if necessary. Cook an additional 5 minutes. Stir in the tortilla chips just before serving.

Tomato Basil Soup

This soup makes a nice first course for a dinner party and is also very good as a sauce served over vegetables, potatoes, or pasta.

PREP: 10 MINUTES | COOK: 1 HOUR 30 MINUTES • SERVES 6 TO 8

2 cans (28 ounces each) diced tomatoes in juice

1½ cups V-8 juice

1 onion, coarsely chopped

4–6 cloves garlic, crushed or minced

1 cup (packed) fresh basil

1 cup soy milk or rice milk (optional)

Freshly ground black pepper

Put the tomatoes and their liquid, V-8 juice, onion, garlic, and basil in a large saucepan. Stir in ½ cup of water. Bring to a boil, reduce heat, cover, and simmer for 1½ hours.

Puree the soup using an immersion blender, or process it in batches in a blender or food processor, returning the soup to the pan.

Stir in the milk, if you are using it, and heat until hot but not quite boiling. Add pepper to taste.

Serve hot.

Potato Chowder

If you purchase frozen, oil-free hash brown potatoes you will have this McDougall Program favorite on the table in no time flat.

PREP: 10 MINUTES | COOK: 30 MINUTES • SERVES 4 TO 6

4 cups vegetable broth

1 onion, chopped

2 ribs celery, chopped

1 leek, white and light green parts only, thinly sliced

6 cups frozen chopped hash brown potatoes

2 cups soy milk or rice milk

$\frac{1}{8}$ teaspoon ground white pepper

2 tablespoons parsley

2 tablespoons dried chives

$\frac{1}{2}$ teaspoon sea salt (optional)

Liquid smoke (optional)

Pour $\frac{1}{2}$ cup of the broth into a large soup pot and add the onion, celery, and leek. Cook until the vegetables soften, about 5 minutes. Add the potatoes and the remaining broth. Bring the soup to a boil, then reduce the heat, cover, and simmer for 20 minutes.

Puree the soup using an immersion blender, or process it in batches in a blender or food processor, returning the soup to the pan.

Stir in the milk, pepper, parsley, chives, the salt if you are using it, and a shake of liquid smoke, if desired. Heat until hot, then serve.

Moroccan Red Lentil Soup

Versions of this lentil soup with tomatoes and chickpeas are served all over Morocco during the festival of Ramadan and to celebrate special occasions throughout the year. This is my interpretation.

We serve it with whole grain flatbread to scoop up the juices, or ladle the soup over brown rice.

1 onion, chopped

4 ribs celery, chopped

6 cups vegetable broth

1½ cups chopped tomatoes

1 cup dried red lentils

1 can (15 ounces) chickpeas, drained and rinsed

1 bay leaf

½ teaspoon ground cinnamon

½ teaspoon ground ginger

½ teaspoon ground turmeric

¼ teaspoon ground coriander

¼ teaspoon freshly ground black pepper

⅓ cup orzo

½ cup chopped cilantro

2 tablespoons fresh lemon juice

Pour ½ cup of water into a large soup pot along with the onion and celery. Cook, stirring occasionally, until the vegetables begin to soften, about 5 minutes. Add the broth, tomatoes, lentils, chickpeas, bay leaf, cinnamon, ginger, turmeric, coriander, and black pepper. Bring to a boil, reduce the heat to a simmer, then cover and simmer until the lentils are tender, about 45 minutes.

Stir in the orzo, cilantro, and lemon juice. Cook 10 minutes longer, until the orzo is al dente.

Serve hot.

Split Pea Vegetable Soup

This thick soup is filled with chunky vegetables for a comforting meal on a cool, rainy day. Mustard powder and a hint of smoked paprika give it an alluring flavor. Serve it on its own, or ladle the soup over brown rice for an even more satisfying meal. This soup will thicken as it cools, so I usually make it early in the day, then let it cool and thicken before reheating and adding the tomatoes and fresh herbs.

2 cups split peas

1 large onion, chopped

3 ribs celery, chopped

2 carrots, chopped

2 cups chopped fingerling potatoes

2 cloves garlic, crushed or minced

2 tablespoons parsley

2 bay leaves

1 teaspoon mustard powder

$\frac{1}{2}$ teaspoon smoked paprika

Freshly ground white pepper

1 large tomato, cut into $\frac{1}{2}$" cubes

$\frac{1}{2}$ cup coarsely chopped fresh cilantro or parsley

Sea salt (optional)

Put the peas in a large soup pot and add 8 cups of water. Bring to a boil over medium heat, then reduce the heat to low and simmer, uncovered, for 20 minutes. Stir in the onion, celery, carrots, potatoes, garlic, parsley, bay leaves, mustard, paprika, and white pepper. Bring back to a boil, reduce the heat, cover, and simmer until all of the vegetables are tender, about 45 minutes. Add the tomato, cilantro or parsley, and sea salt to taste, if desired.

Let rest 5 minutes before ladling into bowls.

Festive dal Soup

In India and throughout Nepal, Pakistan, Sri Lanka, and Bangladesh, split lentils, peas, and beans are used in a variety of thick soups and stews known as dal. This richly flavored and textured soup is great for using up leftover greens. For extra bite, top the dal with your favorite hot sauce.

PREP: 10 MINUTES | COOK: 1 HOUR • SERVES 4

1 onion, chopped

2 cloves garlic, crushed or minced

$1\frac{1}{2}$ teaspoons grated fresh ginger

1 teaspoon smoked paprika

$\frac{1}{2}$ teaspoon ground cumin

$\frac{1}{4}$ teaspoon ground coriander

Freshly ground black pepper

1 cup red lentils

1 can (15 ounces) chickpeas, drained and rinsed

1 can (14.5 ounces) diced tomatoes

2 cups coarsely chopped Yukon Gold potatoes

1 tablespoon fresh lemon juice

1–2 teaspoons sambal oelek (Indonesian chili paste)

2 cups coarsely chopped leafy greens, such as chard, kale, or spinach

Sea salt (optional)

Pour $\frac{1}{4}$ cup water into a large soup pot. Add the onion and garlic and cook over medium heat, stirring occasionally, until the onion softens, about 5 minutes.

Mix in the ginger, paprika, cumin, coriander, and pepper to taste. Add the lentils, chickpeas, tomatoes, potatoes, and 3 cups of water. Bring the soup to a boil, then reduce the heat, cover, and simmer until the lentils are tender, about 50 minutes.

Stir in the lemon juice, 1 teaspoon of the chili paste, and the greens. Cook until the greens are tender, 5 to 7 minutes. Taste and add more chili paste and a bit of sea salt, if desired.

Serve hot.

Quinoa Chowder

This soup is perfect for those cold winter nights that call for something simple and comforting. Fingerlings are long, narrow potatoes that look like pudgy fingers. If you can't find them, cut Yukon Gold or red new potatoes into bite-size chunks.

PREP: 15 MINUTES | COOK: 40 MINUTES • SERVES 6 TO 8

4 cups vegetable broth

$\frac{1}{2}$ cup quinoa, rinsed well in a strainer under cool running water

$2\frac{1}{2}$ cups chopped fingerling potatoes, cut into bite-size pieces

1 large onion, chopped

2–4 cloves garlic, crushed or minced

2 jalapeño peppers, seeded and finely chopped (wear plastic gloves when handling)

2 cups fresh or frozen and thawed corn kernels

4 cups fresh spinach, coarsely chopped

Chili sauce

Freshly ground black pepper

Put the broth, drained quinoa, potatoes, onion, garlic, and jalapeño peppers in a large soup pot along with 2 cups of water. Bring to a boil, reduce the heat, cover, and cook until everything is tender, about 20 minutes. Stir in the corn and cook 15 minutes. Five minutes before the soup is done, stir in the spinach. Just before serving, add some chili sauce and pepper to taste.

Serve hot, with additional chili sauce on the side for those who prefer a little more kick.

BLACK BEAN–CHIPOTLE SLOW-COOKED SOUP

This is the perfect soup for your slow cooker: Pile the ingredients into the pot in the morning and you'll have soup in time for dinner.

PREP: 10 MINUTES | COOK: 8 HOURS • SERVES 8 TO 10

2 cups dried black beans

2 cans (16 ounces each) fire-roasted chopped tomatoes

1 can (4 ounces) chopped green chiles

1 onion, chopped

2 cloves garlic, crushed or minced

1 teaspoon chili powder

1 teaspoon ground cumin

$\frac{1}{4}$ teaspoon crushed red pepper

$\frac{1}{8}$ teaspoon chipotle powder

$\frac{1}{4}$ cup chopped fresh cilantro

Put the beans, tomatoes, chiles, onion, garlic, chili powder, cumin, red pepper, and chipotle powder in a slow cooker. Stir in 6 cups of water. Cover and cook on high for 8 hours.

Serve the soup hot, stirring in the cilantro as you serve it.

Autumn Garden Vegetable Soup

This soup uses a nice variety of vegetables. Feel free to substitute your own favorites.

PREP: 45 MINUTES | COOK: 1 HOUR • SERVES 8

1 onion, chopped

4 cloves garlic, crushed or minced

2 carrots, peeled and sliced into rounds

2 ribs celery, chopped

6 cups vegetable broth

3 cups chopped Roma tomatoes

1 can (15 ounces) cannellini beans, drained and rinsed

1 can (15 ounces) small white beans, drained and rinsed

2 tablespoons regular or reduced-sodium soy sauce

2 cups sliced zucchini

2 cups small cauliflower florets

2 cups thinly sliced green cabbage

2 cups thinly sliced Swiss chard

$1/2$ cup small uncooked pasta

$1/4$ cup fresh basil, cut into fine ribbons

Freshly ground black pepper

Put the onion, garlic, carrots, and celery in a large soup pot and add $1/2$ cup of water. Cook, stirring occasionally, for 5 minutes. Stir in the broth, tomatoes, both types of beans, and the soy sauce. Bring to a boil, then reduce the heat, cover, and cook for 10 minutes. Stir in the zucchini, cauliflower, and cabbage and cook for 15 minutes. Add the chard and pasta and cook until the pasta is tender, about 10 minutes. Stir in the fresh basil and pepper to taste just before serving.

Serve hot.

Sweet Potato Bisque

Either sweet potatoes or yams work well in this soup; yams are the orange-fleshed tubers and will result in a deeper orange bisque.

PREP: 20 MINUTES | COOK: 1 HOUR • SERVES 6 TO 8

1 onion, chopped

4½ cups vegetable broth

2 jalapeño peppers, seeded and chopped (wear plastic gloves when handling)

3 cups coarsely chopped peeled sweet potato or yam

3 carrots, peeled and sliced into rounds

1 cup soy milk or rice milk

1–2 tablespoons fresh basil, cut into fine ribbons

1 tablespoon brown sugar

Dash of ground red pepper (optional)

Put the onion and ½ cup of the broth in a medium saucepan. Cook, stirring occasionally, until the onion softens, about 5 minutes. Add the jalapeños and cook 2 minutes. Add the remaining 4 cups of broth along with the sweet potatoes or yams and carrots. Bring to a boil, reduce the heat, then cover and cook until the vegetables are tender, about 45 minutes.

Puree the soup using an immersion blender, or process it in batches in a blender or food processor, returning the soup to the pan.

Stir in the milk, basil, brown sugar, and ground red pepper, if using. Simmer for about 5 minutes, stirring occasionally.

Serve hot.

Broccoli Bisque

Purchase the broccoli already cut into florets to make quick work of this soup.

PREP: 10 MINUTES | COOK: 20 MINUTES • SERVES 6 TO 8

4 cups broccoli florets

3 cups vegetable broth

2 cups frozen chopped hash brown potatoes

1 onion, chopped

1 teaspoon dried dill weed

2½ cups soy milk or rice milk

1 tablespoon Dijon mustard

Dash of ground white pepper

Put the broccoli, broth, potatoes, onion, and dill weed in a medium saucepan. Bring to a boil, cover, and cook over medium heat for 15 minutes.

Puree the soup using an immersion blender, or process it in batches in a blender or food processor, returning the soup to the pan.

Stir in the milk, mustard, and white pepper. Heat until steaming and serve hot.

MUSHROOM-BARLEY SOUP

Purchasing sliced fresh mushrooms and shredded cabbage will save you some time in making this soup.

Look for the Japanese horseradish known as wasabi in powdered form in natural food stores or Asian markets.

PREP: 10 MINUTES | COOK: 1 HOUR • SERVES 4 TO 6

1 cup pearled barley

1 onion, chopped

1 tablespoon regular or reduced-sodium soy sauce

1 tablespoon parsley

2 teaspoons dill weed

½ teaspoon ground cumin

¼ teaspoon garlic powder

⅛ teaspoon freshly ground black pepper

$^{1}/_{8}$ teaspoon wasabi powder

$^{1}/_{2}$ pound fresh mushrooms, sliced

2 cups shredded cabbage

Put the barley, onion, soy sauce, parsley, dill, cumin, garlic powder, pepper, and wasabi powder in a soup pot and stir in $6^{1}/_{2}$ cups of water. Bring to a boil, then reduce the heat to medium, cover, and cook until the barley is tender, about 30 minutes. Add the mushrooms and cabbage and cook 30 minutes.

Serve hot.

VENTANA LENTIL STEW

This is my version of the revitalizing lentil stew served at the bed and breakfast where we stay when we go windsurfing in La Ventana, Mexico. We sometimes serve this over whole wheat bread or split rolls or ladled over baked potatoes or brown rice.

PREP: 10 MINUTES | COOK: 1 HOUR 15 MINUTES • SERVES 6 TO 8

1 onion, chopped

2 cloves garlic, crushed or minced

1–2 jalapeño peppers, seeded and chopped (wear plastic gloves when handling)

2 cups green lentils

2 cups chopped fingerling potatoes, cut into bite sized pieces

$^{1}/_{4}$–$^{1}/_{2}$ teaspoon chipotle chili powder

2 cups baby spinach leaves or chopped spinach

Hot sauce, for serving

Put the onion, garlic, and jalapeños in a large saucepan along with $^{1}/_{2}$ cup of water. Cook, stirring occasionally, until the onion softens, about 5 minutes. Stir in the lentils, potatoes, $^{1}/_{4}$ teaspoon chipotle powder, and $5^{1}/_{2}$ cups more water. Cover and bring the soup to a boil, then reduce the heat and simmer until the lentils are soft, about 1 hour. Stir in the spinach and cook 5 minutes. Add additional chili powder to taste.

Serve hot in bowls, with hot sauce on the side.

Pumpkin Stew in a Pumpkin

This recipe takes a little more work than most, but it makes an impressive presentation and is truly delicious. We love it as a holiday centerpiece and dinner. I suggest using one of the many gourmet pumpkin varieties rather than the regular Halloween-type pumpkin, because the flesh in the gourmet pumpkins is much more flavorful and less stringy. Some suggestions are Lumina (white skin), Jarrahdale (blue-gray skin), and Long Island Cheese (pale gold skin). All of these have a moist, delicious, deep-orange flesh.

Seitan is made from wheat gluten and has a chewy
texture. Look for it in natural food stores.

PREP: 1 HOUR | COOK: 1 HOUR 20 MINUTES • SERVES 8

2 cups vegetable broth

1 onion, chopped

1 red or green bell pepper, coarsely chopped

2 cloves garlic, crushed or minced

2 teaspoons chili powder

2 bay leaves

1½ teaspoons ground oregano

Freshly ground black pepper

3 carrots, scrubbed and cut into 1" pieces

2 ears corn, cut into 1" pieces

2 yams, peeled and cut into large chunks

2 white potatoes, peeled and cut into large chunks

1 bag (10 ounces) frozen petite whole onions

1 can (4 ounces) chopped green chiles

8 ounces seitan, cut into bite-size pieces

1 pumpkin (14–15 pounds)

2 tablespoons pure maple syrup

Put $1/4$ cup of the broth into a large saucepan and add the onion, bell pepper, and garlic. Cook, stirring occasionally, until the onion softens, about 5 minutes. Stir in the chili powder, bay leaves, oregano, and pepper to taste. Cook and stir for 2 minutes. Stir in the remaining $1^3/4$ cups broth and the carrots, corn, yams, potatoes, petite onions, chiles, and seitan. Cook over low heat, covered, for 30 minutes.

While the stew simmers, preheat the oven to 350°F.

Cut the top off the pumpkin, as you would to make a jack-o'-lantern, and set it aside. Use a large spoon to clean out and discard the seeds and strings from inside the pumpkin. Brush the inside of the pumpkin with the maple syrup and replace the top of the pumpkin. Put the pumpkin into a baking dish large enough to hold it and pour $1/2$ inch of water into the bottom. Bake for 30 minutes. Remove the pumpkin top and ladle the hot stew into the pumpkin. Replace the top, then continue to bake for 45 minutes.

To serve, scoop out bits of the pumpkin along with the stew and serve in large bowls.

TUNISIAN SWEET POTATO STEW

Once you have sampled this intoxicating combination of sweet potatoes, peanut butter, and spices you will wonder why you never thought to combine these ingredients. This hearty stew is delicious served over rice or other cooked starches. Couscous is the national dish of Tunisia and the traditional choice in this Northern African country.

PREP: 20 MINUTES | COOK: 40 MINUTES • SERVES 6 TO 8

1 onion, chopped

2 jalapeño peppers, seeded and finely chopped (wear plastic gloves when handling)

2 teaspoons finely chopped fresh ginger

2 cloves garlic, crushed or minced

2 teaspoons ground cumin

$1/2$ teaspoon ground cinnamon

$1/4$ teaspoon crushed red pepper

$1/4$ teaspoon ground coriander

5 cups peeled and coarsely chopped sweet potatoes or yams

2 cans (14.5 ounces each) coarsely chopped tomatoes

2 cans (15 ounces each) chickpeas, drained and rinsed

1 cup green beans, cut into 1" pieces

1½ cups vegetable broth

¼ cup natural peanut butter

¼ cup coarsely chopped fresh cilantro

Put the onion, peppers, ginger, and garlic into a large saucepan. Stir in ⅓ cup water and cook, stirring occasionally, for 5 minutes. Add the cumin, cinnamon, red pepper, and coriander. Cook and stir for 1 minute. Add the sweet potatoes or yams, tomatoes, chickpeas, green beans, vegetable broth, and peanut butter. Bring to a boil, reduce the heat to low, and simmer until the potatoes are tender, about 30 minutes. Stir in the cilantro, then let the stew rest for 2 minutes before serving.

Serve hot.

GLOBAL BEAN STEW

This may be made with other cooked grains, such as bulgur, kasha, millet, or rice, or even with whole wheat couscous (which is not a grain, but a pasta). Most natural food stores sell prepared low-fat hummus, or you can easily make your own by pureeing cooked chickpeas with a small amount of broth, garlic, and salt. You may also substitute chickpeas for the white beans. If you can't find baby potatoes, use larger red potatoes and chop them into bite-sized chunks. If you want to use chard or kale instead of the spinach, it will need to cook about 5 additional minutes. We like this plain in a bowl over brown rice or scooped up with baked tortilla chips.

PREP: 25 MINUTES | COOK: 1 HOUR • SERVES 6

3 cups vegetable broth

1 onion, chopped

2 ribs celery, chopped

2 carrots, chopped

1 green bell pepper, chopped

1 red bell pepper, chopped

3 cloves garlic, minced

2 cups coarsely chopped baby potatoes

2 cans (15 ounces each) cannellini beans, drained and rinsed

1 can (8 ounces) tomato sauce

$1\frac{1}{2}$ cups prepared hummus

$1\frac{1}{2}$ tablespoons parsley

$1\frac{1}{2}$ tablespoons regular or low-sodium soy sauce

1 teaspoon dried basil

$\frac{1}{2}$ teaspoon dried oregano

$\frac{1}{2}$ teaspoon smoked paprika

$\frac{1}{8}$–$\frac{1}{4}$ teaspoon crushed red pepper

$\frac{1}{2}$ cup cooked quinoa

$1\frac{1}{2}$ cups thinly sliced fresh spinach

Place $\frac{1}{2}$ cup of the broth in a large pot. Add the onion, celery, carrots, bell peppers, and garlic. Cook, stirring occasionally, for 10 minutes. Add remaining broth, potatoes, and beans. Bring to a boil, cover, reduce heat, and cook for 30 minutes. Add tomato sauce, hummus, and seasonings. Cook an additional 10 minutes. Add quinoa, mix well, and cook for 5 minutes. Stir in spinach and cook an additional 2 minutes.

CHICKPEA DELIGHT

While this cooks, it will thicken as the yams break apart and become part of the broth. This is a delicious, surprisingly sweet vegetable stew, sure to become a favorite. It can be made ahead and reheated before serving.

PREP: 20 MINUTES | COOK: 50 TO 60 MINUTES • SERVES 8

4 cups vegetable broth

1 onion, chopped

1 carrot, chopped

2 ribs celery, chopped

2 leeks, sliced (white parts only)

2 yams, peeled and cut into chunks

2 cans (15 ounces each) chickpeas, drained and rinsed

2½ cups broccoli florets

1 tablespoon lemon juice

1 tablespoon regular or low-sodium soy sauce

1½ teaspoons pure prepared horseradish

1 teaspoon ground cumin

1 teaspoon ground coriander

Dash of ground red pepper

Dash of Tabasco sauce

Pour 2 cups of the broth in a large pot. Add the onion, carrot, celery, leeks, and yams. Bring to a boil, reduce heat, and cook, uncovered, for 30 minutes. Add the chickpeas, broccoli, remaining vegetable broth, and seasonings. Mix well. Return to a boil, reduce heat, and cook an additional 20 to 30 minutes, stirring occasionally.

Serve over brown rice or other whole grains, whole wheat toast, or potatoes, or in a bowl by itself.

Main Dishes

When people first adopt a starch-based diet, they often fear that it will demand a lot from them in the kitchen. That doesn't need to be the case. If you keep your meals simple as we do, you won't find yourself overwhelmed with piles of vegetables waiting to be chopped or complicated preparations requiring every pan and utensil in the kitchen, hours of work, and burdensome cleanup. In fact, we eat mostly one-dish meals that can be prepared using just one or two pots and pans.

Another frequent misconception is that a complete dinner calls for putting several different dishes on the table. At first, I thought that too. But time has taught me that some of the best meals are composed of a casserole or pot of soup with a simple green salad and a loaf of whole grain bread.

We rely on convenient foods made of simple, fresh ingredients to keep things easy. These are not the convenience foods filled with long lists of chemicals you've never heard of and can't pronounce. Instead, they are typically one- or two-ingredient packaged foods: canned tomatoes, perhaps with a little added basil; canned beans packed in their cooking water; frozen corn kernels; vegetable broth in aseptic containers; prechopped onions and carrots; a bottle of hot sauce. Stocking these foods in your pantry and freezer makes cooking a breeze. When you have them on hand, feel free to substitute your home-cooked equivalents: cooked beans, fresh corn kernels, home-made vegetable stock, and the like. (For more on how to stock your pantry, see Chapter 13.)

The following section includes the dishes we eat day in and day out and also serve to our family, guests, and McDougall Program participants in residence. Most of the recipes can be made ahead and refrigerated for 2 or 3 days before serving, or refrigerated as leftovers for lunch the following day. Many taste great at room temperature, or can also be easily reheated in the oven, in a microwave oven, or in a saucepan on the stovetop.

New Old-Fashioned Tofu Loaf

Served with mashed potatoes (made with vegetable broth or a nondairy milk) and Golden Gravy (page 248), this tofu loaf evokes memories of a favorite comfort food from childhood. Slices of the loaf also make terrific sandwiches.

> If you don't have bread crumbs on hand, process a slice or two of day-old whole wheat bread in a food processor until it is in crumbs. In fact, it's worth processing stale bread when you have it and freezing the crumbs in a zip-top bag to have on hand for recipes.

PREP: 15 MINUTES | COOK: 1 HOUR | COOL: 5 MINUTES • SERVES 6 TO 8

30 ounces firm tofu, drained well and mashed with a fork

1²/₃ cups quick-cooking oats

³/₄ cup whole wheat bread crumbs

¹/₂ cup ketchup or barbecue sauce

¹/₃ cup regular or reduced-sodium soy sauce

2 tablespoons Dijon mustard

2 tablespoons vegetarian Worcestershire sauce

¹/₄ teaspoon garlic powder

¹/₄ teaspoon freshly ground black pepper

Preheat the oven to 350°F. Have on hand a nonstick standard or silicone loaf pan.

Put the tofu into a large bowl and add the remaining ingredients. Mix with your hands to combine everything well.

Turn the mixture into the prepared pan and bake until the top and edges are golden brown, about 1 hour. Transfer the pan to a rack to cool for 5 minutes before serving.

To serve, run a spatula around the sides of the pan to loosen, then invert the loaf onto a serving plate and cut into slices.

Artichoke Paella

Artichokes and brown rice give our take on paella fantastic texture and flavor. A pinch of saffron adds color and an earthiness that perfectly complements the artichokes. Watch out when using it—it stains!

PREP: 30 MINUTES | COOK: 40 MINUTES | REST: 5 MINUTES • SERVES 8

1 cup brown rice

2 cups boiling water

$2^1/_3$ cups vegetable broth

1 onion, chopped

2 cloves garlic, crushed or minced

$3/_4$ cup julienned green bell pepper

$3/_4$ cup julienned red bell pepper

1 package (10 ounces) frozen baby lima beans, thawed

2 small tomatoes, chopped

1 teaspoon dried oregano

$1/_4$ teaspoon sea salt

$1/_8$ teaspoon crushed red-pepper flakes

Pinch of saffron

1 can (15 ounces) water-packed artichoke hearts, drained and cut in halves

1 cup frozen peas, thawed

Put the rice into a bowl and pour the boiling water over it. Cover and let stand for 20 minutes while you prepare the remaining ingredients. After 20 minutes, drain off any excess water and set the rice aside.

Heat the vegetable broth to boiling in a saucepan. Scoop out $1/_3$ cup of the broth into a wok or large skillet with sloping sides. Add the onion and garlic and stir over medium heat until the onion softens slightly, about 3 minutes. Add the green and red peppers, lima beans, and tomatoes and cook, stirring, for 3 minutes. Stir in the oregano, salt, pepper flakes, saffron, and the reserved rice and the remaining hot vegetable broth. Bring to a boil, reduce the heat, cover, and cook for 30 minutes. Stir in the artichokes and peas.

Remove the pan from the heat, cover, and let stand for 5 minutes before serving.

Thai Green Curry Rice

This dish is made with mild Thai green curry paste sold in Asian markets, natural food stores, and some supermarkets. For a spicier variation, substitute red curry paste for the green, or serve hot sauce on the side. For an especially colorful dish, use Thai purple rice in place of the brown rice.

> Coconut extract mixed into rice milk or almond milk makes a flavorful substitution in recipes calling for coconut milk.

PREP: 20 MINUTES | COOK: 12 MINUTES • SERVES 4

$\frac{1}{3}$ cup vegetable broth

1 onion, cut into $\frac{1}{2}$" cubes

1 red bell pepper, cut into $\frac{1}{2}$" cubes

1 yellow bell pepper, cut into $\frac{1}{2}$" cubes

2 cloves garlic, crushed or minced

1–2 tablespoons Thai green curry paste

2 cups coarsely chopped napa cabbage

1 cup broccoli florets

1 cup cauliflower florets

1 cup sugar snap peas

1 tablespoon regular or reduced-sodium soy sauce

4 cups cooked long-grain brown rice

1 tomato, cut into $\frac{1}{2}$" cubes

1 tablespoon coarsely chopped fresh Thai or common (field) basil

1 tablespoon coarsely chopped fresh cilantro

1 cup almond milk or rice milk

1 teaspoon coconut extract

Place the broth in a large saucepan along with the onion, red and yellow peppers, and garlic. Cook over medium heat, stirring occasionally, for 5 minutes. Stir in 1 tablespoon of the curry paste, or up to 2 table-spoons for a spicier dish. Add the cabbage, broccoli, cauliflower, snap peas, and soy sauce. Mix well, cover, reduce the heat to low, and cook until the vegetables are tender, about 5 minutes.

Add the rice, tomato, basil, cilantro, milk, and coconut extract. Stir well, then cook until heated through, 2 to 3 minutes. Serve hot, on plates or in bowls, with chopsticks if you like.

Tamale Pie

This is a great recipe for making a day ahead. Just refrigerate overnight and all you need do the next day is put it into a preheated oven. It will take about the same amount of time, even from the fridge.

PREP: 10 MINUTES | COOK: 1 HOUR | REST: 10 MINUTES • SERVES 4 TO 6

5 cups fresh or frozen and thawed corn kernels

$\frac{1}{2}$ cup masa harina (see page 307)

$\frac{1}{4}$ cup vegetable broth

$\frac{1}{2}$ cup Tofu Sour Cream (page 242)

1 can (4 ounces) chopped green chiles

2 tablespoons chopped roasted red peppers

2 tablespoons chopped black olives

$\frac{1}{4}$ teaspoon salt (optional)

Salsa fresca, Enchilada Sauce (page 246), and/or Guacamole (page 305), for serving

Preheat the oven to 350°F. Have ready a 2-quart baking dish.

Combine the corn, masa, and broth in a food processor and process until smooth. Scrape the mixture into a large bowl and add the Tofu Sour Cream, chiles, peppers, olives, and salt, if using. Mix well.

Turn the mixture into the baking dish. Cover the dish with parchment paper, then with aluminum foil, crimping the edges over the rim of the dish, or cover with a lid. Bake until hot, about 1 hour. Let rest for 10 minutes before serving.

To serve, use a large spoon to scoop the tamale pie onto individual plates. Serve salsa, Enchilada Sauce, and/or Guacamole in bowls on the table to spoon over the top.

Polenta with Black Beans and Mango Salsa

Cooked polenta packaged in rolls makes an easy base for this and other dishes. Look for polenta that is fat free and contains cornmeal, water, and few if any other ingredients other than herbs and spices.

Sliced, packaged polenta can be baked in the oven, as it is here, or cooked on a nonstick griddle until golden on both sides. Polenta is not difficult to make from scratch; use a good-quality dry polenta (coarse cornmeal) and follow the package directions. The finished polenta should be thick enough that the mixing spoon stands up when you plunge it into the pan. To slice it, you will need to form it into rolls or press it into a pan and allow it to cool until it is firm enough to cut.

PREP: 15 MINUTES | COOK: 20 MINUTES • SERVES 6 TO 8

1 package (24 ounces) cooked polenta, cut into $\frac{1}{2}$"-thick slices

$\frac{1}{2}$ cup vegetable broth

1 onion, chopped

1 red bell pepper, chopped

1 orange or yellow bell pepper, chopped

2 cloves garlic, crushed or minced

2 cans (15 ounces each) black beans, drained and rinsed

1 can (15 ounces) crushed tomatoes

1 can (4 ounces) chopped green chiles

1 teaspoon chili powder

1 teaspoon ground cumin

Dash or two of Tabasco or other hot sauce

Freshly ground black pepper

¼ cup chopped fresh cilantro

2 cups Mango Salsa (page 306) or store-bought mango salsa

Preheat the oven to 375°F.

Place the polenta slices on a nonstick baking sheet and bake for 15 minutes.

While the polenta bakes, put the broth, onion, bell peppers, and garlic in a large saucepan. Cook, stirring occasionally, until the vegetables soften, about 5 minutes. Add the black beans, tomatoes, chiles, chili powder, cumin, hot sauce, and black pepper to taste. Cook 10 minutes. Taste and add more hot sauce if you wish. Stir in the cilantro and remove the saucepan from the heat.

To serve, arrange a few slices of polenta on each plate and top with the black bean mixture. Top with the Mango Salsa or serve it in a bowl on the side.

Bean and Corn Enchiladas

We frequently enjoy a simple dinner of mashed pinto beans and salsa tucked into tortillas. I use the leftover beans to make these flavorful enchiladas. You could also use the Smashed Slow-Cooked Beans on page 306.

PREP: 40 MINUTES | COOK: 45 MINUTES • SERVES 6 TO 8

5 cups Enchilada Sauce (page 246)

4 cups cooked pinto beans, smashed

1 cup chopped scallions (green and white parts)

1½ cups fresh or frozen and thawed corn kernels

1 can (2.25 ounces) sliced ripe olives, drained

1–2 tablespoons chopped green chiles (optional)

10 whole wheat tortillas or about 16 corn tortillas

Salsa fresca and Tofu Sour Cream (page 242), for serving

Preheat the oven to 350°F. Spread 1½ cups of enchilada sauce in the bottom of a 13" × 9" or 3-quart baking dish.

In a large bowl, mix together the beans, scallions, corn, olives, and green chiles, if you are using them. Lay a tortilla on a flat surface and spread a thick line of the bean mixture down the center. Roll up the tortilla and place it seam-side down in the baking dish. Repeat with the remaining tortillas, snuggling them close together in the pan. Pour the remaining enchilada sauce evenly over the rolled tortillas.

Cover the dish with parchment paper, then with aluminum foil, crimping the edges over the rim of the dish. Bake for 45 minutes. Let rest for 5 minutes before serving hot.

Serve bowls of salsa and Tofu Sour Cream on the side.

CARIBBEAN RICE

The combination of butternut squash, curry spices, brown and wild rice, and chard gives this dish a unique taste and lots of great texture.

PREP: 15 MINUTES | COOK: 1 HOUR • SERVES 6 TO 8

4 cups vegetable broth

1 onion, chopped

1–2 cloves garlic, crushed or minced

1 can (4 ounces) chopped green chiles

3 cups peeled, chopped butternut squash

2 teaspoons curry powder

1 teaspoon ground coriander

$^1/_2$ teaspoon ground cumin

Freshly ground black pepper

1 cup long-grain brown rice

$^1/_2$ cup wild rice

1 can (15 ounces) kidney beans, drained and rinsed

1 cup chopped Swiss chard

$^3/_4$ cup chopped scallions (green and white parts)

Put $^1/_2$ cup of the broth into a large saucepan and add the onion, garlic, and chiles. Cook, stirring occasionally, until the onion softens, about 5 minutes.

Stir in the squash, curry powder, coriander, cumin, and pepper to taste and cook for 2 minutes. Add both types of rice and the remaining $3^1/_2$ cups broth. Bring to a boil, reduce the heat, cover, and simmer gently until the rice is tender, about 45 minutes. Stir in the beans, chard, and scallions and cook until they are heated through and the chard is tender, about 5 minutes.

Serve hot.

Tex-Mex Potatoes

These baked potato wedges topped with salsa- and chile-laced beans are my idea of the quintessential Mexican meal. Even though the recipe uses canned ingredients, fresh tomato and cilantro keep it tasting fresh.

PREP: 20 MINUTES | COOK: 40 MINUTES • SERVES 6

6 large red potatoes, cut lengthwise into wedges

2 cans (15 ounces each) pinto beans, drained and rinsed

1 cup salsa fresca

1 can (4 ounces) chopped green chiles

1 small onion, chopped

1–2 cloves garlic, crushed or minced

$\frac{1}{2}$ teaspoon chili powder

$\frac{1}{2}$ teaspoon ground cumin

$\frac{1}{4}$ cup chopped fresh cilantro, divided

1 tomato, chopped

$\frac{1}{4}$ cup fresh or frozen and thawed corn kernels

2 scallions (green and white parts), chopped

Tofu Taco Topping (page 242) (optional)

Preheat the oven to 375°F. Place the potatoes on a baking sheet and bake until lightly browned, about 40 minutes.

While the potatoes cook, in a saucepan, stir together the beans, salsa, chiles, onion, garlic, chili powder, cumin, and half of the cilantro. Cook over low heat, stirring occasionally, for 15 minutes.

Stir together the tomato, corn, scallions, and the remaining cilantro in a small bowl.

To serve, arrange the baked potato wedges on a serving platter. Spoon the warm bean mixture over them and top with the fresh tomato mixture. Garnish with several dollops of Tofu Taco Topping, if desired.

Spicy Lima Beans and Cabbage

Using leftover rice and the shredded cabbage available in many supermarkets, this delicious meal comes together in just 15 minutes, start to finish. It is one of our most requested recipes. We serve it with Sriracha hot sauce and warm corn tortillas.

If you don't have these convenient items on hand, shred your own cabbage in a food processor and purchase frozen cooked brown rice, warming it according to package directions. Look for prepared spice mixes such as Mrs. Dash or the Lemony Dill Zest made by Vegetarian Express, or make your own combination of your favorite herbs and spices. To vary this recipe slightly, substitute a bag of frozen, shelled edamame (soybeans) for the lima beans.

PREP: 5 MINUTES | COOK: 10 MINUTES • SERVES 3 TO 4

$2\frac{1}{2}$ cups (16 ounces) frozen lima beans

$2\frac{1}{2}$ cups shredded cabbage

$\frac{1}{4}$ cup vegetable broth

$\frac{1}{2}$ tablespoon regular or reduced-sodium soy sauce

1–2 teaspoons spice mix (see above)

$\frac{1}{2}$–1 teaspoon sambal oelek (Indonesian chili paste)

$1\frac{1}{2}$ cups fresh or frozen and thawed corn kernels

$2\frac{1}{2}$–3 cups cooked brown rice

1 large chopped tomato (optional)

Warm corn tortillas (optional)

Sriracha hot sauce (optional)

Put the lima beans, cabbage, broth, and soy sauce in a large nonstick skillet. Cook, stirring frequently, until the vegetables begin to soften, about 2 minutes. Add the spice mixture and sambal and cook for 3 minutes longer. Add the corn and cook, stirring occasionally, for 2 minutes. Stir in the rice and cook until it is heated through and all of the vegetables are tender. If you are using them, stir in the tomatoes just before serving.

Serve immediately, in individual bowls or family-style on the table, with warm tortillas and Sriracha, if desired.

VEGETABLE SHEPHERD'S PIE

This recipe is perfect for using up leftover mashed potatoes. If you don't have any on hand, boil potatoes until they are quite soft, then mash with a little vegetable broth or soy milk until they are spreadable.

PREP: 35 MINUTES | COOK: 1 HOUR • SERVES 6

3 cups vegetable broth

1 onion, chopped

1 rib celery, chopped

1 green bell pepper, chopped

1 clove garlic, crushed or minced

$\frac{1}{2}$ teaspoon sage leaves

$\frac{1}{2}$ teaspoon ground marjoram

1 tablespoon regular or reduced-sodium soy sauce

1 carrot, thinly sliced

$1\frac{1}{2}$ cups sliced fresh mushrooms

$1\frac{1}{2}$ cups cauliflower florets

1 cup thinly sliced cabbage

1 cup green beans, cut into 1" segments

2 tablespoons cornstarch

Freshly ground black pepper

3 cups mashed potatoes

Paprika, for dusting

Preheat the oven to 350°F.

Put $\frac{1}{2}$ cup of the broth in a large saucepan along with the onion, celery, bell pepper, and garlic. Cook, stirring occasionally, until the vegetables soften, about 5 minutes. Stir in the sage, marjoram, and soy sauce. Add the carrot, mushrooms, cauliflower, cabbage, green beans, and the remaining $2\frac{1}{2}$ cups of vegetable broth. Bring the mixture to a boil, cover, reduce the heat, and simmer for 20 minutes, stirring occasionally.

Put the cornstarch in a small bowl and stir in $\frac{1}{3}$ cup cold water until smooth. Stir into the vegetables and continue to stir until the mixture thickens. Add pepper to taste.

Transfer the mixture to a baking dish and spread the mashed potatoes over the top. Sprinkle the top with paprika. Bake uncovered until the potatoes are hot and slightly browned, about 30 minutes.

Serve immediately.

Yukon Stuffed Peppers

These are great on their own, and even better served with the Marsala Mushroom Sauce on page 248.

PREP: 45 MINUTES | BAKE: 20 MINUTES • SERVES 6

$2\frac{1}{2}$ pounds Yukon Gold potatoes, peeled and cut into chunks

2 cloves garlic

6 bell peppers, top $\frac{1}{2}$" cut off and discarded, halved lengthwise, seeds and large veins removed

$\frac{3}{4}$ cup soy milk

$\frac{1}{3}$ cup chopped scallions (green and white parts)

1 cup fresh or frozen and thawed corn kernels

Salt

Freshly ground black pepper

Preheat the oven to 350°F.

Put the potatoes and garlic in a saucepan and add water to cover them. Bring to a boil, then cook, uncovered, until the potatoes are tender, about 30 minutes.

Bring 1" of water to a boil in a saucepan with a steamer insert. Add the peppers, cover, and steam until tender, about 10 minutes. Arrange the pepper halves cut-side up in a nonstick baking pan.

Drain the cooked potatoes, add the soy milk, and mash well with a potato masher or fork. Stir in the scallions and corn. Season the potatoes to taste with salt and pepper.

Mound the potato filling into the peppers. Bake until the potatoes begin to turn slightly golden, about 20 minutes.

Potato Enchiladas

Use firm, waxy potatoes (not the mealy baking kind) in this Mexican favorite: Yukon Gold, Yellow Finn, or purple potatoes all work well.

PREP: 15 MINUTES | COOK: 50 MINUTES • SERVES 4 TO 6

4 medium-large potatoes, peeled and cut into 1" chunks

1 onion, chopped

1–2 cloves garlic, crushed or minced

¾ cup vegetable broth

2 jalapeño peppers, seeded and finely chopped (wear plastic gloves when handling)

1 teaspoon chili powder

Freshly ground black pepper

1 cup fresh spinach, cut crosswise into thin ribbons

2½ cups Enchilada Sauce (page 246)

8 whole wheat tortillas

Salsa fresca (optional)

Preheat the oven to 350°F. Have ready a nonstick 13" × 9" or 3-quart baking dish.

Boil the potatoes in enough water to cover them until they are almost tender, 5 to 7 minutes. Drain and set aside.

Put the onion and garlic in a large nonstick skillet with ¼ cup of the broth. Cook, stirring frequently, until the onion softens, about 5 minutes. Add the jalapeños and another ¼ cup of the broth and cook 1 minute. Add the chili powder, pepper to taste, the cooked potatoes, and the remaining ¼ cup broth. Mix well, then cook and stir 1 minute. Stir in the spinach, then remove the pan from the heat.

Spread ½ cup of Enchilada Sauce in the bottom of the baking dish. Lay a tortilla on a flat surface and spread about ¼ cup of potato mixture in a line down the center of the tortilla. Roll the tortilla and place it seam-side down in the baking dish. Repeat. Pour the remaining Enchilada Sauce evenly over the rolled, filled tortillas.

Cover the dish and bake for 30 minutes. Serve hot, with salsa on the side, if desired.

THAI-STYLE NOODLES

I have yet to find anyone who does not thoroughly enjoy this dish, regardless of his or her taste in food. It is perfect for hot summer nights.

PREP: 20 MINUTES | COOK: 20 MINUTES • SERVES 4

12 ounces linguine

1/4 cup creamy natural peanut butter

1/4 cup agave nectar

1/4 cup regular or reduced-sodium soy sauce

3 tablespoons rice wine vinegar

1–2 teaspoons sambal oelek (Indonesian chili paste)

1/8 teaspoon sesame oil (optional)

3 tablespoons vegetable broth

1 bunch scallions (green and white parts), chopped

6 cloves garlic, crushed or minced

1 tablespoon finely chopped fresh ginger

1 1/2 cups mung bean sprouts

1 1/2 cups shredded carrots

7 ounces baked seasoned tofu, thinly sliced

Chopped cilantro

Chopped peanuts (optional)

Break the linguine strands in half and drop them into a large pot of boiling water. Cook until tender, about 8 minutes. Drain, transfer to a large serving bowl, and set aside.

In a small bowl, whisk together the peanut butter, agave, soy sauce, vinegar, sambal, and sesame oil, if you are using it, until smooth. Set aside.

Pour the broth into a nonstick skillet and add the scallions, garlic, and ginger. Cook, stirring frequently, until the scallions begin to soften, about 3 minutes. Mix in the peanut butter mixture and cook until hot, about 3 minutes.

Scrape the peanut-scallion mixture over the linguine and toss well to coat the noodles. Add the bean sprouts, carrots, and tofu and toss again.

Serve warm or at room temperature, with bowls of chopped cilantro and peanuts, if desired, for diners to add as they wish.

Baked Macaroni with Creamy Cashew Sauce

Let's face it—an important hurdle in adjusting to a healthy diet is giving up macaroni and cheese. Our stand-in is enriched with a creamy sauce made from blended cashews and topped with bread crumbs. Although I developed the recipe with children in mind, it is mighty popular with the grown-up crowd, too.

PREP: 15 MINUTES | COOK: 30 MINUTES • SERVES 6 TO 8

12 ounces whole grain macaroni

1¼ cups raw cashews

¼ cup nutritional yeast

2½ tablespoons chopped pimientos

1 tablespoon fresh lemon juice

2 teaspoons white miso paste

1 teaspoon onion powder

¼ teaspoon salt

⅓ cup whole wheat bread crumbs

Preheat the oven to 350°F.

Bring a large pot of water to a boil. Add the macaroni and cook just until al dente, about 6 minutes, depending on the type used. Drain, transfer to a large bowl, and set aside.

Combine the cashews with ½ cup water in a food processor and process until nearly smooth. Add the yeast, pimientos, lemon juice, miso paste, onion powder, salt, and an additional ¾ cup water. Process for several minutes, scraping down the sides of the bowl as needed, until the mixture is completely smooth.

Pour the cashew mixture over the pasta and stir to combine. Transfer the mixture to a 2-quart covered baking dish and sprinkle the bread crumbs over the top. Cover the baking dish and bake for 30 minutes, until the sauce is bubbling.

Serve hot.

Tofu Lasagna

This is the lasagna that I have been making for my family for many years. This recipe uses no soy cheese, which makes it lower in fat but still "creamy" and delicious. Make sure to let it rest for at least 45 minutes before serving so it "sets up" nicely.

PREP: 30 MINUTES | COOK: 1 HOUR | REST: 45 MINUTES • SERVES 6 TO 8

Prepare the tofu ricotta before assembling the lasagna.

TOFU RICOTTA

1 package (12.3 ounces) silken tofu, drained in a fine-mesh strainer

1 package (16 ounces) fresh water-packed tofu, drained in a fine-mesh strainer

$\frac{1}{4}$ cup nutritional yeast

$\frac{1}{4}$ cup lemon juice

$\frac{1}{4}$ cup soy milk

1 tablespoon parsley

1 teaspoon dried basil

1 teaspoon dried oregano

$\frac{1}{2}$ teaspoon garlic powder

$\frac{1}{4}$ teaspoon salt

Freshly ground black pepper

Combine all ingredients in a food processor until smooth. Set aside.

LASAGNA

10 ounces frozen chopped spinach, thawed and squeezed dry (see sidebar on opposite page)

Tofu Ricotta

2 jars (25 ounces each) fat-free pasta sauce

8 ounces no-boil lasagna noodles (see sidebar on opposite page)

No-Parmesan Cheese (page 249)

Add the spinach to the Tofu Ricotta and stir well to mix.
Preheat the oven to 350°F.

Pour about 1 cup of the pasta sauce into the bottom of a 13" × 9" baking dish. Place a single layer of noodles over the sauce. Spread half of the tofu mixture over the noodles. Pour another cup or so of the pasta sauce over the tofu mixture and spread evenly. Add another layer of noodles and spread the remaining tofu mixture over them. Pour another cup or so of sauce over the tofu and spread evenly. Top with another layer of noodles and another cup or so of the sauce, making sure all the noodles are covered. Sprinkle the top with No-Parmesan Cheese. Cover with parchment paper, then aluminum foil, crimping the edges under the baking dish top to seal the top well. Bake for 1 hour. Let rest for at least 45 minutes before cutting.

For a more spinach-flavored lasagna, use 20 ounces of spinach, thawed and squeezed dry. Do not mix with the tofu; instead, layer it over the tofu mixture before covering with the sauce. To add more vegetables to the sauce, sauté some onions and mushrooms in a dry nonstick pan until softened, about 5 minutes. Add this to the pasta sauce before using in the recipe. Other vegetables may also be added as desired. Another delicious option is to thinly slice some zucchini length-wise and lay these strips over the tofu in each layer. No-boil lasagna noodles are available in most super-markets and natural food stores. Use whole grain varieties whenever possible. For a fantastic gluten-free option to the wheat lasagna noodles, use Tinkyada brown rice lasagna noodles. There are many varieties of lasagna noodles that do not need to be boiled ahead of time before using in recipes.

Soy-Glazed Soba with Crispy Tofu and Vegetables

Use whatever seasonal vegetables you enjoy with these flavorful buckwheat noodles paired with marinated tofu that has been sautéed until crispy and tossed with a flavorful Asian-style sauce.

PREP: 30 MINUTES | COOK: 20 MINUTES • SERVES 3 TO 4

$1/4$ cup regular or reduced-sodium soy sauce, plus more for coating noodles

$1^1/2$ tablespoons agave nectar

Dash of sesame oil

1 package (10 ounces) extra-firm tofu, drained and cut into $1/2$" cubes

1 pound asparagus, trimmed and cut into 1" pieces

$1^1/2$ cups snow peas, trimmed

1 package (about 9.5 ounces) soba (buckwheat noodles)

Dash of soy sauce

1 tablespoon mirin

$1/2$ tablespoon rice wine vinegar

1 clove garlic, crushed or minced

2 teaspoons cornstarch

Dash of sesame oil or chili oil (optional)

Pinch of crushed red pepper (optional)

Sriracha hot sauce (optional)

In a medium bowl, stir together the soy sauce, agave nectar, and sesame oil. Add the tofu and stir gently to coat. Let stand for 10 minutes, stirring occasionally.

Heat a large nonstick skillet over medium heat. Use a slotted spoon to transfer the tofu cubes to the skillet and sauté, turning occasionally with a spatula, until the tofu browns on all sides. Reserve the marinade. Remove the skillet from the heat and set it aside.

Bring a large pot of water to a boil. Add the asparagus and snow peas and cook for 2 minutes. Use a large slotted spoon to transfer the vegetables to the pan of tofu. Return the water to a boil and add the soba noodles. Cook until tender, 4 to 5 minutes. Drain and transfer the noodles to a large bowl and add the tofu and vegetables to the bowl. Splash noodles and vegetables with a dash of soy sauce and toss to mix.

Transfer the remaining tofu marinade to a saucepan and stir in the mirin, vinegar, and garlic. In a small bowl, stir the cornstarch with 1 tablespoon of cold water until smooth, then add to the saucepan. Slowly bring the mixture to a boil, stirring constantly. Cook until the sauce thickens, 1 to 2 minutes. Stir in the oil and crushed red pepper, if you are using them. Pour the sauce over the noodles and stir gently to mix and coat everything evenly.

Serve warm or at room temperature, with Sriracha on the side, if desired.

Spinach Fettuccine with Pesto

You can get a head start on this dish by preparing the tofu pesto up to a day ahead and refrigerating it in an airtight container. When you are ready to make the dish, just boil the pasta, toss in the sauce, and serve.

PREP: 15 MINUTES | COOK: 10 MINUTES • SERVES 6

14 ounces spinach fettuccine

2 bags (6 ounces each) triple-washed baby spinach

1 cup (packed) coarsely chopped fresh basil

2 cloves garlic, crushed or minced

1 package (12.3 ounces) silken tofu, drained in a fine-mesh strainer

¼ teaspoon salt

Freshly ground black pepper or ground white pepper

1½ cups halved cherry tomatoes

Bring a large pot of water to a boil. Add the pasta, stir, and cook until barely tender, about 8 minutes. Stir in the spinach and cook until wilted, about 1 minute. Drain and transfer to a serving bowl.

Briefly combine the basil and garlic in a food processor. Add the tofu, salt, and $1/4$ cup water. Process until very smooth, stopping several times to scrape down the sides of the processor bowl. Add pepper to taste. Set aside.

Pour the tofu pesto over the pasta and toss well to coat. Add the cherry tomatoes and toss again. Serve immediately.

MUSHROOM STROGANOFF

Three types of mushrooms give this pasta great texture and earthy flavor. Feel free to substitute your own favorite mushroom varieties.

PREP: 15 MINUTES | COOK: 20 MINUTES • SERVES 6

1 pound fettuccine or spaghetti

1 onion, cut in half lengthwise, then cut crosswise into thin slices

3 cups sliced button mushrooms

2 cups sliced shiitake mushrooms

1 cup sliced oyster mushrooms

1 cup vegetable broth

1 cup soy milk

3 tablespoons regular or reduced-sodium soy sauce

2 tablespoons white wine (optional)

Dash of ground red pepper

Freshly ground black pepper

2 tablespoons cornstarch

Bring a large pot of water to a boil. Add the pasta and cook until al dente, about 8 minutes. Drain the pasta and transfer it to a serving bowl. Set aside.

While the pasta cooks, put the onion in a large nonstick skillet and add $1/3$ cup of water. Cook, stirring occasionally, until the onion softens, about 3 minutes. Add all three types of mushrooms and cook about 3 minutes. Add the broth, soy milk, soy sauce, wine (if using), red pepper, and black pepper to taste. Cook over medium heat, stirring occasionally, until the mushrooms are tender, about 12 minutes.

In a small bowl, whisk the cornstarch with $\frac{1}{4}$ cup cold water. Add the cornstarch mixture to the skillet and cook, stirring, until the sauce thickens. Toss the mushroom sauce with the pasta and serve immediately.

POTATO GNOCCHI WITH BUTTERNUT SQUASH AND ASPARAGUS

Your effort in preparing this recipe will be amply rewarded when you taste the finished dish. The squash and asparagus mixture can be prepared ahead and warmed just before serving, making quick work of finishing the dish.

PREP: 30 MINUTES | BAKE: 1 HOUR • SERVES 6 TO 8

1 butternut or other winter squash (2–3 pounds), cut into several large pieces, seeds and strings scraped out and discarded

1 onion, chopped

4 large cloves garlic, crushed or minced

8 asparagus spears, round ends trimmed, cut into $1\frac{1}{2}$" pieces

2 packages (16 ounces each) potato gnocchi

2 cups spinach

$\frac{1}{2}$ cup toasted pine nuts

Small bunch basil leaves, rolled up and cut crosswise into thin ribbons

Salt

Freshly ground black pepper

Preheat the oven to 350°F.

Put the squash pieces into a baking dish large enough to hold them and pour 1 cup of water into the dish. Bake until the squash is easily pierced with a fork, about 1 hour. Let cool, then cut away and discard the skin and cut the squash into bite-size chunks. Set aside.

While the squash bakes, put the onion and garlic in a large skillet with $\frac{1}{4}$ cup of water. Cook, stirring occasionally, until the onion softens, about 5 minutes. Add the asparagus and a bit more water, if needed. Cook until the asparagus is just tender, 2 to 3 minutes. Add the squash pieces. Set aside.

Bring a large pot of water to a boil. Add the gnocchi, stir, and cook until they rise to the top, 3 to 4 minutes. Add the spinach, stir, then drain the gnocchi and spinach and transfer to a warm serving bowl.

Add the cooked squash mixture to the gnocchi along with the pine nuts and basil. Toss to combine everything well. Season with salt and pepper to taste.

Serve immediately.

Pasta with Walnut-Herb Sauce

Look for the Indonesian chili paste known as sambal oelek in Asian groceries or in the Asian aisle of your supermarket. It gives this pasta a hint of heat, which you can intensify by adding more.

PREP: 30 MINUTES | COOK: 11 TO 12 MINUTES • SERVES 6 TO 8

2 cups vegetable broth

2 cups walnuts

⅓ cup (packed) parsley, large stems removed

⅓ cup (packed) fresh cilantro, large stems removed (optional)

3 teaspoons fresh lemon juice

4 cloves garlic, crushed or minced

2 teaspoons sambal oelek (Indonesian chili paste)

Salt

Freshly ground black pepper

16 ounces corkscrew pasta

3 cups broccoli florets

1 cup red bell pepper strips

1 cup yellow bell pepper strips

1 pound mushrooms, cut into bite-size pieces

1 cup halved cherry tomatoes

Combine the broth, nuts, parsley, cilantro (if using), lemon juice, garlic, and sambal in a blender until very smooth. Add salt, pepper, and additional sambal to taste. Set aside.

Bring a large pot of water to a boil. Add the pasta and cook for 5 minutes. Add the broccoli and peppers and cook 4 to 5 minutes. Add the mushrooms and cook for 2 minutes.

Drain the pasta and vegetables and transfer them to a serving bowl. Pour in the walnut sauce and toss to coat everything evenly. Add the tomatoes and mix again.

Serve warm, at room temperature, or chilled.

Baked Penne Florentine

Our grandson, Jaysen, loves this pasta as much as I do. I give my plate a kick with a squirt of Sriracha hot sauce. To make the dish ahead, refrigerate the covered dish for up to 1 day and add 15 minutes to the baking time.

PREP: 30 MINUTES | COOK: 45 MINUTES | REST: 5 MINUTES • SERVES 6 TO 8

8 ounces penne pasta

1 package (10 ounces) frozen chopped spinach, thawed and squeezed dry

$\frac{1}{4}$ cup vegetable broth

1 onion, chopped

$\frac{1}{2}$ cup raw cashews

1 can (15 ounces) white beans, drained and rinsed

1 tablespoon regular or reduced-sodium soy sauce

1 tablespoon white miso paste

2 teaspoons fresh lemon juice

$\frac{1}{4}$ teaspoon mustard powder

$\frac{1}{4}$ teaspoon ground red pepper

$\frac{1}{2}$ cup whole wheat bread crumbs

Preheat the oven to 350°F. Have ready a 3-quart baking dish that has a cover.

Bring a large pot of water to a boil. Add the pasta, stir, and cook until just tender, about 8 minutes. Drain and transfer the pasta to a large bowl. Add the spinach and mix well. Set aside.

Heat the broth and onion in a nonstick skillet, stirring occasionally, until the onion softens, about 5 minutes. Set aside.

Process the cashews in a food processor until they are as fine as possible. Add ¾ cup of water and blend until smooth. Add the cooked onion and the beans, soy sauce, miso, lemon juice, mustard, red pepper, and 1 cup water; process until the sauce is very smooth.

Pour the sauce over the pasta and mix well. Transfer the mixture to the baking dish, sprinkle the bread crumbs evenly over the top, cover, and bake for 45 minutes.

Let rest for 5 minutes before serving.

On the Side

Often, it's the little things that make a meal memorable. These recipes provide flavorful accompaniments to other recipes in the book, or can be put together with a salad, soup, or another side dish as the main event. Many are perfect as dips or snacks, as well.

GUACAMOLE

We suggest enjoying this high-fat treat as a condiment with other recipes. For faster weight loss, avoid avocados and other high-fat foods such as nuts, seeds, and olives, or reserve them for special occasions and use them in very small quantities. A little bit goes a long way.

> To store leftover guacamole, put it into the smallest container into which it will fit and press plastic film directly over the surface so that there is no air between the covering and the avocado. Alternatively, cover the surface with salsa to help prevent it from browning. Either way, refrigerate the guacamole and use within a day or two.

PREP: 5 MINUTES • MAKES ABOUT 1½ CUPS

4 ripe avocados, cut in half and seeded

1 tomato, chopped

⅛ cup canned chopped green chiles

Squeeze of fresh lime juice

Dash of Tabasco sauce

Scoop the avocados from their skins into a bowl and mash well with a fork. Add the tomato, chiles, lime juice, and Tabasco and mix well.

Mango Salsa

We use this tropical salsa in our Polenta with Black Beans and Mango Salsa (page 286), and it is also a great condiment for other Mexican-style dishes. For a snack, try rolling up a warm corn tortilla and using it to scoop up some of this flavorful salsa.

PREP: 10 MINUTES | CHILL: 1 HOUR • MAKES 2 CUPS

2 cups peeled, chopped ripe mango

$\frac{1}{2}$ cup finely chopped onion

$\frac{1}{2}$ cup finely chopped red bell pepper

1 fresh jalapeño pepper, seeded and finely chopped (wear plastic gloves when handling)

1 small clove garlic, crushed or minced

1 tablespoon apple cider vinegar

Salt

Freshly ground black pepper

Put the mango, onion, bell pepper, jalapeño, garlic, and vinegar in a bowl. Add 1 tablespoon of warm tap water and stir to combine. Add salt and pepper to taste.

Cover and refrigerate at least 1 hour or up to 1 week before serving.

Smashed Slow-Cooked Beans

These versatile beans are perfect for rolling up into tortillas with Guacamole (page 305) and salsa fresca or Mango Salsa (above) for a quick snack or lunch. You can tuck lettuce, tomatoes, raw or cooked vegetables, or whatever else you like in there, too, to make a burrito. For extra flourish, put the rolled burrito on a plate and smother with Enchilada Sauce (page 246). The beans also make a great side dish with other entrees. I make a big batch to have beans on hand for recipes and snacking.

> Don't limit yourself to pintos; these are also delicious
> made with cranberry beans or Peruvian Mayocoba
> beans, two of our favorite varieties.

2–3 cups dry pinto beans, rinsed and picked over

1 large onion, coarsely chopped

4–6 cloves garlic

Salt (optional)

Place the beans, onion, and garlic in a slow cooker and add water to cover by about 2". Set the cooker on high and let cook for 8 to 10 hours.

If any water remains after cooking, pour most of it off and save it to use in soups or stocks if you wish.

Mash the beans, onion, and garlic with an electric hand mixer, potato masher, or fork. Season with a little salt, if you wish.

Refrigerate leftover beans in an airtight container for up to 4 days, or freeze. If frozen, thaw the beans in their container overnight in the refrigerator. The beans can be reheated in a microwave oven or in a saucepan over low heat—stir and add a bit of water if needed to prevent scorching.

CORN TORTILLAS

During our McDougall Adventures in Costa Rica, the "tortilla lady" prepares fresh corn tortillas for our every meal. The recipe for making them yourself is simple, though forming the tortillas takes a bit of practice. A tortilla press is the easiest way, but they can also be done by hand.

> Masa harina is a type of corn flour used for making tortillas and tamales. Look for it in Latin markets or in your supermarket's ethnic foods aisle. Store masa harina in a tightly sealed bag in the freezer to keep it fresh.

PREP: 30 MINUTES | REST: 20 MINUTES | COOK: 20 MINUTES • MAKES 16

2 cups masa harina

1¼ cups hot water

In a large bowl, stir together the masa harina and water. Knead the dough with your hands for several minutes until it is smooth. Cover with plastic wrap and let rest for 20 minutes.

Divide the dough into 16 equal pieces and roll each piece into a ball. While you form one tortilla, keep the remaining balls covered with plastic wrap.

Flatten a ball between two pieces of waxed paper or plastic wrap with a rolling pin, by pressing down with a heavy skillet, or using a tortilla press. You are looking for a circle that is about 5" in diameter and about $^1/_{16}$" thick.

Heat a nonstick skillet over medium heat until a drop of water bounces on the skillet when you flick your wet hands over it.

Peel off the waxed paper or plastic wrap and place the tortilla in the hot pan. Cook until it browns lightly on one side, then flip over and lightly brown the second side. Place the tortilla in a cloth-lined basket, cover, and repeat with the remaining dough balls.

The tortillas are best shortly after they are made.

Southwest Red Potatoes

This is a delicious way to eat one of my favorite starches. The seasonings can be adjusted slightly to suit your tastes. For example, if you don't like spicy foods, eliminate the red-pepper flakes. If you are not fond of cumin, just leave it out. Use different oil-free dressings to change the flavor.

PREP: 10 MINUTES | COOK: 15 MINUTES • SERVES 4

2 pounds red potatoes, cut into chunks

$^1/_4$ cup chopped scallions

$^1/_4$ cup oil-free salad dressing

$^3/_4$ teaspoon chili powder

$^1/_2$–$^3/_4$ teaspoon ground cumin

$^1/_8$ teaspoon red-pepper flakes (optional)

In a large pot, add potatoes and water, cover, and boil for about 20 minutes, or just barely fork tender. Drain. Whisk together the remaining ingredients including red-pepper flakes, if using, and place in a nonstick frying pan. Add potatoes and cook until coated with spices, about 5 minutes.

Slow-Cooked Pizza Potatoes

With just a little prep earlier in the day, these potatoes will be all ready in the slow cooker when the dinner bell rings. All you need to round out the meal is a fresh vegetable or a green salad. Thinly slice the potatoes using a mandoline or a knife. (We leave the skins on.) You can use any combination of toppings—I've suggested a few of our favorites. They will be ready in 6 hours but can cook up to 8 hours if you wish to make them in the morning and return to them after a day of work.

PREP: 20 MINUTES | COOK: 6 TO 8 HOURS • SERVES 6 TO 8

4 cups jarred or homemade marinara or pizza sauce

4 cups thinly sliced potatoes

2–3 cups toppings (any combination of sliced onions, mushrooms, bell peppers, tomatoes, frozen or water-packed artichoke hearts, black olives, spinach, or your own favorites)

Put the sauce in a bowl and stir in ¼ cup water. Set aside.

Layer half of the potatoes in the bottom of a slow cooker. Layer toppings over the potatoes. Pour half of the sauce over the toppings. Top with the remaining potatoes and then the remaining sauce. Cook on the lowest setting for at least 6 or up to 8 hours.

Serve hot.

Rainbow Rice

We serve this colorful rice dish alongside beans, with a big salad, or with the Tex-Mex Potatoes (page 289). It's also a great accompaniment to the Bean and Corn Enchiladas (page 287). Cilantro and spinach give it a burst of fresh flavor.

PREP: 15 MINUTES | COOK: 50 MINUTES • SERVES 4

1 onion, chopped

1 bell pepper, chopped

½ cup chopped scallions (white and green parts)

1–2 cloves garlic, crushed or minced

2 cups vegetable broth

1 cup long-grain brown rice

1 can (4 ounces) chopped green chiles

1 jar (4 ounces) chopped pimientos

1¼ cups fresh or frozen and thawed corn kernels

1 tablespoon parsley

1 teaspoon ground cumin

2 cups (packed) chopped fresh spinach

¼ cup chopped fresh cilantro

Freshly ground black pepper

Put the onion, bell pepper, scallions, and garlic in a large saucepan and add ⅓ cup of water. Cook, stirring occasionally, until the vegetables soften slightly, about 3 minutes.

Stir in the broth, rice, chiles, pimientos, corn, parsley, and cumin. Bring to a boil, cover, reduce the heat, and simmer until the rice is tender, about 45 minutes. Stir in the spinach, cilantro, and black pepper to taste and cook for about 2 minutes.

Serve hot.

Sweet Endings

Dessert is the punctuation that makes a meal feel complete. We often enjoy a simple piece of fresh fruit for dessert, but so long as you stick with sweets that have little or no fat, there's no harm for most people in occasionally indulging in a dessert that leaves you feeling satisfied. These recipes also provide a way to enjoy special holidays and occasions with family and friends without feeling left out.

BANANA BREAD

Bananas provide the sweet and starchy base for this moist and delicious bread. Substituting white whole wheat or even regular whole wheat flour for the pastry flour yields a slightly denser but perfectly delicious result.

PREP: 25 MINUTES | COOK: 1 HOUR | COOL: 1 HOUR • SERVES 8 TO 10

1 tablespoon Ener-G Egg Replacer

$^3/_4$ cup soy milk

1 tablespoon fresh lemon juice

1 cup mashed ripe bananas

$^3/_4$ cup granulated sugar or Sucanat

$^1/_3$ cup Sunsweet Lighter Bake

1 teaspoon pure vanilla extract

$1^1/_4$ cups whole wheat pastry flour

1 cup unbleached all-purpose flour

1 teaspoon baking powder

1 teaspoon baking soda

1 teaspoon ground cinnamon

$^1/_8$ teaspoon salt

$^1/_4$ cup chopped walnuts

Preheat the oven to 350°F. Have on hand a 9" × 5" nonstick loaf pan or a flexible silicone pan.

In a small bowl, whisk the Egg Replacer with $^1/_4$ cup warm water until frothy. Pour the soy milk into another small bowl and whisk in the lemon juice. (The mixture will thicken as it sits.) In another small bowl, mix together the bananas, sugar, Lighter Bake, and vanilla. Set the three bowls aside.

In a medium bowl, whisk together the whole wheat pastry and all-purpose flours, baking powder, baking soda, cinnamon, and salt until well combined. Stir in the walnuts.

Use a spatula to mix the Egg Replacer, banana mixture, and soy milk mixture into the flour mixture just until everything is combined. Pour and spread the batter into the loaf pan and bake until a wooden pick inserted in the center comes out clean, about 1 hour. Set the pan on a rack until it is completely cool, about 1 hour.

To unmold the bread from a nonstick pan, run a butter knife around the sides of the pan to loosen the loaf, then invert the loaf directly onto the wire rack. If using a flexible silicone pan, bend and flex the sides of the pan all around to loosen the loaf, then invert to release it.

Cut into slices after the loaf is completely cool.

BANANA ICE CREAM

This quick ice "cream" is the perfect way to use up extra bananas. When your bananas are ripe but you don't feel like eating them, peel them, break them into pieces, and store them in an airtight container or zip-top bag in the freezer.

To vary the flavor, add a handful of frozen berries or a tablespoon of fat-free cocoa powder along with the bananas.

If you have a Champion Juicer you can make soft-serve banana ice cream the way we do: by simply pushing frozen bananas through the juicer.

PREP: 10 MINUTES • SERVES 2

2 frozen bananas, peeled

Soy milk

Combine the frozen bananas in a food processor with just enough soy milk to get them moving. Process until smooth. Serve in small bowls, topped with fruit, if desired.

CHOCOLATE BROWNIES

We serve these brownies topped with vanilla soy ice cream on the first night of every McDougall Program. They are a rich treat best reserved for special occasions. We especially like them cold from the fridge, so we sometimes make them ahead, cut and arrange them on a platter, cover tightly with plastic wrap, and refrigerate for a day before serving them. Leftovers can be refrigerated for up to 3 days, but I doubt they'll be around that long.

PREP: 15 MINUTES | COOK: 30 MINUTES | COOL: 30 MINUTES • MAKES 9

2 tablespoons Ener-G Egg Replacer

1 cup unbleached all-purpose flour

$^2/_3$ cup Wonderslim Wondercocoa Fat-Free Cocoa Powder

1 teaspoon baking powder

1 teaspoon baking soda

$^1/_4$ teaspoon salt

$^1/_4$ cup chopped cashews or walnuts (optional)

1 cup Sunsweet Lighter Bake

1 cup granulated sugar

1 teaspoon pure vanilla extract

Preheat the oven to 350°F.

In a small bowl, whisk the Egg Replacer with $^1/_2$ cup warm water until frothy. Set aside.

In a medium bowl, whisk together the flour, cocoa, baking powder, baking soda, and salt. Stir in the nuts, if using. Set aside.

In a small bowl, whisk together the Lighter Bake, sugar, and vanilla. Stir in the Egg Replacer. Stir this mixture into the flour mixture just until the ingredients are combined.

Spread the batter evenly into a nonstick or silicone 8" × 8" baking pan, smoothing the top. Bake until a wooden pick inserted in the center comes out clean, about 30 minutes.

Set the pan on a rack until cool, about 30 minutes. Cut the brownies into 3 equal strips in one direction, then 3 in the other, to make 9 brownies. (If using a silicone pan, flex and invert the pan to release the brownies onto a platter before cutting them.)

SPECIAL OCCASION CHOCOLATE CAKE

Some occasions demand a cake, and this is a perfectly delicious solution.

PREP: 15 MINUTES | COOK: 25 MINUTES |COOL: 30 MINUTES • SERVES 9 TO 12

1$\frac{1}{2}$ cups unbleached all-purpose flour

1 cup Sucanat

$\frac{3}{4}$ cup Wonderslim Wondercocoa Fat-Free Cocoa Powder

1 teaspoon baking soda

1$\frac{1}{4}$ cups chocolate soy milk

6 ounces vanilla soy yogurt

1 tablespoon Sunsweet Lighter Bake

1 teaspoon pure vanilla extract

$\frac{1}{4}$ cup slivered almonds (optional)

Chocolate Frosting (opposite) (optional)

Preheat the oven to 375°F. Have on hand an 8" × 8" nonstick or silicone baking pan.

In a mixing bowl, whisk together the flour, Sucanat, cocoa, and baking soda.

In a small bowl, whisk together the soy milk, yogurt, Lighter Bake, and vanilla until very smooth. Stir into the flour mixture until well blended. Stir in the nuts if you are using them.

Spread the batter into the baking pan and smooth the top. Bake until a wooden pick inserted into the center comes out clean, about 25 minutes. Set the pan on a rack to cool for at least 30 minutes.

To unmold the cake from a nonstick pan, run a butter knife around the sides of the pan to loosen it, then invert the cake directly onto a flat serving plate. If using a flexible silicone pan, bend and flex the sides of the pan all around to loosen the cake before inverting it.

If you are using it, spread the frosting over the cake before cutting. Cut the cake into thirds in both directions to make 9 squares, or into thirds in one direction and quarters in the other to make 12.

Chocolate Frosting

This quick frosting will make any birthday celebrant feel special indeed. It can also be used to frost brownies.

PREP: 3 MINUTES • MAKES ENOUGH TO FROST AN 8" × 8" CAKE

2 cups confectioners' sugar

$\frac{1}{4}$ cup Wonderslim Wondercocoa Fat-Free Cocoa Powder

$\frac{1}{4}$–$\frac{1}{3}$ cup soy milk

$\frac{1}{4}$ teaspoon pure vanilla extract

In a bowl, whisk together the confectioners' sugar and cocoa. Stir in $\frac{1}{4}$ cup of the soy milk and the vanilla, mixing until smooth. Continue to add soy milk, a little at a time, to reach a spreadable consistency.

Carrot Cake

This cake is extremely moist and full of great flavor from carrots, dates, and spices.

PREP: 30 MINUTES | COOK: 10 MINUTES | BAKE: 45 MINUTES • SERVES 12

1 cup grated carrots

1 cup raisins

$\frac{1}{2}$ cup agave nectar

$\frac{1}{4}$ cup chopped dates

1 teaspoon ground cinnamon

1 teaspoon ground allspice

$\frac{1}{2}$ teaspoon ground nutmeg

$\frac{1}{2}$ teaspoon ground cloves

$\frac{3}{4}$ cup unbleached all-purpose flour

$^3/_4$ cup whole wheat flour

$^1/_2$ cup bran

1 teaspoon baking soda

$^1/_2$ cup chopped walnuts (optional)

Preheat the oven to 350°F.

Put the carrots, raisins, agave, dates, cinnamon, allspice, nutmeg, and cloves in a large saucepan. Add 1$^3/_4$ cups water, stir, and bring to a boil. Reduce the heat, cover, and simmer, stirring occasionally, until the carrots and dates are completely soft, about 10 minutes. Remove from the heat and set aside to cool.

In a medium bowl, whisk together the all-purpose and whole wheat flours, bran, and baking soda. Stir in the cooled carrot mixture until evenly combined. Stir in the walnuts, if you are using them.

Spread the batter evenly into a nonstick or silicone 9" × 9" baking pan and smooth the top. Bake until a wooden pick inserted in the center comes out clean, about 45 minutes.

Serve the cake warm or at room temperature.

APPLE CRISP

This crisp is an everyday dessert you don't need to feel bad about eating, even after a midweek dinner or as an afternoon treat. I use Granny Smith or another firm apple, such as Braeburn or Pippin, to make this crisp so that the apples retain a little crunch even after they are baked. Avoid Delicious or McIntosh apples in this one, as they will turn to mush and won't have much flavor.

PREP: 20 MINUTES | COOK: 40 TO 50 MINUTES • SERVES 4 TO 6

4 large firm apples, peeled and sliced

$^1/_2$ cup raisins or currants

1 tablespoon fresh lemon juice

1 teaspoon ground cinnamon

$^3/_4$ cup Grape-Nuts cereal

$^3/_4$ cup rolled oats

$^1\!/_2$ cup pure maple syrup

$^2\!/_3$ cup apple juice

1 teaspoon cornstarch

Preheat the oven to 350°F.

Put the apple slices, raisins, lemon juice, and $^1\!/_2$ teaspoon of the cinnamon in an 8" × 8" nonstick or silicone baking pan. Stir to coat everything evenly.

In a small bowl, mix the cereal, oats, and remaining $^1\!/_2$ teaspoon cinnamon. Stir in the maple syrup, then spread the topping evenly over the apples.

In a small bowl, whisk together the apple juice and cornstarch. Pour evenly over the apples and topping.

Bake the crisp until the apples are crisp-tender, 40 to 50 minutes. Serve warm or at room temperature.

PEACH-OATMEAL CRISP

Vary this simple recipe to make a crisp from whatever fruit is ripe and in season. Use preserves that match or complement the fruit; for example, I sometimes use sliced fresh strawberries in place of the peaches and strawberry preserves in place of the apricot. When served warm, the crisp is lovely with a scoop of vanilla soy ice cream.

PREP: 15 TO 20 MINUTES | BAKE: 45 MINUTES| COOL: 15 MINUTES • SERVES 8

$^1\!/_3$ cup apricot preserves

2 teaspoons fresh lemon juice

$^1\!/_8$ teaspoon grated nutmeg

4 cups sliced peaches (about 8)

3 tablespoons all-purpose flour

$^1\!/_2$ cup quick-cooking oats

2 tablespoons medium ground cornmeal

2 tablespoons pure maple syrup

1 teaspoon pure vanilla extract

Preheat the oven to 375°F.

In a medium bowl, stir together the preserves, lemon juice, and nutmeg. Add the peaches and mix gently to coat them evenly. Sprinkle the flour over the top and mix again. Transfer the fruit to an ungreased 9" pie pan and bake until the fruit is very tender, about 30 minutes.

While the fruit bakes, stir together the oats and cornmeal in a small bowl. Stir together the maple syrup and vanilla and pour them over the oat mixture; mix well.

Remove the crisp from the oven and reduce the heat to 350°F. Use your fingertips to crumble and scatter the oat mixture over the fruit. Bake for 15 minutes.

Let the crisp cool for at least 15 minutes before scooping out servings with a large spoon into individual bowls. It can be served either warm or at room temperature.

DECADENT CHOCOLATE PUDDING

When we serve this rich-tasting yet lean chocolate pudding on the last day of the McDougall Program, our participants are always surprised to learn that it is made only with soy milk—no rich cream or even silken tofu. They are also delighted to find out how easy it will be to recreate at home. Clearly, there will be no deprivation as they get started with their new regimen.

PREP: 5 MINUTES | COOK: 10 MINUTES | CHILL: 2 HOURS • SERVES 4 TO 6

$^3/_4$ cup granulated sugar

$^1/_2$ cup Wonderslim Wondercocoa Fat-Free Cocoa Powder

3 tablespoons cornstarch

3 cups soy milk

$1^1/_2$ teaspoon pure vanilla extract

In a medium saucepan, whisk together the sugar, cocoa, cornstarch, and soy milk until very smooth. Bring to a boil over medium-low heat, then simmer, stirring gently but constantly, until the pudding thickens.

Remove from the heat and stir in the vanilla. Pour the pudding into a serving bowl, or into 4 to 6 individual dessert bowls. Cover with plastic wrap and refrigerate until very cold, at least 2 hours or up to 1 day. Serve cold.

Resources

Champion Juicer
www.championjuicer.com

Ener-G Egg Replacer
www.ener-g.com/egg-replacer.html

Sunsweet Lighter Bake (butter and oil replacement)
http://store.sunsweet.com
/merchant2/merchant
.mvc?Screen=PROD&Store
_Code=store&Product
_Code=260

White Whole Wheat Flour
www.bobsredmill.com
www.kingarthurflour.com

Wonderslim Wondercocoa Fat-Free Cocoa Powder
www.thebetterhealthstore.com
/Wonderslim-Wondercocoa
-Fat-Free-1can-6-Oz

Salsa Fresca
Fresh salsa is available for purchase in most supermarkets.

Previous McDougall National Bestsellers

The McDougall Plan

McDougall's Medicine: A Challenging Second Opinion

The McDougall Health-Supporting Cookbook, Volume 1

The McDougall Health-Supporting Cookbook, Volume 2

The McDougall Program: 12 Days to Dynamic Health

The McDougall Program for Maximum Weight Loss

The New McDougall Cookbook

The McDougall Program for Women

The McDougall Program for a Healthy Heart: A Life-Saving Approach to Preventing and Treating Heart Disease

The McDougall Quick & Easy Cookbook: Over 300 Delicious Low-Fat Recipes You Can Prepare in Fifteen Minutes or Less

Dr. McDougall's Digestive Tune-Up

REFERENCES

NOTE: Unless otherwise indicated, all of the information on the nutritional values of foods was obtained from:

Pennington JA, Bowes A, Church H. *Bowes & Church's Food Values of Portions Commonly Used.* 17th ed. (Philadelphia and New York: Lippincott Williams & Wilkins, 1998).

Chapter 1. Starch: The Traditional Diet of People

1. Weiss E, Wetterstrom W, Nadel D, Bar-Yosef O. The broad spectrum revisited: evidence from plant remains. *Proc Natl Acad Sci USA.* 2004 Jun 29; 101 (26): 9551–55.

2. Deacon HJ. Planting an idea: An archeology of stone age gatherers in South Africa. *S Afr Archaeol Bull* 48: 86–93, 1993.

3. Revedin A, Aranguren B, Becattini R, Longo L, Marconi E, Lippi MM, Skakun N, Sinitsyn A, Spiridonova E, Svoboda J. Thirty thousand-year-old evidence of plant food processing. *Proc Natl Acad Sci USA.* 2010 Nov 2; 107 (44): 18815–19.

4. Mercader J. Mozambican grass seed consumption during the Middle Stone Age. *Science.* 2009 Dec 18; 326 (5960): 1680–83.

5. Henry AG, Brooks AS, Piperno DR. Microfossils in calculus demonstrate consumption of plants and cooked foods in Neanderthal diets (Shanidar III, Iraq; Spy I and II, Belgium). *Proc Natl Acad Sci USA.* 2011 Jan 11; 108 (2): 486–91.

6. Eades M and Eades M. *Protein Power: The High-Protein/Low Carbohydrate Way to Lose Weight, Feel Fit, and Boost Your Health—in Just Weeks!* (New York: Bantam, 1996).

7. Allam AH, Thompson RC, Wann LS, et al. Atherosclerosis in ancient Egyptian mummies: the Horus study. *JACC Cardiovasc Imaging.* 2011 Apr; 4 (4): 315–27.

8. David AR, Kershaw A, Heagerty A. Atherosclerosis and diet in ancient Egypt. *Lancet.* 2010 Feb 27; 375 (9716): 718–19.

9. Guardians.net/hawass/hatshepsut/search_for_hatshepsut.htm

10. Gerloni A, Cavalli F, Costantinides F, Costantinides F, et al. Dental status of three Egyptian mummies: radiological investigation by multislice computerized tomography. *Oral Surg Oral Med Oral Pathol Oral Radiol Endod.* 2009 Jun; 107 (6): e58–64.

11. Kuksis A, Child P, Myher JJ, et al. Bile acids of a 3200-year-old Egyptian mummy. *Can J Biochem.* 1978 Dec; 56 (12):1141–48.

12. Boano R, Fulcheri E, Martina MC, et al. Neural tube defect in a 4000-year-old Egyptian infant mummy: a case of meningocele from the museum of anthropology and ethnography of Turin (Italy). *Eur J Paediatr Neurol.* 2009 Nov; 13 (6): 481–87.

13. Macko SA, Engel MH, Andrusevich V, et al. Documenting the diet in ancient human populations through stable isotope analysis of hair. *Philos Trans R Soc Lond B Biol Sci.* 1999 Jan 29; 354 (1379): 65–75.

14. Durant W. *The Story of Civilization Vol III: Caesar and Christ.* (New York: Simon and Schuster, 1944).

15. Curry A. The gladiator's diet. *Archeology* 2008 Nov/Dec 61. www.archaeology.org/0811/abstracts/gladiator.html.

16. Perry GH, Dominy NJ, Claw KG, Lee AS, et al. Diet and the evolution of human amylase gene copy number variation. *Nat Genet.* 2007 Oct; 39 (10): 1256–60.

17. News.bbc.co.uk/2/hi/6983330.stm

18. Flatt JP. Carbohydrate balance and body-weight regulation. *Proc Nutr Soc.* 1996 Mar; 55 (1B): 449-65.

19. Zerodisease.com/archive/Dietary_Goals_For_The_United_States.pdf

20. Chopra M, Galbraith S, Darnton-Hill I. A global response to a global problem: the epidemic of overnutrition. *Bull World Health Organ.* 2003 Jan 23; 80: 952-58.

21. Hossain P, Kawar B, El Nahas M. Obesity and diabetes in the developing world—a growing challenge. *N Engl J Med.* 2007 Jan 18; 356 (3): 213-15.

22. www.fao.org/docrep/010/a0701e/a0701e00.htm

Chapter 2. People Passionate about Starches Are Healthy and Beautiful

1. Bujnowski D, Xun P, Daviglus ML, et al. Longitudinal association between animal and vegetable protein intake and obesity among men in the United States: the Chicago Western Electric Study. *J Am Diet Assoc.* 2011 Aug; 111 (8): 1150-55.e1.

2. Webcenters.netscape.compuserve.com/homerealestate/package.jsp?name=fte /thinnestpeople/thinnestpeople

3. Rolls BJ. The role of energy density in the overconsumption of fat. *J Nutr.* 2000 Feb; 130 (2S Suppl): 268S-271S.

4. Blundell JE, Lawton CL, Cotton JR, Macdiarmid JI. Control of human appetite: implications for the intake of dietary fat. *Annu Rev Nutr.* 1996; 16: 285-319.

5. Rolls BJ, Kim-Harris S, Fischman MW, et al. Satiety after preloads with different amounts of fat and carbohydrate: implications for obesity. *Am J Clin Nutr.* 1994 Oct; 60 (4): 476-87.

6. Hellerstein MK. De novo lipogenesis in humans: metabolic and regulatory aspects. *Eur J Clin Nutr.* 1999 Apr; 53 Suppl 1: S53-65.

7. Acheson KJ, Schutz Y, Bessard T, et al. Glycogen storage capacity and de novo lipogenesis during massive carbohydrate overfeeding in man. *Am J Clin Nutr.* 1988 Aug; 48 (2): 240-47.

8. Minehira K, Bettschart V, Vidal H, et al. Effect of carbohydrate overfeeding on whole body and adipose tissue metabolism in humans. *Obes Res.* 2003 Sep; 11 (9): 1096-1103.

9. McDevitt RM, Bott SJ, Harding M, et al. De novo lipogenesis during controlled overfeeding with sucrose or glucose in lean and obese women. *Am J Clin Nutr.* 2001 Dec; 74 (6): 737-46.

10. Dirlewanger M, di Vetta V, Guenat E, et al. Effects of short-term carbohydrate or fat overfeeding on energy expenditure and plasma leptin concentrations in healthy female subjects. *Int J Obes Relat Metab Disord.* 2000 Nov; 24 (11): 1413-18.

11. McDevitt RM, Bott SJ, Harding M, et al. De novo lipogenesis during controlled overfeeding with sucrose or glucose in lean and obese women. *Am J Clin Nutr.* 2001 Dec; 74 (6): 737-46.

12. Danforth E Jr. Diet and obesity. *Am J Clin Nutr.* 1985 May; 41 (5 Suppl): 1132-45.

13. Hellerstein MK. No common energy currency: de novo lipogenesis as the road less traveled. *Am J Clin Nutr.* 2001 Dec; 74 (6): 707-8.

14. Tappy L. Metabolic consequences of overfeeding in humans. *Curr Opin Clin Nutr Metab Care.* 2004 Nov; 7 (6): 623-8.

15. Levine JA. Non-exercise activity thermogenesis (NEAT). *Best Pract Res Clin Endocrinol Metab.* 2002 Dec; 16 (4): 679-702.

16. Mickelsen O, Makdani DD, Cotton RH, Titcomb ST, Colmey JC, Gatty R. Effects of a high fiber bread diet on weight loss in college-age males. *Am J Clin Nutr.* 1979 Aug; 32(8): 1703-9.

17. Thomas LH, Jones PR, Winter JA, Smith H. Hydrogenated oils and fats: the presence of chemically-modified fatty acids in human adipose tissue. *Am J Clin Nutr.* 1981 May; 34 (5): 877–86.

18. London SJ, Sacks FM, Caesar J, et al. Fatty acid composition of subcutaneous adipose tissue and diet in postmenopausal US women. *Am J Clin Nutr.* 1991 Aug; 54 (2): 340–45.

19. Baylin A, Kabagambe EK, Siles X, Campos H. Adipose tissue biomarkers of fatty acid intake. *Am J Clin Nutr.* 2002 Oct; 76 (4): 750–57.

20. Brevik A, Veierød MB, Drevon CA, Andersen LF. Evaluation of the odd fatty acids 15:0 and 17:0 in serum and adipose tissue as markers of intake of milk and dairy fat. *Eur J Clin Nutr.* 2005 Dec; 59 (12): 1417–22.

21. McDougall J. Effects of a low-carbohydrate diet. *Mayo Clin Proc.* 2004 Mar; 79 (3): 431.

22. Reif A, Lesch KP. Toward a molecular architecture of personality. *Behav Brain Res.* 2003 Feb 17; 139 (1–2): 1–20.

23. Noblett KL and Coccaro EF. Molecular genetics of personality. *Curr Psychiatry Rep.* 2005 Mar; 7 (1): 73–80.

Chapter 3. Five Major Poisons Found in Animal Foods

1. Brenner BM. Dietary protein intake and the progressive nature of kidney disease: the role of hemodynamically mediated glomerular injury in the pathogenesis of progressive glomerular sclerosis in aging, renal ablation, and intrinsic renal disease. *N Engl J Med.* 1982 Sep 9; 307 (11): 652–59.

2. Meyer TW. Dietary protein intake and progressive glomerular sclerosis: the role of capillary hypertension and hyperperfusion in the progression of renal disease. *Ann Intern Med.* 1983 May; 98 (5 Pt 2): 832–38.

3. Hansen HP. Effect of dietary protein restriction on prognosis in patients with diabetic nephropathy. *Kidney Int.* 2002 Jul; 62 (1): 220–28.

4. Biesenbach G. Effect of mild dietary protein restriction on urinary protein excretion in patients with renal transplant fibrosis. *Wien Med Wochenschr.* 1996; 146 (4): 75–8.

5. Pedrini MT. The effect of dietary protein restriction on the progression of diabetic and nondiabetic renal diseases: a meta-analysis. *Ann Intern Med.* 1996 Apr 1; 124 (7): 627–32.

6. Cupisti A. Vegetarian diet alternated with conventional low-protein diet for patients with chronic renal failure. *J Ren Nutr.* 2002 Jan; 12 (1): 32–7.

7. Bianchi GP. Vegetable versus animal protein diet in cirrhotic patients with chronic encephalopathy. A randomized cross-over comparison. *J Intern Med.* 1993 May; 233 (5): 385–92.

8. Hegsted M, Schuette SA, Zemel MB, Linkswiler HM. Urinary calcium and calcium balance in young men as affected by level of protein and phosphorus intake. *J Nutr.* 1981 Mar; 111 (3): 553–62.

9. Flegal KM, Carroll MD, Ogden CL, Curtin LR. Prevalence and trends in obesity among US adults, 1999–2008. *JAMA.* 2010 Jan 20; 303 (3): 235–41.

10. Danforth E Jr. Diet and obesity. *Am J Clin Nutr.* 1985 May; 41 (5 Suppl): 1132–45.

11. Schrauwen P. High-fat diet, muscular lipotoxicity and insulin resistance. *Proc Nutr Soc.* 2007 Feb; 66 (1): 33–41.

12. Yecies JL and Manning BD. Chewing the fat on tumor cell metabolism. *Cell.* 2010 Jan 8; 140 (1): 28–30.

13. Behrman EJ and Gopalan V. Cholesterol and plants. *J. Chem. Educ.* 2005; 82 (12): 1791.

14. Subramanian S and Chait A. The effect of dietary cholesterol on macrophage accumulation in adipose tissue: implications for systemic inflammation and atherosclerosis. *Curr Opin Lipidol.* 2009 Feb; 20 (1): 39–44.

15. Morin RJ, Hu B, Peng SK, Sevanian A. Cholesterol oxides and carcinogenesis. *J Clin Lab Anal.* 1991; 5 (3): 219–25.

16. Cacciapuoti F. Hyper-homocysteinemia: a novel risk factor or a powerful marker for cardiovascular diseases? Pathogenetic and therapeutical uncertainties. *J Thromb Thrombolysis.* 2011 Jul; 32 (1): 82–8.

17. Cellarier E. Methionine dependency and cancer treatment. *Cancer Treat Rev.* 2003 Dec; 29 (6): 489–99.

18. Levine J. Fecal hydrogen sulfide production in ulcerative colitis. *Am J Gastroenterol.* 1998 Jan; 93 (1): 83–7.

19. Remer T. Influence of diet on acid-base balance. *Semin Dial.* 2000 Jul–Aug; 13 (4): 221–26.

20. Frassetto L. Diet, evolution and aging—the pathophysiologic effects of the post-agricultural inversion of the potassium-to-sodium and base-to-chloride ratios in the human diet. *Eur J Nutr.* 2001 Oct; 40 (5): 200–13.

21. Remer T. Potential renal acid load of foods and its influence on urine pH. *J Am Diet Assoc.* 1995 Jul; 95 (7): 791–97.

22. Barzel US. Excess dietary protein can adversely affect bone. *J Nutr.* 1998 Jun; 128 (6): 1051–53.

23. Jajoo R, Song L, Rasmussen H, et al. Dietary acid-base balance, bone resorption, and calcium excretion. *J Am Coll Nutr.* 2006 Jun; 25 (3): 224–30.

24. Maurer M. Neutralization of Western diet inhibits bone resorption independently of K intake and reduces cortisol secretion in humans. *Am J Physiol Renal Physiol.* 2003 Jan; 284 (1): F32–40.

25. Wilhelm B, Rajié A, Greig JD, et al. The effect of hazard analysis critical control point programs on microbial contamination of carcasses in abattoirs: a systematic review of published data. *Foodborne Pathog Dis.* 2011 Sep; 8 (9): 949–60.

26. Wilhelm B, Rajié A, Waddell L, et al. Prevalence of zoonotic or potentially zoonotic bacteria, antimicrobial resistance, and somatic cell counts in organic dairy production: current knowledge and research gaps. *Foodborne Pathog Dis.* 2009 Jun; 6 (5): 525–39.

Chapter 4. Spontaneous Healing on a Starch-Based Diet

For detailed discussions and scientific references on multiple diseases please refer to my Web site, www.drmcdougall.com. The Hot Topics and the Search feature provide efficient means to locate discussions of relevant materials. Refer also to the previous McDougall books for discussions on a variety of illnesses and their management.

Chapter 5. The USDA and the Politics of Starch

1. www.gpo.gov/fdsys/pkg/FR-2011-01-13/pdf/2011-485.pdf

2. www.fns.usda.gov/wic/benefitsandservices/foodpkgregs.htm

3. www.foodcircles.missouri.edu/CRJanuary05.pdf

4. www.omorganics.org/page.php?pageid=131&contentid=123

5. Herman J. Saving U.S. dietary advice from conflicts of interest. *Food and Drug Law Journal* (2010); 65(2): 284–316. www.drmcdougall.com/misc/2010nl/jul/sc%20herman.indd.pdf

6. www.drmcdougall.com/misc/2010other/guidelines.htm

7. www.cnpp.usda.gov/DGAs2010-PolicyDocument.htm

8. www.pcrm.org/search/?cid=2512

9. www.pcrm.org/search/?cid=1395

10. www.pcrm.org/search/?cid=2543

11. www.pcrm.org/search/?cid=137

Chapter 6. We Are Eating the Planet to Death

1. Horrigan L, Lawrence RS, Walker P. How sustainable agriculture can address the environmental and human health harms of industrial agriculture. *Environ Health Perspect.* 2002 May; 110 (5): 445–56.

2. Pimentel D and Pimentel M. Sustainability of meat-based and plant-based diets and the environment. *Am J Clin Nutr.* 2003 Sep; 78 (3 Suppl): 660S–63S.

3. Hossain P, Kawar B, El Nahas M. Obesity and diabetes in the developing world—a growing challenge. *N Engl J Med.* 2007 Jan 18; 356 (3): 213–15.

4. www.climaterealityproject.org

5. Godlee F. How on earth do we combat climate change? *BMJ* 2011; 343:d6789.

6. ftp.fao.org/docrep/fao/010/a0701e/a0701e00.pdf

7. www.newscientist.com/article/dn10786

8. www.51percent.org

9. www.vegetariantimes.com/features/archive_of_editorial/667

10. www.businessweek.com/magazine/content/10_46/b4203103862097.htm

11. Pimentel D and Pimentel M. Sustainability of meat-based and plant-based diets and the environment. *Am J Clin Nutr.* 2003 Sep; 78 (3 Suppl): 660S–663S.

12. www.populationpress.org/essays/essay-pimentel.html

13. www.web4water.com/library/view_article.asp?id=3902&channel=4

14. www.usatoday.com/news/world/2010-09-09-1Achinaonechild09_ST_N.htm

15. www.unicef.org/media/files/Tracking_Progress_on_Child_and_Maternal_Nutrition_EN_110309.pdf

16. www.waldeneffect.org/blog/Calories_per_acre_for_various_foods

17. www.time.com/time/magazine/article/0,9171,1879192,00.html

Chapter 7. When Friends Ask: Where Do You Get Your Protein?

1. Millward DJ. The nutritional value of plant-based diets in relation to human amino acid and protein requirements. *Proc Nutr Soc.* 1999 May; 58 (2): 249–60.

2. Mazess RB. Bone mineral content of North Alaskan Eskimos. *Am J Clin Nutr.* 1974 Sep; 27 (9): 916–25.

3. Carpenter K. A short history of nutritional science: part 2 (1885–1912). *J Nutr.* 2003 Apr; 133 (4): 975–84.

4. Chittenden RH. *Physiological economy in nutrition, with special reference to the minimal protein requirement of the healthy man. An experimental study.* (New York: Frederick A. Stokes Company, 1904).

5. Calloway DH. Sweat and miscellaneous nitrogen losses in human balance studies. *J Nutr.* 1971 Jun; 101 (6): 775–86.

6. Hegsted DM. Minimum protein requirements of adults. *Am J Clin Nutr.* 1968 May; 21 (5): 352–27.

7. Dole V. Dietary treatment of hypertension: clinical and metabolic studies of patients on the rice-fruit diet. *J Clin Invest.* 1950; 29: 1189–1206.

8. Osborne T. Amino-acids in nutrition and growth. *J Bio Chem.* 1914; 17: 325–49.

9. Rose W. Comparative growth of diet containing ten and nineteen amino acids, with further observation upon the role of glutamic and aspartic acid. *J Bio Chem.* 1948; 176: 753–62.

10. Bicker M. The protein requirement of adult rats in terms of the protein contained in egg, milk, and soy flour. *J Nutr.* 1947; 34: 491.

11. Bell G. *Textbook of Physiology and Biochemestry,* 4th ed. (Baltimore: Williams and Wilkins, 1959) 12.

12. Reeds PJ. Protein nutrition of the neonate. *Proc Nutr Soc.* 2000 Feb; 59 (1): 87–97.

13. Rose W. The amino acid requirement of adult man. *Nutr Abst Rev.* 1957; 27: 63–67.

14. McDougall J. *The McDougall Plan.* (El Monte, Calif.: New Win Publishing, 1983), 95–109.

15. Jean Mayer USDA/Human Nutrition Research Center on Aging at Tufts University School of Medicine: www.thedoctorwillseeyounow.com/content/nutrition/art2059.html

16. Tufts University Medical School: http://www.quackwatch.com/03HealthPromotion/vegetarian.html

17. www.hsph.harvard.edu/nutritionsource/protein.html

18. Northwestern University: http://www.feinberg.northwestern.edu/nutrition/factsheets/protein.html

19. St Jeor S, Howard B, Prewitt E. Dietary protein and weight reduction: a statement for healthcare professionals from the Nutrition Committee of the Council on Nutrition, Physical Activity, and Metabolism of the American Heart Association. *Circulation.* 2001; 104: 1869–74.

20. McDougall J. Plant foods have a complete amino acid composition. *Circulation.* 2002 Jun 25; 105 (25): e197; author reply e197.

21. McDougall J. Misinformation on plant proteins. *Circulation.* 2002 Nov 12; 106 (20): e148; author reply e148.

22. Millward DJ. Protein requirements. *Encyclopedia of Nutrition.* (Salt Lake City: Academic Press, 1998), 1661–68.

23. Personal Communication with John McDougall, MD on July 10, 2003.

24. www.heart.org/HEARTORG/GettingHealthy/NutritionCenter/Vegetarian-Diets_UCM_306032_Article.jsp

25. Kon S. XXXV. The value of whole potato in human nutrition. *Biochemical J.* 1928; 22: 258–60.

26. Lopez de Romana G, Graham GG, Mellits ED, MacLean WC Jr. Utilization of the protein and energy of the white potato by human infants. *J Nutr.* 1980 Sep; 110 (9): 1849–57.

27. Lopez de Romana G. Fasting and postprandial plasma free amino acids of infants and children consuming exclusively potato protein. *J Nutr.* 1981 Oct; 111 (10): 1766–71.

Chapter 8. When Friends Ask: Where Do You Get Your Calcium?

1. www.dairycheckoff.com

2. www.nationaldairycouncil.org/NationalDairyCouncil/Health/Digest/dcd69-1Page1.htm

3. www.dairycheckoff.com/DairyCheckoff/AboutUs/HowTheDairyCheckoffWorks/How-The-Dairy-Checkoff-Works

4. www.unistraw.com/fastfacts

5. Walker AR. Osteoporosis and calcium deficiency. *Am J Clin Nutr.* 1965 Mar; 16: 327–36.

6. Smith RW Jr and Rizek J. Epidemiologic studies of osteoporosis in women of Puerto Rico and southeastern Michigan with special reference to age, race, national origin, and to other related and associated findings. *Clin Orthop Relat Res.* 1966 Mar–Apr; 45: 31–48.

7. Wynn E, Krieg MA, Lanham-New SA, Burckhardt P. Postgraduate symposium: Positive influence of nutritional alkalinity on bone health. *Proc Nutr Soc.* 2010 Feb; 69 (1): 166–73.

8. Paterson CR. Calcium requirements in man: a critical review. *Postgrad Med J.* 1978 Apr; 54 (630): 244–48.

9. Walker AR. The human requirement of calcium: should low intakes be supplemented? *Am J Clin Nutr.* 1972 May; 25 (5): 518–30.

10. Irwin MI and Kienholz EW. A conspectus of research on calcium requirements of man. *J Nutr* 1973; 103: 1020–95.

11. Sellers EA, Sharma A, Rodd C. Adaptation of Inuit children to a low-calcium diet. *CMAJ.* 2003 Apr 29; 168 (9): 1141–43. *CMAJ.* 2003 Sep 16; 169 (6): 542; author reply 542–43.

12. www.drmcdougall.com/misc/2007nl/feb/whenfriendsask.htm

13. Thacher TD and Abrams SA. Relationship of calcium absorption with 25(OH)D and calcium intake in children with rickets. *Nutr Rev.* 2010 Nov; 68 (11): 682–88.

14. Winzenberg T, Shaw K, Fryer J, Jones G. Effects of calcium supplementation on bone density in healthy children: meta-analysis of randomised controlled trials. *BMJ.* 2006 Oct 14; 333 (7572): 775.

15. Lanou AJ, Berkow SE, Barnard ND. Calcium, dairy products, and bone health in children and young adults: a reevaluation of the evidence. *Pediatrics.* 2005 Mar; 115 (3): 736–43.

16. Weinsier RL and Krumdieck CL. Dairy foods and bone health: examination of the evidence. *Am J Clin Nutr.* 2000 Sep; 72 (3): 681–89.

17. Recker RR and Heaney RP. The effect of milk supplements on calcium metabolism, bone metabolism and calcium balance. *Am J Clin Nutr.* 1985 Feb; 41 (2): 254–63.

18. Lanou AJ. Bone health in children. *BMJ.* 2006 Oct 14; 333 (7572): 763–64.

19. Abelow BJ, Holford TR, Insogna KL. Cross-cultural association between dietary animal protein and hip fracture: a hypothesis. *Calcif Tissue Int.* 1992 Jan; 50 (1): 14–18.

20. Frassetto LA. Worldwide incidence of hip fracture in elderly women: relation to consumption of animal and vegetable foods. *J Gerontol A Biol Sci Med Sci.* 2000 Oct; 55 (10): M585–92.

21. Remer T. Potential renal acid load of foods and its influence on urine pH. *J Am Diet Assoc.* 1995 Jul; 95 (7): 791–97.

22. Barzel US. Excess dietary protein can adversely affect bone. *J Nutr.* 1998 Jun; 128 (6): 1051–53.

23. Maurer M. Neutralization of Western diet inhibits bone resorption independently of K intake and reduces cortisol secretion in humans. *Am J Physiol Renal Physiol.* 2003 Jan; 284 (1): F32–40.

24. Welch AA, Bingham SA, Reeve J, Khaw KT. More acidic dietary acid-base load is associated with reduced calcaneal broadband ultrasound attenuation in women but not in men: results from the EPIC-Norfolk cohort study. *Am J Clin Nutr.* 2007 Apr; 85 (4): 1134–41.

25. Frassetto L. Diet, evolution and aging—the pathophysiologic effects of the post-agricultural inversion of the potassium-to-sodium and base-to-chloride ratios in the human diet. *Eur J Nutr.* 2001 Oct; 40 (5): 200–13.

26. Wynn E, Krieg MA, Lanham-New SA, Burckhardt P. Postgraduate symposium: Positive influence of nutritional alkalinity on bone health. *Proc Nutr Soc.* 2010 Feb; 69 (1): 166–73.

27. Ahn J, Albanes D, Peters U, et al. Prostate, Lung, Colorectal, and Ovarian Trial Project Team. Dairy products, calcium intake, and risk of prostate cancer in the prostate, lung, colorectal, and ovarian cancer screening trial. *Cancer Epidemiol Biomarkers Prev.* 2007 Dec; 16 (12): 2623–30.

28. Endogenous Hormones and Breast Cancer Collaborative Group. Insulin-like growth factor 1 (IGF1), IGF binding protein 3 (IGFBP3), and breast cancer risk: pooled individual data analysis of 17 prospective studies. *Lancet Oncol.* 2010; 11: 530–42.

29. Yu H and Rohan T. Role of the insulin-like growth factor family in cancer development and progression. *J Natl Cancer Inst.* 2000 Sep 20; 92 (18): 1472–89.

30. Cadogan J, Eastell R, Jones N, Barker ME. Milk intake and bone mineral acquisition in adolescent girls: randomised, controlled intervention trial. *BMJ*. 1997 Nov 15; 315 (7118): 1255–60.

31. Heaney RP, McCarron DA, Dawson-Hughes B, et al. Dietary changes favorably affect bone remodeling in older adults. *J Am Diet Assoc*. 1999 Oct; 99 (10): 1228–33.

32. Bartley J and McGlashan SR. Does milk increase mucus production? *Med Hypotheses*. 2010 Apr; 74 (4): 732–34.

33. Guggenmos J, Schubart AS, Ogg S, et al. Antibody cross-reactivity between myelin oligodendrocyte glycoprotein and the milk protein butyrophilin in multiple sclerosis. *J Immunol*. 2004 Jan 1; 172 (1): 661–68.

34. Panush RS, Stroud RM, Webster EM. Food-induced (allergic) arthritis. Inflammatory arthritis exacerbated by milk. *Arthritis Rheum*. 1986 Feb; 29 (2): 220–26.

35. Benkhedda K, L'abbé MR, Cockell KA. Effect of calcium on iron absorption in women with marginal iron status. *Br J Nutr*. 2010 Mar; 103 (5): 742–48.

36. Prince RL, Devine A, Dhaliwal SS, Dick IM. Effects of calcium supplementation on clinical fracture and bone structure: results of a 5-year, double-blind, placebo-controlled trial in elderly women. *Arch Intern Med*. 2006 Apr 24; 166 (8): 869–75.

37. Tang BM, Eslick GD, Nowson C, et al. Use of calcium or calcium in combination with vitamin D supplementation to prevent fractures and bone loss in people aged 50 years and older: a meta-analysis. *Lancet*. 2007 Aug 25; 370 (9588): 657–66.

38. Reid IR, Bolland MJ, Grey A. Effect of calcium supplementation on hip fractures. *Osteoporos Int*. 2008 Aug; 19 (8): 1119–23.

39. Warensjö E, Byberg L, Melhus H, et al. Dietary calcium intake and risk of fracture and osteoporosis: prospective longitudinal cohort study. *BMJ*. 2011 May 24; 342: d1473. doi: 10.1136/bmj.d1473.

40. Sebastian A, Harris ST, Ottaway JH, et al. Improved mineral balance and skeletal metabolism in postmenopausal women treated with potassium bicarbonate. *N Engl J Med*. 1994 Jun 23; 330 (25): 1776–81.

41. Bolland MJ, Avenell A, Baron JA, et al. Effect of calcium supplements on risk of myocardial infarction and cardiovascular events: meta-analysis. *BMJ*. 2010 Jul 29; 341: c3691. doi: 10.1136/bmj.c3691).

42. Wong S. Recalls of foods and cosmetics due to microbial contamination reported to the U.S. Food and Drug Administration. *J Food Prot*. 2000 Aug; 63 (8): 1113–16.

43. Chapman PA. Sources of Escherichia coli O157 and experiences over the past 15 years in Sheffield, UK. *Symp Ser Soc Appl Microbiol*. 2000; (29): 51S–60S.

44. Lund BM. Pasteurization of milk and the heat resistance of Mycobacterium avium subsp. paratuberculosis: a critical review of the data. *Int J Food Microbiol*. 2002 Jul 25; 77 (1–2):135–45.

45. USDA/APHIS. Bovine Leukosis Virus (BLV) on U.S. Dairy Operations, 2007. www .aphis.usda.gov/animal_health/nahms/dairy/downloads/dairy07/Dairy07_is_BLV.pdf

46. Michigan Dairy Review: Bovine Leukosis Virus Update I: Prevalence, Economic Losses, and Management. www.msu.edu/~mdr/vol14no1/erskine.html

47. Buehring GC, Philpott SM, Choi KY. Humans have antibodies reactive with Bovine leukemia virus. *AIDS Res Hum Retroviruses*. 2003 Dec; 19 (12): 1105–13.

48. McClure HM, Keeling ME, Custer RP, et al. Erythroleukemia in two infant chimpanzees fed milk from cows naturally infected with the bovine C-type virus. *Cancer Res*. 1974 Oct; 34 (10): 2745–57.

49. McDougall J. Marketing milk and disease. www.nealhendrickson.com/mcdougall /030500pudairyanddisease.htm

Chapter 9. Confessions of a Fish Killer

1. Worm B, Barbier EB, Beaumont N, et al. Impacts of biodiversity loss on ocean ecosystem services. *Science.* 2006 Nov 3; 314 (5800): 787–90.

2. Plourde M, Cunnane SC. Extremely limited synthesis of long chain polyunsaturates in adults: implications for their dietary essentiality and use as supplements. *Appl Physiol Nutr Metab.* 2007 Aug; 32 (4): 619–34.

3. Tu WC, Cook-Johnson RJ, James MJ, Mühlhäusler BS, Gibson RA. Omega-3 long chain fatty acid synthesis is regulated more by substrate levels than gene expression. *Prostaglandins Leukot Essent Fatty Acids.* 2010 Aug; 83 (2): 61–8.

4. Harnack K, Andersen G, Somoza V. Quantitation of alpha-linolenic acid elongation to eicosapentaenoic and docosahexaenoic acid as affected by the ratio of n6/n3 fatty acids. *Nutr Metab (Lond).* 2009 Feb 19; 6: 8.

5. Langdon JH. Has an aquatic diet been necessary for hominin brain evolution and functional development? *Br J Nutr.* 2006 Jul; 96 (1): 7–17.

6. Welch AA, Shakya-Shrestha S, Lentjes MA, et al. Dietary intake and status of n-3 polyunsaturated fatty acids in a population of fish-eating and non-fish-eating meat-eaters, vegetarians, and vegans and the precursor-product ratio (corrected) of alpha-linolenic acid to long-chain n-3 polyunsaturated fatty acids: results from the EPIC-Norfolk cohort. *Am J Clin Nutr.* 2010 Nov; 92 (5): 1040–51.

7. Sanders TA. DHA status of vegetarians. *Prostaglandins, Leukotrienes,* and *Essential Fatty Acids.* 2009 Aug–Sep; 81 (2–3): 137–41.

8. www.nap.edu/openbook.php?record_id=10490&page=471

9. Sanders TA. Essential fatty acid requirements of vegetarians in pregnancy, lactation, and infancy. *Am J Clin Nutr.* 1999 Sep; 70 (3 Suppl): 555S–59S.

10. Krüger E, Verreault R, Carmichael PH, et al. Omega-3 fatty acids and risk of dementia: the Canadian study of health and aging. *Am J Clin Nutr.* 2009 Jul; 90 (1): 184–92.

11. Devore EE, Grodstein F, van Rooij FJ, et al. Dietary intake of fish and omega-3 fatty acids in relation to long-term dementia risk. *Am J Clin Nutr.* 2009 Jul; 90 (1): 170–76.

12. Beezhold BL, Johnston CS, Daigle DR. Vegetarian diets are associated with healthy mood states: a cross-sectional study in Seventh Day Adventist adults. *Nutr J.* 2010 Jun 1; 9:26.

13. Krüger E, Verreault R, Carmichael PH, et al. Omega-3 fatty acids and risk of dementia: the Canadian study of health and aging. *Am J Clin Nutr.* 2009 Jul; 90 (1): 184–92.

14. Devore EE, Grodstein F, van Rooij FJ, et al. Dietary intake of fish and omega-3 fatty acids in relation to long-term dementia risk. *Am J Clin Nutr.* 2009 Jul; 90 (1): 170–76.

15. Giem P, Beeson WL, Fraser GE. The incidence of dementia and intake of animal products: preliminary findings from the Adventist Health Study. *Neuroepidemiology.* 1993; 12 (1): 28–36.

16. Smithers LG, Gibson RA, Makrides M. Maternal supplementation with docosahexaenoic acid during pregnancy does not affect early visual development in the infant: a randomized controlled trial. *Am J Clin Nutr.* 2011 Jun; 93 (6): 1293–99.

17. Huston MC. The role of mercury and cadmium heavy metals in vascular disease, hypertension, coronary heart disease, and myocardial infarction. *Altern Ther Health Med.* 2007 Mar–Apr; 13 (2): S128–33.

18. Guallar E, Sanz-Gallardo MI, van't Veer P, et al. Heavy Metals and Myocardial Infarction Study Group. Mercury, fish oils, and the risk of myocardial infarction. *N Engl J Med.* 2002 Nov 28; 347 (22): 1747–54.

19. Virtanen JK, Voutilainen S, Rissanen TH, et al. Mercury, fish oils, and risk of acute coronary events and cardiovascular disease, coronary heart disease, and all-cause mortality in men in eastern Finland. *Arterioscler Thromb Vasc Biol.* 2005 Jan; 25 (1): 228–33.

20. Davidson MH, Hunninghake D, Maki KC, et al. Comparison of the effects of lean red meat vs lean white meat on serum lipid levels among free-living persons with hypercholesterolemia: a long-term, randomized clinical trial. *Arch Intern Med.* 1999 Jun 28; 159 (12): 1331–38.

21. Harris WS, Dujovne CA, Zucker M, Johnson B. Effects of a low saturated fat, low cholesterol fish oil supplement in hypertriglyceridemic patients. A placebo-controlled trial. *Ann Intern Med.* 1988 Sep 15; 109 (6): 465–70.

22. Wilt TJ, Lofgren RP, Nichol KL, et al. Fish oil supplementation does not lower plasma cholesterol in men with hypercholesterolemia. Results of a randomized, placebo-controlled crossover study. *Ann Intern Med.* 1989 Dec 1; 111 (11): 900–05.

23. Hooper L, Thompson RL, Harrison RA, et al. Risks and benefits of omega 3 fats for mortality, cardiovascular disease, and cancer: systematic review. *BMJ.* 2006 Apr 1; 332 (7544): 752–60.

24. Cundiff DK, Lanou AJ, Nigg CR. Relation of omega-3 fatty acid intake to other dietary factors known to reduce coronary heart disease risk. *Am J Cardiol.* 2007 May 1; 99 (9): 1230–33.

25. Burr ML, Ashfield-Watt PA, Dunstan FD, et al. Lack of benefit of dietary advice to men with angina: results of a controlled trial. *Eur J Clin Nutr.* 2003 Feb; 57 (2): 193–200.

26. Senges J. Omega-3 fatty acids on top of modern therapy after acute myocardial infarction (OMEGA). Report presented at American College of Cardiology Annual Meeting, March 30, 2009, Orlando, Florida. www.theheart.org/article/957205.do

27. Kromhout D, Giltay EJ, Geleijnse JM; Alpha Omega Trial Group. N-3 fatty acids and cardiovascular events after myocardial infarction. *N Engl J Med.* 2010 Nov 18; 363 (21): 2015–26.

28. Galan P, Kesse-Guyot E, Czernichow S, et al; SU.FOL.OM3 Collaborative Group. Effects of B vitamins and omega 3 fatty acids on cardiovascular diseases: a randomised placebo controlled trial. *BMJ.* 2010 Nov 29; 341: c6273. doi: 10.1136/bmj.c6273.

29. Kowey PR, Reiffel JA, Ellenbogen KA, et al. Efficacy and safety of prescription omega-3 fatty acids for the prevention of recurrent symptomatic atrial fibrillation: a randomized controlled trial. *JAMA.* 2010 Dec 1; 304 (21): 2363–72.

30. Sacks FM, Stone PH, Gibson CM, et al. Controlled trial of fish oil for regression of human coronary atherosclerosis. HARP Research Group. *J Am Coll Cardiol.* 1995 Jun; 25 (7): 1492–98.

31. Jenkins DJ, Sievenpiper JL, Pauly D, et al. Are dietary recommendations for the use of fish oils sustainable? *CMAJ.* 2009 Mar 17; 180 (6): 633–37.

32. Insull W Jr, Lang PD, Hsi BP, Yoshimura S. Studies of arteriosclerosis in Japanese and American men. I. Comparison of fatty acid composition of adipose tissue. *J Clin Invest.* 1969 Jul; 48 (7): 1313–27.

33. Robertson W. The effect of high animal protein intake on the risk of calcium stone-formation in the urinary tract. *Clin Sci (Lond).* 1979 Sep; 57 (3): 285–88.

34. Dyerberg J, Bang HO. Haemostatic function and platelet polyunsaturated fatty acids in Eskimos. *Lancet.* 1979 Sep 1; 2 (8140): 433–35.

35. Meydani SN, Lichtenstein AH, Cornwall S, et al. Immunologic effects of national cholesterol education panel step-2 diets with and without fish-derived N-3 fatty acid enrichment. *J Clin Invest.* 1993 Jul; 92 (1): 105–13.

36. Stripp C, Overvad K, Christensen J, et al. Fish intake is positively associated with breast cancer incidence rate. *J Nutr.* 2003 Nov; 133 (11): 3664–69. *Cancer Res.* 1998 Aug 1; 58 (15): 3312–19.

37. Klieveri L, Fehres O, Griffini P, et al. Promotion of colon cancer metastases in rat liver by fish oil diet is not due to reduced stroma formation. *Clin Exp Metastasis.* 2000; 18 (5): 371–77.

38. Roodhart JM, Daenen LG, Stigter EC, et al. Mesenchymal stem cells induce resistance to chemotherapy through the release of platinum-induced fatty acids. *Cancer Cell.* 2011 Sep 13; 20 (3): 370–83.

39. Rice TW, Wheeler AP, Thompson BT, et al; NHLBI ARDS Clinical trials network. Enteral omega-3 fatty acid, gamma-linolenic acid, and antioxidant supplementation in acute lung injury. *JAMA.* 2011 Oct 12; 306 (14): 1574–81.

40. Hendra TJ, Britton ME, Roper DR, et al. Effects of fish oil supplements in NIDDM subjects. Controlled study. *Diabetes Care.* 1990 Aug; 13 (8): 821–9.

41. Djouss Ä L, Gaziano JM, Buring JE, Lee IM. Dietary omega-3 fatty acids and fish consumption and risk of type 2 diabetes. *Am J Clin Nutr.* 2011 Jan; 93 (1): 143–50.

42. Olsen SF, Osterdal ML, Salvig JD, et al. Duration of pregnancy in relation to fish oil supplementation and habitual fish intake: a randomised clinical trial with fish oil. *Eur J Clin Nutr.* 2007 Aug; 61 (8): 976–85.

43. Olsen SF, Hansen HS, Sorensen TI, et al. Intake of marine fat, rich in (n-3)-polyunsaturated fatty acids, may increase birthweight by prolonging gestation. *Lancet.* 1986 Aug 16; 2 (8503): 367–69.

44. Ju H, Chadha Y, Donovan T, O'Rourke P. Fetal macrosomia and pregnancy outcomes. *Aust N Z J Obstet Gynaecol.* 2009 Oct; 49 (5): 504–9.

45. Joensen F, Olsen SF, Holm T, Joensen HD. Perinatal deaths in the Faroe Islands during 1986–95. *Acta Obstet Gynecol Scand.* 2000 Oct; 79 (10): 834–38.

46. Olsen SF, Samuelsen S, Joensen HD. A clinico-pathological classification of perinatal deaths in the Faroe Islands. *Br J Obstet Gynaecol.* 1995 May; 102 (5): 389–92.

47. Friedland RP, Petersen RB, Rubenstein R. Bovine spongiform encephalopathy and aquaculture. *J Alzheimers Dis.* 2009 Jun; 17 (2): 277–79.

48. Bell JG, Henderson RJ, Tocher DR, et al. Substituting fish oil with crude palm oil in the diet of Atlantic salmon (Salmo salar) affects muscle fatty acid composition and hepatic fatty acid metabolism. *J Nutr.* 2002 Feb; 132 (2): 222–30.

49. Weaver KL, Ivester P, Chilton JA, et al. The content of favorable and unfavorable polyunsaturated fatty acids found in commonly eaten fish. *J Am Diet Assoc.* 2008 Jul; 108 (7): 1178–85.

50. Lund V, Mejdell CM, Rocklinsberg H, et al. Expanding the moral circle: farmed fish as objects of moral concern. *Dis Aquat Organ.* 2007 May 4; 75 (2): 109–18.

Chapter 10. The Fat Vegan

1. Spence LA, Lipscomb ER, Cadogan J, et al. The effect of soy protein and soy isoflavones on calcium metabolism in postmenopausal women: a randomized crossover study. *Am J Clin Nutr.* 2005 Apr; 81 (4): 916–22.

2. Roughead ZK, Hunt JR, Johnson LK, et al. Controlled substitution of soy protein for meat protein: effects on calcium retention, bone, and cardiovascular health indices in postmenopausal women. *J Clin Endocrinol Metab.* 2005 Jan; 90 (1): 181–89.

3. Kerstetter JE, Wall DE, O'Brien KO, et al. Meat and soy protein affect calcium homeostasis in healthy women. *J Nutr.* 2006 Jul; 136 (7): 1890–95.

4. Arjmandi BH, Khalil DA, Smith BJ, et al. Soy protein has a greater effect on bone in postmenopausal women not on hormone replacement therapy, as evidenced by reducing bone resorption and urinary calcium excretion. *J Clin Endocrinol Metab.* 2003 Mar; 88 (3): 1048–54.

5. Khalil DA, Lucas EA, Juma S, et al. Soy protein supplementation increases serum insulin-like growth factor-I in young and old men but does not affect markers of bone metabolism. *J Nutr.* 2002 Sep; 132 (9): 2605–8.

6. Sauer LA, Blask DE, Dauchy RT. Dietary factors and growth and metabolism in experimental tumors. *J Nutr Biochem.* 2007 Oct; 18 (10): 637–49.

7. Griffini P. Dietary omega-3 polyunsaturated fatty acids promote colon carcinoma metastasis in rat liver. *Cancer Res.* 1998 Aug 1; 58 (15): 3312–19.

8. Coulombe J, Pelletier G, Tremblay P, et al. Influence of lipid diets on the number of metastases and ganglioside content of H59 variant tumors. *Clin Exp Metastasis.* 1997 Jul; 15 (4): 410–17.

9. Klieveri L. Promotion of colon cancer metastases in rat liver by fish oil diet is not due to reduced stroma formation. *Clin Exp Metastasis.* 2000; 18 (5): 371–77.

10. Thiäbaut AC, Kipnis V, Chang SC, et al. Dietary fat and postmenopausal invasive breast cancer in the National Institutes of Health-AARP Diet and Health Study cohort. *J Natl Cancer Inst.* 2007 Mar 21; 99 (6): 451–62.

11. Ferrari R and Rapezzi C. The Mediterranean diet: a cultural journey. *Lancet.* 2011 May 1; 377 (9779): 1730–31.

12. Keys A. Mediterranean diet and public health: personal reflections. *Am J Clin Nutr.* 1995 Jun; 61 (6 Suppl): 1321S–23S.

13. Brown JM, Shelness GS, Rudel LL. Monounsaturated fatty acids and atherosclerosis: opposing views from epidemiology and experimental animal models. *Curr Atheroscler Rep.* 2007 Dec; 9 (6): 494–500.

14. Blankenhorn DH, Johnson RL, Mack WJ, et al. The influence of diet on the appearance of new lesions in human coronary arteries. *JAMA.* 1990 Mar 23–30; 263 (12): 1646–52.

15. Felton CV, Crook D, Davies MJ, Oliver MF. Dietary polyunsaturated fatty acids and composition of human aortic plaques. *Lancet.* 1994 Oct 29; 344 (8931): 1195–96.

16. Sanders TA, de Grassi T, Miller GJ, Humphries SE. Dietary oleic and palmitic acids and postprandial factor VII in middle-aged men heterozygous and homozygous for factor VII R353Q polymorphism. *Am J Clin Nutr.* 1999; 69: 220–25.

17. Larsen LF, Bladbjerg EM, Jespersen J, Marckmann P. Effects of dietary fat quality and quantity on postprandial activation of blood coagulation factor VII. *Arterioscler Thromb Vasc Biol.* 1997 Nov; 17 (11): 2904–9.

18. Friedman M, Rosenman RH, Byers SO. Serum lipids and conjunctival circulation after fat ingestion in men exhibiting type-A behavior patterns. *Circulation.* 1964 Jun; 29: 874–86.

19. Friedman M, Byers SO, Rosenman RH. Effect of unsaturated fats upon lipemia and conjunctival circulation. A study of coronary-prone (pattern A) men. *JAMA.* 1965 Sep 13; 193: 882–86.

20. Kuo P, Whereat AF, Horwitz O. The effect of lipemia upon coronary and peripheral arterial circulation in patients with essential hyperlipemia. *Am J Med.* 1959 Jan; 26 (1): 68–75.

21. Natoli S and McCoy P. A review of the evidence: nuts and body weight. *Asia Pac J Clin Nutr.* 2007; 16 (4): 588–97.

22. Sacks FM, Lichtenstein A, Van Horn L, et al; American Heart Association Nutrition Committee. Soy protein, isoflavones, and cardiovascular health: an American Heart Association Science Advisory for professionals from the Nutrition Committee. *Circulation.* 2006 Feb 21; 113 (7): 1034–44.

23. Cassileth BR and Vickers AJ. Soy: an anticancer agent in wide use despite some troubling data. *Cancer Invest.* 2003; 21 (5): 817–18.

24. Lu L. Effects of soya consumption for one month on steroid hormones in premenopausal women: implications for breast cancer risk reduction. *Cancer Epidemiol Biomarkers Prev.* 1996 Jan; 5 (1): 63–70.

25. Divi R. Anti-thyroid isoflavones from soybean: isolation, characterization, and mechanisms of action. *Biochem Pharmacol.* 1997 Nov 15; 54 (10): 1087–96.

26. Doerge DR and Sheehan DM. Goitrogenic and estrogenic activity of soy isoflavones. *Environ Health Perspect.* 2002 Jun; 110 Suppl 3: 349–53.

27. Yellayi S. The phytoestrogen genistein induces thymic and immune changes: a human health concern? *Proc Natl Acad Sci USA.* 2002 May 28; 99 (11): 7616–21.

28. Zoppi G. Immunocompetence and dietary protein intake in early infancy. *J Pediatr Gastroenterol Nutr.* 1982; 1 (2): 175–82.

29. Zoppi G. Gammaglobulin level and soy-protein intake in early infancy. *Eur J Pediatr.* 1979 Apr 25; 131 (1): 61–9.

30. Zoppi G. Diet and antibody response to vaccinations in healthy infants. *Lancet.* 1983 Jul 2; 2 (8340): 11–14.

31. Fort P. Breast and soy-formula feedings in early infancy and the prevalence of autoimmune thyroid disease in children. *J Am Coll Nutr.* 1990 Apr; 9 (2): 164–67.

32. Alexandersen P. Ipriflavone in the treatment of postmenopausal osteoporosis: a randomized controlled trial. *JAMA.* 2001 Mar 21; 285 (11): 1482–88.

33. White LR, Petrovitch H, Ross GW, et al. Brain aging and midlife tofu consumption. *J Am Coll Nutr.* 2000 Apr; 19 (2): 242–55.

34. Reddy ST. Effect of low-carbohydrate high-protein diets on acid-base balance, stone-forming propensity, and calcium metabolism. *Am J Kidney Dis.* 2002 Aug; 40 (2): 265–74.

35. Jenkins DJ, Kendall CW, Vidgen E, et al. Effect of high vegetable protein diets on urinary calcium loss in middle-aged men and women. *Eur J Clin Nutr.* 2003 Feb; 57 (2): 376–82.

36. Yu H. Role of the insulin-like growth factor family in cancer development and progression. *J Natl Cancer Inst.* 2000 Sep 20; 92 (18): 1472–89.

37. Bartke A, Chandrashekar V, Dominici F, et al. Insulin-like growth factor 1 (IGF-1) and aging: controversies and new insights. *Biogerontology.* 2003; 4 (1): 1–8.

38. Miller RA. Genetic approaches to the study of aging. *J Am Geriatr Soc.* 2005 Sep; 53 (9 Suppl): S284–86.

39. Holzenberger M. The GH/IGF-I axis and longevity. *Eur J Endocrinol.* 2004 Aug; 151 Suppl 1: S23–7.

40. Sutter NB, Bustamante CD, Chase K, et al. A single IGF1 allele is a major determinant of small size in dogs. *Science.* 2007 Apr 6; 316 (5821): 112–15.

41. Samaras TT, Elrick H, Storms LH. Is height related to longevity? *Life Sci.* 2003 Mar 7; 72 (16): 1781–1802.

42. Siegel-Itzkovich J. Health committee warns of potential dangers of soya. *BMJ.* 2005 Jul 30; 331 (7511): 254.

43. Turck D. Soy protein for infant feeding: what do we know? *Curr Opin Clin Nutr Metab Care.* 2007 May; 10 (3): 360–65.

44. www.wholesoystory.com/newsletters/FrenchWARNING.pdf

45. www.babycareadvice.com/babycare/general_help/article.php?id=43

Chapter 11. Just to Be on the Safe Side: Stay Away from Supplements

1. Bjelakovic G, Nikolova D, Simonetti RG, Gluud C. Antioxidant supplements for prevention of mortality in healthy participants and patients with various diseases. *Cochrane Database Syst Rev.* 2008 Apr 16; (2): CD007176.

2. Bjelakovic G, Nikolova D, Simonetti RG, Gluud C. Antioxidant supplements for preventing gastrointestinal cancers. *Cochrane Database Syst Rev.* 2008 Jul 16; (3): CD004183.

3. Peto R, Doll R, Buckley JD, Sporn MB. Can dietary beta-carotene materially reduce human cancer rates? *Nature.* 1981 Mar 19; 290 (5803): 201–8.

4. Bjelke E. Dietary vitamin A and human lung cancer. *Int J Cancer.* 1975 Apr 15; 15 (4): 561–65.

5. The Alpha-Tocopherol, Beta Carotene Cancer Prevention Study Group. The effect of vitamin E and beta carotene on the incidence of lung cancer and other cancers in male smokers. *N Engl J Med.* 1994 Apr 14; 330 (15): 1029–35.

6. Omenn GS, Goodman GE, Thornquist MD, et al. Effects of a combination of beta carotene and vitamin A on lung cancer and cardiovascular disease. *N Engl J Med.* 1996 May 2; 334 (18): 1150–55.

7. Pietrzik K. Antioxidant vitamins, cancer, and cardiovascular disease. *N Engl J Med.* 1996 Oct 3; 335 (14): 1065–66.

8. Bjelakovic G and Gluud C. Vitamin and mineral supplement use in relation to all-cause mortality in the Iowa Women's Health Study. *Arch Intern Med.* 2011 Oct 10; 171 (18): 1633–34.

9. Redberg RF. Vitamin supplements: more cost than value: comment on "dietary supplements and mortality rate in older women." *Arch Intern Med.* 2011 Oct 10; 171 (18): 1634–35.

10. Lee JE and Chan AT. Fruit, vegetables, and folate: cultivating the evidence for cancer prevention. *Gastroenterology.* 2011 Jul; 141 (1): 16–20.

11. Lippman SM, Klein EA, Goodman PJ, et al. Effect of selenium and vitamin E on risk of prostate cancer and other cancers: the Selenium and Vitamin E Cancer Prevention Trial (SELECT). *JAMA.* 2009; 301: 39–51.

12. Klein EA, Thompson IM Jr, Tangen CM, et al. Vitamin E and the risk of prostate cancer. The Selenium and Vitamin E Cancer Prevention Trial (SELECT). *JAMA.* 2011 Oct 12; 306 (14): 1549–56.

13. Heart Protection Study Collaborative Group. MRC/BHF Heart Protection Study of antioxidant vitamin supplementation in 20,536 high-risk individuals: a randomised placebo-controlled trial. *Lancet.* 2002 Jul 6; 360 (9326): 23–33.

14. Rapola JM, Virtamo J, Ripatti S, et al. Randomised trial of alpha-tocopherol and beta-carotene supplements on incidence of major coronary events in men with previous myocardial infarction. *Lancet.* 1997 Jun 14; 349 (9067): 1715–20.

15. Mursu J, Robien K, Harnack LJ, et al. Dietary Supplements and Mortality Rate in Older Women: The Iowa Women's Health Study. *Arch Intern Med.* 2011 Oct 10; 171 (18): 1625–33.

16. Lonn E, Bosch J, Yusuf S, et al; HOPE and HOPE-TOO Trial Investigators. Effects of long-term vitamin E supplementation on cardiovascular events and cancer: a randomized controlled trial. *JAMA.* 2005 Mar 16; 293 (11): 1338–47.

17. Lange H, Suryapranata H, De Luca G, et al. Folate therapy and in-stent restenosis after coronary stenting. *N Engl J Med.* 2004 Jun 24; 350 (26): 2673–81.

18. Bønaa KH, Njølstad I, Ueland PM, et al; NORVIT Trial Investigators. Homocysteine lowering and cardiovascular events after acute myocardial infarction. *N Engl J Med.* 2006 Apr 13; 354 (15): 1578–88.

19. Albert CM, Cook NR, Gaziano JM, et al. Effect of folic acid and B vitamins on risk of cardiovascular events and total mortality among women at high risk for cardiovascular disease: a randomized trial. *JAMA.* 2008 May 7; 299 (17): 2027–36.

20. Durga J, Bots ML, Schouten EG, et al. Effect of 3 y of folic acid supplementation on the progression of carotid intima-media thickness and carotid arterial stiffness in older adults. *Am J Clin Nutr.* 2011 May; 93 (5): 941–49.

21. Study of the Effectiveness of Additional Reductions in Cholesterol and Homocysteine (SEARCH) Collaborative Group, Armitage JM, Bowman L, Clarke RJ, et al. Effects of homocysteine-lowering with folic acid plus vitamin B₁₂ vs placebo on mortality and major morbidity in myocardial infarction survivors: a randomized trial. *JAMA*. 2010 Jun 23; 303 (24): 2486–94.

22. House AA, Eliasziw M, Cattran DC, et al. Effect of B-vitamin therapy on progression of diabetic nephropathy: a randomized controlled trial. *JAMA*. 2010 Apr 28; 303 (16): 1603–9.

23. Sanders KM, Stuart AL, Williamson EJ, et al. Annual high-dose oral Vitamin D and falls and fractures in older women: a randomized controlled trial. *JAMA*. 2010 May 12; 303 (18): 1815–22.

24. Graat JM, Schouten EG, Kok FJ. Effect of daily vitamin E and multivitamin-mineral supplementation on acute respiratory tract infections in elderly persons: a randomized controlled trial. *JAMA*. 2002 Aug 14; 288 (6): 715–21.

Vitamin D References:

25. Pittas AG, Chung M, Trikalinos T, et al. Systematic review: Vitamin D and cardiometabolic outcomes. *Ann Intern Med*. 2010 Mar 2; 152 (5): 307–14.

26. Grey A, Bolland MJ, Reid IR. Vitamin D supplementation. *Arch Intern Med*. 2010 Mar 22; 170 (6): 572–73.

27. Glerup H, Mikkelsen K, Poulsen L, et al. Commonly recommended daily intake of vitamin D is not sufficient if sunlight exposure is limited. *J Internal Med*. 2000; 247: 260–68.

28. Holick MF. Vitamin D: a millenium perspective. *J Cell Biochem*. 2003; 88: 296–307.

29. Reichrath J. The challenge resulting from positive and negative effects of sunlight: how much solar UV exposure is appropriate to balance between risks of vitamin D deficiency and skin cancer? *Prog Biophys Mol Biol*. 2006 Sep; 92 (1): 9–16.

30. Reusch J, Ackermann H, Badenhoop K. Cyclic changes of vitamin D and PTH are primarily regulated by solar radiation: 5-year analysis of a German (50 degrees N) population. *Horm Metab Res*. 2009 May; 41 (5): 402–7.

31. Salamone LM, Dallal GE, Zantos D, et al. Contributions of vitamin D intake and seasonal sunlight exposure to plasma 25-hydroxyvitamin D concentration in elderly women. *Am J Clin Nutr*. 1994 Jan; 59 (1): 80–86.

32. Vieth R. Vitamin D supplementation, 25-hydroxyvitamin D concentrations, and safety. *Am J Clin Nutr*. 1999; 69: 84256.

33. Holick MF. Sunlight Dilemma: risk of skin cancer or bone disease and muscle weakness. *Lancet*. 2001; 357: 46.

34. Wolpowitz D and Gilchrest BA. The vitamin D questions: how much do you need and how should you get it? *J Am Acad Dermatol*. 2006 Feb; 54 (2): 301–17.

35. Lucas RM, Repacholi MH, McMichael AJ. Is the current public health message on UV exposure correct? *Bull World Health Organ*. 2006 Jun; 84 (6): 485–91.

36. Wharton JR and Cockerell CJ. The sun: a friend and enemy. *Clin Dermatol*. 1998 Jul–Aug; 16 (4): 415–19.

37. Porojnicu A, Robsahm TE, Berg JP, Moan J. Season of diagnosis is a predictor of cancer survival. Sun-induced vitamin D may be involved: a possible role of sun-induced Vitamin D. *J Steroid Biochem Mol Biol*. 2007 Mar; 103 (3–5): 675–78.

38. Robsahm TE, Tretli S, Dahlback A, Moan J. Vitamin D₃ from sunlight may improve the prognosis of breast-, colon- and prostate cancer (Norway). *Cancer Causes Control*. 2004 Mar; 15 (2): 149–58.

39. Zhou W, Suk R, Liu G, et al. Vitamin D is associated with improved survival in early-stage non-small cell lung cancer patients. *Cancer Epidemiol Biomarkers Prev.* 2005 Oct; 14 (10): 2303–9.

40. Berwick M, Armstrong BK, Ben-Porat L, et al. Sun exposure and mortality from melanoma. *J Natl Cancer Inst.* 2005 Feb 2; 97 (3):195–99.

41. Holick MF. Vitamin D: importance in the prevention of cancers, type 1 diabetes, heart disease, and osteoporosis. *Am J Clin Nutr.* 2004 Mar; 79 (3): 362–71.

42. Parry J, Sullivan E, Scott AC. Vitamin D sufficiency screening in preoperative pediatric orthopaedic patients. *J Pediatr Orthop.* 2011 Apr–May; 31 (3): 331–33.

43. Lee JH, Gadi R, Spertus JA, et al. Prevalence of vitamin D deficiency in patients with acute myocardial infarction. *Am J Cardiol.* 2011 Mar 23.

44. Long AN, Ray MM, Nandikanti D, et al. Prevalence of 25-hydroxyvitamin D deficiency in an urban general internal medicine academic practice. *Tenn Med.* 2011 Jan; 104 (1): 45–6, 52.

45. Gómez-Alonso C, Naves-Díaz ML, Fernández-Martín JL, et al. Vitamin D status and secondary hyperparathyroidism: the importance of 25-hydroxyvitamin D cut-off levels. *Kidney Int Suppl.* 2003 Jun; (85): S44–48.

46. Rosen CJ. Vitamin D insufficiency. *N Engl J Med.* 2011 Jan 20; 364 (3): 248–54.

47. Binkley N, Novotny R, Krueger D, et al. Low vitamin D status despite abundant sun exposure. *J Clin Endocrinol Metab.* 2007 Jun; 92 (6): 2130–35.

48. Pramyothin P, Techasurungkul S, Lin J, et al. Vitamin D status and falls, frailty, and fractures among postmenopausal Japanese women living in Hawaii. *Osteoporos Int.* 2009 Nov; 20 (11): 1955–62.

49. Abrams SA. Vitamin D requirements in adolescents: what is the target? *Am J Clin Nutr.* 2011 Mar; 93 (3): 483–84.

50. Shaw N. Vitamin D and bone health in children. *BMJ.* 2011 Jan 25; 342: d192. doi: 10.1136/bmj.d192.

51. Schneider S and Kramer H. Who uses sunbeds? A systematic literature review of risk groups in developed countries. *J Eur Acad Dermatol Venereol.* 2010 Jun; 24 (6): 639–48.

52. Tangpricha V, Turner A, Spina C, et al. Tanning is associated with optimal vitamin D status (serum 25-hydroxyvitamin D concentration) and higher bone mineral density. *Am J Clin Nutr.* 2004; 80: 1645–49.

53. Treatment of vitamin D deficiency with UV light in patients with malabsorption syndromes: a case series. *Photodermatol Photoimmunol Photomed.* 2007 October; 23 (5): 179–85.

54. Heikkinen AM, Tuppurainen MT, Niskanen L, et al. Long-term vitamin D₃ supplementation may have adverse effects on serum lipids during postmenopausal hormone replacement therapy. *Eur J Endocrinol.* 1997 Nov; 137 (5): 495–502.

55. Tuppurainen M, Heikkinen AM, Penttilä I, Saarikoski S. Does vitamin D₃ have negative effects on serum levels of lipids? A follow-up study with a sequential combination of estradiol valerate and cyproterone acetate and/or vitamin D3. *Maturitas.* 1995 Jun; 22 (1): 55–61.

56. Heikkinen AM, Tuppurainen MT, Niskanen L, et al. Long-term vitamin D₃ supplementation may have adverse effects on serum lipids during postmenopausal hormone replacement therapy. *Eur J Endocrinol.* 1997 Nov; 137 (5): 495–502.

57. Tuohimaa P, Tenkanen L, Ahonen M, et al. Both high and low levels of blood vitamin D are associated with a higher prostate cancer risk: a longitudinal, nested case-control study in the Nordic countries. *Int J Cancer.* 2004 Jan 1; 108 (1): 104–8.

58. Marshall TG. Vitamin D discovery outpaces FDA decision making. *Bioessays.* 2008 Feb; 30 (2): 173–82.

59. Meyer G and Köpke S. Vitamin D and falls. Information on harm is missing. *BMJ.* 2009 Oct 28; 339: b4395. doi: 10.1136/bmj.b4395.

60. Hsia J, Heiss G, Ren H, et al. 2007 Women's Health Initiative. Calcium/vitamin D supplementation and cardiovascular events. *Circulation.* 2007; 115: 846–54.

61. Byers T. Anticancer vitamins du jour—the ABCED's so far. *Am J Epidemiol.* 2010 Jul 1; 172 (1): 1–3.

62. Holick MF, Biancuzzo RM, Chen TC, et al. Vitamin D_2 is as effective as vitamin D_3 in maintaining circulating concentrations of 25-hydroxyvitamin D. *J Clin Endocrinol Metab.* 2008; 93 (3): 677–81.

Vitamin B$_{12}$ References:

63. Stabler SP and Allen RH. Vitamin B$_{12}$ deficiency as a worldwide problem. *Annu Rev Nutr.* 2004; 24: 299–326.

64. Herbert V. Vitamin B$_{12}$: Plant sources, requirements, and assay. *Am J Clin Nutr.* 1988 Sep; 48 (3 Suppl): 852–58.

65. Koebnick C, Hoffmann I, Dagnelie PC, et al. Long-term ovo-lacto vegetarian diet impairs vitamin B$_{12}$ status in pregnant women. *J Nutr.* 2004 Dec; 134 (12): 3319–26.

66. Albert MJ, Mathan VI, Baker SJ. Vitamin B$_{12}$ synthesis by human small intestinal bacteria. *Nature.* 1980 Feb 21; 283 (5749): 781–82.

67. Butler CC, Vidal-ALaball J, Cannings-John R, et al. Oral vitamin B$_{12}$ versus intramuscular vitamin B$_{12}$ for vitamin B$_{12}$ deficiency: a systematic review of randomized controlled trials. *Fam Pract.* 2006 Jun; 23 (3): 279–85.

68. Vidal-Alaball J, Butler CC, Cannings-John R, et al. Oral vitamin B$_{12}$ versus intramuscular vitamin B$_{12}$ for vitamin B$_{12}$ deficiency. *Cochrane Database Syst Rev.* 2005 Jul 20; (3): CD004655.

69. Freeman AG. Hydroxocobalamin versus cyanocobalamin. *J R Soc Med.* 1996 Nov; 89 (11): 659.

70. Watanabe F, Takenaka S, Kittaka-Katsura H, et al. Characterization and bioavailability of vitamin B$_{12}$-compounds from edible algae. *J Nutr Sci Vitaminol (Tokyo).* 2002 Oct; 48 (5): 325–31.

71. Watanabe F. Vitamin B$_{12}$ sources and bioavailability. *Exp Biol Med (Maywood).* 2007 Nov; 232 (10): 1266–74.

72. Watanabe F, Takenaka S, Katsura H, Masumder SA, Abe K, Tamura Y, Nakano Y. Dried green and purple lavers (Nori) contain substantial amounts of biologically active vitamin B$_{12}$ but less of dietary iodine relative to other edible seaweeds. *J Agric Food Chem.* 1999 Jun; 47 (6): 2341–43.

73. Croft MT, Lawrence AD, Raux-Deery E, et al. Algae acquire vitamin B$_{12}$ through a symbiotic relationship with bacteria. *Nature.* 2005 Nov 3; 438 (7064): 90–93.

Chapter 12. Salt and Sugar: The Scapegoats of the Western Diet

Salt References:

1. Moyer MW. It's time to end the war on salt. *Sci Am.* 2011 July; 304 (7): 24.

2. Fodor JG, Whitmore B, Leenen F, Larochelle P. Lifestyle modifications to prevent and control hypertension. 5. Recommendations on dietary salt. Canadian Hypertension Society, Canadian Coalition for High Blood Pressure Prevention and Control, Laboratory Centre for Disease Control at Health Canada, Heart and Stroke Foundation of Canada. *CMAJ.* 1999 May 4; 160 (9 Suppl): S29–34.

3. Hooper L, Bartlett C, Davey Smith G, Ebrahim S. Advice to reduce dietary salt for prevention of cardiovascular disease. *Cochrane Database Syst Rev.* 2004; (1): CD003656.

4. Cohen HW, Hailpern SM, Alderman MH. Sodium Intake and Mortality Follow-Up in the Third National Health and Nutrition Examination Survey (NHANES III). *Gen Intern Med.* 2008 Sep; 23 (9): 1297–1302.

5. Adrogué HJ and Madias NE. Sodium and potassium in the pathogenesis of hypertension. *N Engl J Med.* 2007 May 10; 356 (19): 1966–78.

6. Hollenberg NK, Martinez G, McCullough M, et al. Aging, acculturation, salt intake, and hypertension in the Kuna of Panama. *Hypertension.* 1997 Jan; 29 (1 Pt 2): 171–76.

7. Craig WJ. Health effects of vegan diets. *Am J Clin Nutr.* 2009 May; 89 (5): 1627S–33S.

8. Cohen HW, Hailpern SM, Alderman MH. Salt intake and cardiovascular mortality. *Am J Med.* 2007 Jan; 120 (1): e7.

9. Stolarz-Skrzypek K, Kuznetsova T, Thijs L, et al. European Project on Genes in Hypertension (EPOGH) Investigators. Fatal and nonfatal outcomes, incidence of hypertension, and blood pressure changes in relation to urinary sodium excretion. *JAMA.* 2011 May 4; 305 (17): 1777–85.

10. Taylor RS, Ashton KE, Moxham T, et al. Reduced dietary salt for the prevention of cardiovascular disease: a meta-analysis of randomized controlled trials (Cochrane review). *Am J Hypertens.* 2011 Aug; 24 (8): 843–53. doi: 10.1038/ajh.2011.115.

11. Graudal NA, Hubeck-Graudal T, Jürgens G. Effects of low-sodium diet vs. high-sodium diet on blood pressure, renin, aldosterone, catecholamines, cholesterol, and triglyceride (Cochrane Review). *Am J Hypertens.* 2012 Jan; 25 (1): 1–15. doi: 10.1038/ajh.2011.210.

12. L. Dahl. Salt intake and salt need. *N Engl J Med.* 1958 Jun 12; 258 (24): 1205–8.

Sugar References:

13. Bolton-Smith C and Woodward M. Dietary composition and fat to sugar ratios in relation to obesity. *Int J Obes Relat Metab Disord.* 1994 Dec; 18 (12): 820–28.

14. Janket SJ, Manson JE, Sesso H, et al. A prospective study of sugar intake and risk of type 2 diabetes in women. *Diabetes Care.* 2003 Apr; 26 (4): 1008–15.

15. Kitagawa T. Increased incidence of non-insulin dependent diabetes mellitus among Japanese schoolchildren correlates with an increased intake of animal protein and fat. *Clin Pediatr (Phila).* 1998 Feb; 37 (2): 111–15.

16. Llanos G. Diabetes in the Americas. *Bull Pan Am Health Organ.* 1994 Dec; 28 (4): 285–301.

17. Egede LE and Dagogo-Jack S. Epidemiology of type 2 diabetes: focus on ethnic minorities. *Med Clin North Am.* 2005 Sep; 89 (5): 949–75, viii.

18. ADA recommends high carbohydrate intake: http://www.diabetes.org/diabetes -research/summaries/anderson-carbs.jsp

19. Kiehm TG, Anderson JW, Ward K. Beneficial effects of a high carbohydrate, high fiber diet on hyperglycemic diabetic men. *Am J Clin Nutr.* 1976 Aug; 29 (8): 895–99.

20. Jenkins DJ, Kendall CW, Marchie A, Jenkins AL, Augustin LS, Ludwig DS, Barnard ND, Anderson JW. Type 2 diabetes and the vegetarian diet. *Am J Clin Nutr.* 2003 Sep; 78 (3 Suppl): 610S–16S.

21. Barnard ND, Cohen J, Jenkins DJ, et al. A low-fat vegan diet improves glycemic control and cardiovascular risk factors in a randomized clinical trial in individuals with type 2 diabetes. *Diabetes Care.* 2006 Aug; 29 (8): 1777–83.

22. Poppitt SD, Keogh GF, Prentice AM, et al. Long-term effects of ad libitum low-fat, high-carbohydrate diets on body weight and serum lipids in overweight subjects with metabolic syndrome. *Am J Clin Nutr.* 2002 Jan; 75 (1): 11–20.

23. Teff KL, Elliott SS, Tschop M, et al. Dietary fructose reduces circulating insulin and leptin, attenuates postprandial suppression of ghrelin, and increases triglycerides in women. *J Clin Endocrinol Metab.* 2004 Jun; 89 (6): 2963–72.

24. Jequier E and Bray GA. Low-fat diets are preferred. *Am J Med.* 2002 Dec 30; 113 Suppl 9B: 41S–46S.

25. Saris WH. Glycemic carbohydrate and body weight regulation. *Nutr Rev.* 2003 May; 61 (5 Pt 2): S10–16.

26. Anderson GH and Woodend D. Effect of glycemic carbohydrates on short-term satiety and food intake. *Nutr Rev.* 2003 May; 61 (5 Pt 2): S17–26.

27. Holt SH, Miller JC, Petocz P, Farmakalidis E. A satiety index of common foods. *Eur J Clin Nutr.* 1995 Sep; 49 (9): 675–90.

28. Hawley JA. Effect of meal frequency and timing on physical performance. *Br J Nutr.* 1997 Apr; 77 Suppl 1: S91–103.

29. Walton P. Glycaemic index and optimal performance. *Sports Med.* 1997 Mar; 23 (3): 164–72.

30. Vidon C. Effects of isoenergetic high-carbohydrate compared with high-fat diets on human cholesterol synthesis and expression of key regulatory genes of cholesterol metabolism. *Am J Clin Nutr.* 2001 May; 73 (5): 878–84.

31. Schaefer EJ. Body weight and low-density lipoprotein cholesterol changes after consumption of a low-fat ad libitum diet. *JAMA.* 1995 Nov 8; 274 (18): 1450–55.

32. Schwarz JM, Linfoot P, Dare D, Aghajanian K. Hepatic de novo lipogenesis in normoinsulinemic and hyperinsulinemic subjects consuming high-fat, low-carbohydrate and low-fat, high-carbohydrate isoenergetic diets. *Am J Clin Nutr.* 2003 Jan; 77 (1): 43–50.

33. Welsh JA, Sharma A, Abramson JL, Vaccarino V, Gillespie C, Vos MB. Caloric sweetener consumption and dyslipidemia among US adults. *JAMA.* 2010 Apr 21; 303 (15): 1490–97.

34. Reiser S, Hallfrisch J, Michaelis OE 4th, et al. Isocaloric exchange of dietary starch and sucrose in humans. I. Effects on levels of fasting blood lipids. *Am J Clin Nutr.* 1979 Aug; 32 (8): 1659–69.

35. Hudgins LC, Seidman CE, Diakun J, Hirsch J. Human fatty acid synthesis is reduced after the substitution of dietary starch for sugar. *Am J Clin Nutr.* 1998 Apr; 67 (4): 631–39.

36. Bantle JP, Raatz SK, Thomas W, Georgopoulos A. Effects of dietary fructose on plasma lipids in healthy subjects. *Am J Clin Nutr.* 2000 Nov; 72 (5): 1128–34.

37. Zero DT. Sugars—the arch criminal? *Caries Res.* 2004 May–Jun; 38 (3): 277–85.

38. Cox TM. The genetic consequences of our sweet tooth. *Nat Rev Genet.* 2002 Jun; 3 (6): 481–87.

GENERAL INDEX

Protein
  amino acids in, 89, 92, 93–94, 94–95
  in animal foods, 35, 38, 39, 39, 40, 99
  misconceptions about, 92–93, 100, 101
  consumption of
    advertising influencing, 84
    debates about, 83
  fear of deficiency of, from starch-based
    diet, 100–101
  overconsumption of, 70
  in plant foods, 35, 38, 39, 40, 40, 89, 92,
    94–95, 94–95, 98–99, 99
  misconceptions about, 95–100, 96
  recommended daily requirement for, 88–89,
    89
  early studies on, 85–88, 92–94
  toxic effects of, 41

Refrigerated foods, stocking, 198
Rheumatoid arthritis. See Inflammatory
    arthritis, spontaneous healing from

Salads, buying ingredients for, 201
Salt. See also Sodium restriction
  for adjusting to starch-based diet, 171–72, 194
  how to season foods with, 199, 210
  instinct to eat, 175–76, 183
  in processed foods, 176–77, 176
  recommended consumption of, 177
  taste buds for, 171, **172**
  value associated with, 173
Sauces, 178, 189, 194
School lunches, USDA recommendations for,
    59–60, **60**
Seasonings, 189, 193–94, 199. See also Salt;
    Spices; specific herbs
7-Day Sure-Start Plan, x, xx, 189
  menu plan for, 211–13, 217–18
  preparing for, 207–11
Shelf-stable foods, for pantry, 197–98
Smoking, 34–35, 46–47, 152, 153
Snack foods, stocking, 200
Sodium restriction
  problems with, 172–75, 183–84
  for salt-sensitive people, 177–78
Soil depletion, myth of mineral deficiencies
    from, 156–57
Soy foods
  in Asian diet, 141
  changing recommendations about, 144–45
  fake, 134–35, 140–41, 142–44, 144, 210
  healthiest choices of, 196, 210, 212
Soy protein isolates, 134–35, 142–45, 144

Spices, 184, 193–94, 199
Spontaneous healing. See Healing, spontaneous
Starch(es). See also Starch-based diet; Starch
    Solution
  affordability of, 61
  benefits of, 14–16
  composition of, 4, 6–7
  converted to body fat, myth about, 22, 24–25
  for detoxification, 43
  in "Eat More Starch" Challenge, 24–25
  examples of, 7, 7, 8, 190
  in healthy populations, 8, **9**, 10, 12, 20
  importance of, in human history, 3, 7–8
  in Mediterranean diet, 135
  misconceptions about, 20, 23
  nonfood uses of, 13
  in plan for maximum weight loss, 216
  rarity of sickness from, 38
  in 7-Day Sure-Start Plan, 210, 212
  USDA Dietary Guidelines and, 59, 60, 61,
    63, 64, 65
Starch-based diet. See also Starch(es); Starch
    Solution; Vegan diet
  benefits of, ix, xv, xvii, xviii, xix, 6, 17, 20,
    26, 33, 45, 46, 57, 68, 78, 79, 145–46,
    149 (see also Star McDougallers;
    Success stories)
  cost savings from, 203, 205–6, 205, 206
  ease of meal preparation with, 281
  fear of protein deficiency from, 100–101
  salt and sugar for adjusting to, 171–72,
    178–79, 184, 194
  satiety from, vii, 8, 15, 21–22, 139
  simplicity of, 15
  as solution to global problems, 17, 69, 77, 78–79
  studies on, xvi–xvii
"Starchivores," humans as, 8, 12–14
Starch Solution, vii, ix–x, xviii. See also
    Starch(es); Starch-based diet; Vegan diet
  alternatives to cooking for, 201–2
  benefits of, viii, ix, x, 17, 27, 79, 79 (see also
    Star McDougallers; Success stories)
  cardinal rule of, 189
  dealing with others' concerns about, 187–88
  dining out guidelines for, 202
  expected results from, 69, 187
  food groups in, **5**
  guidelines for starting
    choosing cookware, 200
    doctor approval, 208, 209
    food preparation, 193–94
    kitchen and pantry staples, 194–200
    7-Day Sure-Start Plan (see 7-Day
      Sure-Start Plan)
    substitutions for foods to be avoided, 195
    what to eat and what to avoid, 188–83

Recipe Index

Underscored page references indicate boxed text and tables.
Boldface references indicate illustrations and photographs.